HOSPITAL CARE
IN NEW YORK CITY

HOSPITAL CARE
IN NEW YORK CITY

THE ROLES OF VOLUNTARY
AND MUNICIPAL HOSPITALS

By HERBERT E. KLARMAN

NEW YORK AND LONDON 1963

COLUMBIA UNIVERSITY PRESS

PUBLISHED FOR

HOSPITAL COUNCIL OF GREATER NEW YORK, INC.

3 EAST 54 STREET, NEW YORK 22, NEW YORK

A nonprofit organization incorporated to coordinate and improve the hospital and health services
of New York City and to plan the development
of these services in relation to community needs

HOSPITAL COUNCIL OF GREATER NEW YORK

HOSPITAL COUNCIL OF GREATER NEW YORK

COMMITTEE TO STUDY RELATIONS BETWEEN MUNICIPAL AND VOLUNTARY HOSPITAL SYSTEMS

ALVIN C. EURICH, *Chairman*

GEORGE BUGBEE

CARROLL J. DICKSON

JAMES FELT

MORRIS A. JACOBS, M.D.

CLOYD LAPORTE

PETER MARSHALL MURRAY, M.D.

HAYDEN C. NICHOLSON, M.D.

MISS HARRIET I. PICKENS

THOMAS J. ROSS

* NATHAN S. SACHS

MARTIN R. STEINBERG, M.D.

JOSEPH P. WALSH

* Deceased

STAFF

HAYDEN C. NICHOLSON, M.D.
Executive Director

HERBERT E. KLARMAN
Associate Director

SIGMUND L. FRIEDMAN
Staff Consultant

FRANCISCA K. THOMAS
Senior Research Associate

ROBERT R. MURPHY
Research Associate

JOSEPH P. PETERS
Staff Consultant

MARGARET A. COLEMAN
Research Associate

DOROTHY A. WOODHEAD
Statistical Assistant

DOROTHY L. WILLIAMS
Librarian

NADIA DENISSOFF

JOHN H. FRAZIER

JOAN GREENBERG

JOSE GONZALEZ

MARIANNE J. JACKER

LEO J. MORÓN

VERNA R. MORÓN

CLAIRE M. MORRISSETTE

FOREWORD

This book on hospital care in New York City was completed just prior to the reorganization of the Hospital Council of Greater New York into the Hospital Review and Planning Council of Southern New York. (The manuscript was edited for the last time and completely retyped early in March, 1962, while the new organization was formally established a few weeks later.) We thought it important to have the book published, because it serves several purposes rather well. I commend it as a summary of trends in hospital care during the generation in which the original Hospital Council was active in New York; as a statement and discussion of the prominent issues in hospital care in the late 1950s and early 1960s; as a factual base for the future planning of hospital care in New York; and as a prototype of the variety and levels of information and analysis that may be required to achieve effective planning in the enlarged fourteen-county area served by the new Hospital Review and Planning Council.

The Hospital Council of Greater New York was founded in 1938 as a voluntary nonprofit agency to guide the coordinated development of hospital facilities in accordance with measured needs and was unique among hospital organizations in this country for many years. Its corporate members were not hospitals or physicians but civic and professional organizations. The board of directors consisted of individual citizens who were concerned with the provision of adequate hospital services and had some knowledge in the field but who were selected mostly for their objectivity and independence of judgment. Although without official powers or sanctions, the Hospital Council's board derived its authority from the respect that the community accorded to its studies and recommendations. Government manifested its regard when New York State asked the Hospital Council to serve as its local agent in the administration of the Hill-Burton program and incorporated *The Master Plan for Hospitals and Related Facilities for New York City* into the State's plan.

The Hospital Council employed a full-time professional staff, drawn from a variety of academic disciplines, to gather data and analyze them. The Board of Directors usually relied on a standing or special committee to provide detailed and continued guidance to the staff, always reserving a full and detailed review of recommendations. For this study we were fortunate to have a special committee of distinguished board members, including officers, headed by Alvin Eurich.

New York City has been fortunate in its long tradition of partnership of voluntary and municipal hospitals in caring for the sick poor in their wards and outpatient departments. The question was whether numerous changes in medical care, technology, finances, and medical education had changed the conditions conducive to effective cooperation. If so, there was an urgent need for study and appropriate remedial action.

The idea of a study of the roles of the voluntary and municipal hospitals in New York City—their relationships, their problems, and their prospects—first emerged in the summer of 1955, shortly after Dr. Hayden C. Nicholson came to the Hospital Council as Executive Director.

After the Board of Directors voted in November 1955 to conduct a broad study of the roles of voluntary and municipal hospitals, a committee was appointed and an outline of study was developed. The sections outlining the study's objectives and a statement of issues, current and long-range, were submitted for endorsement to several organizations, including the New York Academy of Medicine, the Department of Hospitals of the City of New York, the Greater New York Hospital Association, and the United Hospital Fund. They promptly gave their endorsement and proferred their help. It was not until the winter of 1959 that it became possible to free the Associate Director, Dr. Klarman, to devote himself to this study exclusively. Within two months Dr.

Eurich's committee started to meet at frequent intervals to review and criticize the several sections of the report as they were prepared and circulated by the staff.

Most of the report was completed by the summer of 1960, when a summary was prepared. The chapters dealing with population and hospital services were written in the fall of 1960. In December, 1960, the Hospital Council's report *New York City and Its Hospitals* was published, incorporating major findings and recommendations. The basic report was then edited, with some of the chapters rewritten in part or in full, in response to criticisms by experts and friends. The summer and fall of 1961 saw further editing of text and checking of tables, but there was no attempt to up-date information beyond December, 1960.

The result of all this work is a big book, much bigger than we had anticipated or desired. It would not, however, have been possible to present the large volume of data collected and analyzed in a book with significantly fewer pages. In its present form the book may be considered a successor volume to the Hospital Survey for New York (1935–37) and the New York State Hospital Study (1948–49), as a benchmark for future research in this field. The many headings—center, side, and paragraph—and a detailed index should be of some assistance to the reader.

As a layman, I claim no competence in handling data or in technical analysis. What does impress me is the light that the judicious selection and presentation of data can shed on problem areas that are otherwise difficult to understand. Why were the hospitals in New York so dissatisfied with the Blue Cross payment formula which, when adopted in 1948, seemed so objective, so fair, so automatic in application? Why have municipal hospitals experienced increasing difficulty in attracting medical staff? Why is the patient load in hospital wards so high in New York City when more than 70 percent of the population has some form of hospital care insurance?

I have mentioned the Hospital Council's report *New York City and Its Hospitals*. That report, not this book, presents the official views of the Hospital Council. We are pleased to sponsor this book for the wealth of statistical materials it presents and for the qualities of technique and analysis applied to the data. However, the opinions and suggestions are those of Dr. Klarman and not of the Hospital Council.

Finally, it is my pleasant duty to acknowledge the contributions that various organizations and individuals have made toward this book. The very size of the book speaks for Dr. Klarman's industry. Dr. Nicholson was constantly available to Dr. Klarman and kept the chairman and me informed of what was taking place. Dr. Eurich led the committee in an extensive review of the text, raising questions and suggesting improvements. I leave it to Dr. Klarman to list his helpers and critics.

The United Hospital Fund and the New York Foundation made special grants toward publication of this book. However, the staff's salaries and supplies were paid from the Hospital Council's regular budget. Once again, I take the opportunity to express our appreciation of the continuing financial support offered by the United Hospital Fund, the Greater New York Fund, Associated Hospital Service, Federation of Jewish Philanthropies, Federation of Protestant Welfare Agencies, Catholic Charities of the Archdiocese of New York, Catholic Charities of the Diocese of Brooklyn, and the Medical Societies of the Counties of New York, Bronx, Kings, and Richmond and the State of New York. Such support has enabled the Hospital Council to work with independence and freedom from financial worries.

THOMAS J. ROSS

July 3, 1962   *President*

PREFACE

As a result of this comprehensive study, the principles that guide the physical development of hospitals in a community may never be quite the same again. Even in a city as well endowed with medical resources as New York City, we can no longer take for granted the availability of physicians, nurses, and interns and residents to staff hospitals. We can no longer assume that a liberal tradition of free care is enough to provide needed services without improved hospital management and leadership. We know that money is important, not in and of itself, but because its unequal distribution among hospitals means unequal capacities to command the real physical and personnel resources required for high quality medical care. Even when money is centrally collected, its distribution must be governed by priorities: what is spent for one purpose cannot be spent for another.

Many of us who were active in this study believe that it has meaning, perhaps even direct applicability, outside New York City. This is certainly true of the basic principles of operation, of the technical innovations, and may even be true of some of the findings. The data on finances, on means of paying for the care of the indigent, on changes in graduate medical education, on staffing of the nursing service, and on hospital utilization can at least serve other large cities as bases for comparison. Wherever there is more than a single hospital serving a community and where differences exist in their ownership and in sources of support, the discussion of hospital management, regionalization, and coordination of services, and of methods of payment employed by Blue Cross and government will be relevant.

The task of the study committee was to guide the staff in its work, to report to the board of directors about progress and problems, and to screen the manuscript before it reached the board for final review and approval. The relationship between the chairman and the Executive Director of the Hospital Council has been particularly close, and I wish to express here my deep appreciation of Dr. Nicholson's many kindnesses and his constant, willing, and discerning help. The report accurately reflects the Hospital Council's aim to base policy recommendations on fact rather than on surmise, however authoritative the latter's source may be.

It is often not possible to have all the evidence needed for reaching decisions, but we tried to gather a large part of it by paying close attention to problems that are just emerging and by anticipating their probable importance. Thus this study is problem-oriented, and to the extent that some emerging problems were missed the study has gaps. For example, it is now clear that the development of proprietary hospitals should have received more attention than it did. On the other hand, absence of data and discussion on community planning for hospital care in the traditional sense—need for and availability of suitable physical facilities plus provision for their geographic distribution—is a deliberate omission. The Hospital Council knows a great deal about physical facilities and intended to learn more in a special study designed as a forerunner to the revision of its *Master Plan*. We felt that we knew too little about other elements of the hospital scene, including programs of care, staffing, finances, and organization. Accordingly, these were emphasized in this study of the roles of voluntary and municipal hospitals.

I have been impressed by the economy with which the voluminous and diverse data were compiled. There were very few special surveys conducted for this study, and none was on a large scale. Most of the data were obtained from the records and reports that agencies prepared for routine administrative purposes. Where data were incomplete or suspect, estimates were developed. Methods of making estimates are described in the appendixes.

The book contains innovations in technique, some of which may have lasting value. For example, the *bed turnover rate* is employed both as an additional measure of hospital use and in relation to the two older indexes of hospital use, rate of occupancy and length of stay. In fact, the new measure is defined in terms of the other two. *An index of obsolescence* of physical plant is employed, which assumes that the only useful way of comparing the status of several physical plants is to compare the relative size of expenditures required to bring each to a satisfactory condition. There is no shorter way to obtain commensurability among hospital plants or among departments in the same hospital. The discussion of *rates of occupancy* by type of accommodation suggests that such rates should be viewed with great caution and that no policy conclusions can be drawn from them without concrete knowledge of the ways in which patients are distributed in an institution. The analysis of *increases in hospital* cost employs the usual data by major departmental groupings. But instead of examining rates of increase in each grouping, the author looks at the percentage distribution of the increase in cost among the several departmental groupings.

Dr. Klarman makes numerous suggestions for further research. I should like to call attention especially to the discussion on measuring the quality of care and how difficult that is in practice. The suggestion is made that a large sum of money, as much as one million dollars, be spent in an attempt to evaluate and compare the quality of care furnished in several types of hospital. Such a study could well lead to more efficient, economical, and higher quality hospital care.

Mr. Ross has noted how long this study took. One of the factors involved, both irritating and exhilarating, was the constant changing in the relative importance of issues. As described in the Introduction, some issues declined in urgency (sometimes because they were resolved) while others assumed importance, or even emerged for the first time, during the investigation. But the study took as long as it did mainly because of its size and scope. It takes time to gather data, even more to conduct interviews, and still more to digest what is learned and to write it down. The extent to which additional staff may be substituted for calendar time soon reaches the point of diminishing returns. In a planning organization like the Hospital Council, arrangements for staffing such a study present a further difficulty. If new, temporary staff is hired, it takes longer to get under way and there is no transfer of learning to the regular operations of the organization upon completion of the study. If permanent staff is to be used, provision must be made for divesting them of other duties. In retrospect, it would seem that perhaps the best arrangement is a judicious mixture of regular and special staffs.

It remains for me to acknowledge the assistance received by the chairman from the members of the committee—and especially from Mr. Ross, President of the Council—who added the review of this manuscript to their heavy regular schedules. In addition, I should like to single out the contribution of Mr. George Bugbee, chairman of the Master Plan Committee, who initially was not a regular member of the committee. His broad and practical knowledge of research in hospital and medical care, of hospital administration, and of area-wide planning made his contribution to the deliberations of a distinguished committee so exceptional as to warrant special commendation.

ALVIN C. EURICH

July 31, 1962   *Chairman of Committee*

ACKNOWLEDGMENTS

This book could be written only because many people—more than 200—gave freely of their time, knowledge and judgment. Mine was the task of bringing together the information they supplied and the explanations they suggested, and then of selecting among alternative hypotheses.

It is not practicable to thank by name every person who contributed to this volume. Here I should like to list those who provided substantial bodies of data, spent considerable time talking to me, or read and criticized drafts of chapters.

One person, Mrs. Francisca K. Thomas, did all these things. She was my teacher and guide from the day I joined the staff of the Hospital Council in the fall of 1949 to the time of her retirement in the summer of 1960. For this study she developed the basic data for several chapters, particularly Chapters 5 and 8. She read the first draft of the entire manuscript, made numerous criticisms, and rewrote a good part of Chapter 10.

Other colleagues on the staff of the Hospital Council made specific contributions, in addition to reading the drafts of various chapters as they appeared. Dr. Hayden C. Nicholson's background as a medical educator is reflected in Chapter 6, and his comments influenced the discussion in Chapters 11 and 21. Joseph P. Peters did the initial analysis of the data for Chapter 6 and prepared memoranda for the historical sections of Chapters 14 and 15. Chapter 8 reflects Dr. Sigmund L. Friedman's contributions to the evaluation of physical plant, and his comments influenced the revision of Chapter 10. Miss M. Ann Coleman's work on services for ambulatory patients and for long-term patients appears in Chapter 2. Robert W. Murphy, first as a resident, worked on the data for

Chapter 20 and, later as a staff member, helped with Chapter 19. Mrs. Dorothy A. Woodhead supervised or herself performed most of the large-scale tabulations and took special pains to assure the accuracy of tables and uniformity of headings. Leonard Zeitz performed the tabulations on inpatients in Chapters 2 and 3, and John H. Frazier did the tabulations for Chapters 1 and 17. Howard H. Moses, as a resident, did additional tabulations for the revision of Chapter 19.

Among those who taught me what I have learned about the financial and management aspects of the voluntary and municipal hospitals in New York City the names of Edward Bauer of the United Hospital Fund of New York and Jacob Levine of the New York City Department of Hospitals are foremost. On innumerable occasions they accompanied their statistical reports with detailed descriptions of the underlying report forms and with patient explanations of the meaning of individual accounts.

I also had the privilege of witnessing the deliberations of several groups involved in planning the development of better hospital care in New York City. For ten years I regularly attended the monthly meetings of the board of directors of the Hospital Council and for twelve years the meetings of its Master Plan Committee. In 1958–59, as technical consultant to the study director, I attended the meetings of the subcommittee on hospitals and health agencies of the study committee of Federation of Jewish Philanthropies of New York; and in 1961–62, serving as its consultant on medical care for the aged, I attended the meetings of the Interdepartmental Health Council of the City of New York. Frequently I attended the monthly meetings of the Greater New York Hospital Association, which shares a floor with the Hospital Council and the United Hospital Fund.

The meetings of Dr. Eurich's special committee were, of course, a source of criticism, stimulus, and advice. I also wish to acknowledge the help received from several members of the committee in their individual capacities, namely, George Bugbee, Dr. Peter Marshall Murray, and Dr. Martin R. Steinberg. Among other board members, Dr. George Baehr explored certain aspects of Chapter 9, and Milton Bluestein's thinking influenced the argument in Chapter 11. Dr. George Reader of the Master Plan Committee discussed with me medical education and the quality of care.

A number of persons, besides Messrs. Bauer and Levine, went well beyond the call of duty in furnishing basic data and in responding to repeated requests for additional information and interpretation. Among them are: James C. Ingram and Harry Sesan of the Associated Hospital Service of New York; Dr. Blanche Bernstein and Florence E. Cuttrell of the Community Council of Greater New York; Dr. Eli Ginzberg and Dr. Peter Rogatz of the subcommittee on hospitals and health agencies of the study committee of Federation of Jewish Philanthropies of New York; Dr. Paul M. Densen, Carl L. Erhardt, Dr. George James, Mrs. Frieda Greenstein Nelson, and Louis Weiner of the New York City Department of Health; Dr. Herman E. Bauer, Robert J. Carlin, Dr. Marta Fraenkel, Dr. Harvey Gollance, and Miss Dorothy Weddige of the Department of Hospitals; Henry J. Rosner and Harry Sussman of the New York City Department of Welfare; Henry Cohen and Marvin D. Roth of the New York City Office of the City Administrator; Grant Adams and Charles G. Roswell of the United Hospital Fund; William J. Dann and Daniel I. Rosen of the United States Veterans Administration; and Dr. C. Rufus Rorem of the Hospital Planning Association of Allegheny County, Pittsburgh, Pennsylvania.

The following furnished unpublished data, tabulations, punch cards, or completed questionnaires: Dr. Frank G. Dickinson, Dr. Leonard W. Martin, Dr. John C. Nunemaker, and Dr. Walter S. Wiggins of the American Medical Association; Mrs. Agnes W. Brewster of the United States Department of Health, Education, and Welfare; Mrs. Eva Balamuth and Sam Shapiro of the Health Insurance Plan of Greater New York; Charles M. Royle of the Hospital Association of New York State; Herbert H. Rosenberg of the National Institutes of Health; Mrs. Evelyn S. Mann and Louis Winnick of the New York City Department of City Planning; Henry G. McCormick of the New York City Office of the Comptroller; Mrs. Gladys Webbink of the New York State Department of Labor; Dr. Alvin I. Goldfarb and Robert E. Patton of the New York State Department of Mental Hygiene; Peter Kasius, Dr. David M. Schneider, and Miss Sadie Zuchovitz of the New York

State Department of Social Welfare; and Arthur H. Jette of the United Community Funds and Councils of America.

At different stages the manuscript was read in its entirety by Mrs. Marian Weinart and by Jacqueline Mueller. Both made editorial changes and suggested deletions.

The manuscript was dictated to Mrs. Nadia Denissoff and Miss Claire M. Morrissette. Between them they did all the typing or saw to it that it was done, again and again. Mrs. Denissoff also produced many of the memoranda that underlie the study and designed the tables for typing. Miss Morrissette spent many a Saturday and Sunday and holiday taking dictation and typing. They read proof, as did at various stages Messrs. Murphy and Moses and Leonard S. Machtinger.

Much of the work on this book was done outside regular office hours. For this contribution of time I am indebted to my wife and children.

To all those named above, and to the many not named, I offer my sincere thanks. As always, I am responsible for the final product. The defects of this volume, and perhaps even some of its good points, are mine.

August 1, 1962   HERBERT E. KLARMAN

CONTENTS

TABLES

HOSPITAL CARE
IN NEW YORK CITY

INTRODUCTION

The study of the relations between the voluntary and municipal hospitals in New York City was intended to develop a body of facts and judgments that might help to appraise alternative policies and programs. By the summer of 1955 certain evidences of strain had appeared, suggesting serious weaknesses in the traditional pattern of providing hospital care for the people of New York City. It was hoped that a systematic inquiry might detect some of these weaknesses at an early stage and make possible preventive or mitigating action; in situations where curative action was called for, such an inquiry might offer the opportunity to formulate a coordinated program, rather than a series of discrete measures.

Illustrative of the strains visible at the time were the continued, marked rise in the cost of hospital care; a lag in the daily rate paid by the City to voluntary hospitals for the care of public charge inpatients; the decision by several voluntary hospitals to terminate their participation in the city's emergency ambulance service; the unilateral action by the City in distributing among hospitals the declining number of patients with tuberculosis; a decline in the availability of patients for teaching purposes; and persistence of the shortage in registered (professional) nurses.

The scope of study, as originally envisioned, was both broad and limited. It was limited at least in the sense that the total volume of hospital services needed by the people of the city was not to be the object of study but would be determined according to accepted principles of master planning. Although a review of these principles was then contemplated for the near future, it was to take the form of a separate project.

The scope of study was broad in that it was to attempt to assess in each hospital system the adequacy of available resources to perform its share of the total task. The respective roles of the voluntary and municipal hospital systems were to be ascertained by comparing the characteristics of patients served as well as trends in the volume of services rendered. Appraisal of resources was to include the availability of money and of real resources, such as key personnel and physical plant, and also their organization and coordination.

The questions to be raised in the proposed study seemed so basic that endorsement and support from allied organizations were considered essential. Endorsement was sought and received from the New York Academy of Medicine, Department of Hospitals of the City of New York, Greater New York Hospital Association, and United Hospital Fund. Much help was forthcoming from these organizations and from others, notably the following: Associated Hospital Service of New York; Department of Health, City of New York; Department of Welfare, City of New York; Health Insurance Plan of Greater New York; Office of the Comptroller, City of New York; New York State Hospital Association; New York State Department of Social Welfare; American Hospital Association; American Medical Association; National Institutes of Health; United States Public Health Service; Social Security Administration; Veterans Administration; hospital councils in metropolitan areas throughout the country; and, most important, many hospitals in New York City.

In the original outline of the study the questions at issue were divided into immediate (those that "face us today") and long range (subjects "likely to arise"), depending on their relative urgency at the time. The questions follow.

Questions That Face Us Today

1. Methods of effecting changes in the distribution of public charge inpatients between voluntary and municipal hospitals
2. Selective admission policies and practices of voluntary hospitals
3. Admission policies and practices of municipal hospitals
4. Problems in the equitable distribution of a given patient

load between voluntary and municipal hospitals, including methods of transferring nonemergency patients who can pay for their care from municipal to voluntary hospitals

5. The effect of hospital care insurance and other factors on the availability of beds and patients for teaching and research

6. Flexibility in using hospital facilities in response to medical advances and other changes

7. Bases for setting City rates for the care of public charges in voluntary hospitals

8. Consideration by the City of New York of payment for outpatient department care in voluntary hospitals

9. State reimbursement of the City's expenditures for hospital care

Other Subjects That Are Likely to Arise

1. The respective roles of voluntary and municipal hospitals in the provision of the several types of care, for example, general, long term, psychiatric, and tuberculosis

2. Equitable distribution of patients for teaching among qualified voluntary and municipal hospitals

3. If governmental responsibility for financing a certain program is accepted, criteria for determining whether the City should buy services from voluntary hospitals or provide them in its own hospitals

4. Consideration of other methods, additional to those now in use, whereby the City might contribute to the income of voluntary hospitals for operating or capital purposes

5. The City's policies and practices in approving for payment patients in voluntary hospitals

6. Division of ward patients between voluntary and municipal hospitals during an economic downturn

7. Care of private patients in municipal hospitals (in all of them or in major teaching institutions only)

8. Factors entering into the continuing availability of top management personnel for municipal hospitals

9. Means by which hospital staff appointments for practicing physicians can be integrated between the two groups of hospitals.

In the course of the study certain of these issues were resolved in full or in part. For example, the City's decision to allow Sea View Hospital to close by stages postponed for several years the urgency of the problem of allocating tuberculosis patients among the hospitals. Similarly, a first step was taken in the fall of 1958 to pay voluntary hospitals for the care of outpatients when a fee of $5 per visit was authorized for recipients of public assistance.

Conversely, certain issues that did not seem pressing at the outset came to the fore. Examples are proposals that facilities for private patients be provided in certain nonuniversity municipal hospitals and measures to assure the continuing availability of top management personnel to municipal hospitals.

Finally, some issues emerged and assumed importance during the study that did not even appear in the outline. Examples are the inability of some hospitals to recruit graduates of American and Canadian medical schools as interns and residents, attrition of the attending staffs of certain municipal hospitals, and increasing evidence of obsolescence of physical plant in both hospital systems.

Ultimately, the scope of study was fixed not by the initial list of questions but by the basic objective of the study. This was stated in the outline: "It is the purpose of the Hospital Council in this study to try to determine the facts as they are and by analyzing their implications objectively to contribute to an understanding of the conditions under which this joint, cooperative use of [voluntary and municipal] hospital facilities in New York City can best be fostered and improved."

The Hospital Council has proceeded on the assumption that voluntary and municipal hospitals will continue to operate in New York City side by side and that cooperative behavior among hospitals is more likely than separate, unrelated action or competition to further the goal of an adequate volume of hospital care of good quality provided at economical cost, "without gaps and without waste." There was no question about the goal. The problem was how to promote the goal and a complementary set of relationships between the two hospital systems.

It was decided to try to develop as complete and accurate a picture as possible of the hospital scene in New York City and of the various influences shaping it. This was to be supported by a study of trends over a generation or longer. It was also decided to compare the pattern and experience of New York City with those in other parts of the country, both to validate judgments regarding probable future developments and to illustrate policies and practices that have been tested elsewhere and found to be workable.

The book is organized in three parts:

I. Background. This section contains chapters on trends in the population of New York City and on certain characteristics of the population that bear most directly on the use of hospitals; trends in hospital service; characteristics of patients in the two hospital systems; and some of the reasons why patients with hospital care insurance continue to seek care in the ward.

II. Resources and Organization. The chapters in this section deal, in order, with physicians as members of the attending staff, including a discussion of hospital staff appointments in the two hospital systems and of trends in the number of practicing physicians in New York City; availability of American-educated and foreign-educated physicians as interns and residents, including a discussion of the teaching role of the hospital; staffing of the nursing service, including discussion of the private duty nurse in the hospital and of nursing education; trends in the suitability of physical plant and in expenditures for hospital construction; selected problems in hospital management, with special emphasis on the location of responsibility and authority in government hospitals; methods and problems in appraising the quality of care in hospitals, including the contribution of medical education and research; and alternative proposals for coordinating hospitals in New York City, both to effect economies and to improve service.

III. Financing Hospital Care. This section deals, in order, with trends in total expenditures for hospital care in New York City and in the distribution of the total by source of income and by hospital ownership; trends in the income of voluntary hospitals; the net deficit and surplus position of voluntary hospitals in recent years; trends in income of municipal hospitals; the role of government, with particular reference to reimbursement of the City by the State of New York and by the federal government; the role of Blue Cross and its subscribers in the hospital's economy; trends in income from philanthropic sources; factors in rising hospital cost and selected comparisons between certain types of cost; how hospital care is financed in the United States as a whole and in other large cities of the country, in comparison with New York City; and a discussion of certain proposals for improving hospital finances in New York City.

For convenience each chapter has its own summary. A general summary of the findings of this report and their implications for policy was presented by the Hospital Council in December, 1960.[1]

Part I. BACKGROUND

1 POPULATION, INCOME, AND HEALTH INSURANCE

The amount and types of hospital service used are determined by the size of population and by certain of its characteristics, such as age, socioeconomic status, and health insurance enrollment. It is known, for example, that the aged use more hospital care than other groups do. To some degree, however, aging is associated with changes in marital status, and the one factor may in part obscure the effects of the other. Financial status and educational level may be associated with differences in the amount of hospital care used and are most certainly associated with differences in the type of hospital accommodation sought—private, semiprivate, or ward. Persons with voluntary health insurance generally use more hospital care than those without insurance, but the opposite has been reported when health insurance is combined with group medical practice. In any event, insured persons are more likely than uninsured persons to occupy private (including semiprivate) accommodations.

For purposes of this study it suffices to note that the important problem facing New York City today and for the foreseeable future is not the total volume of hospital facilities and services but their distribution—by pay status, type of accommodation, hospital ownership, type of program, and geographic location. The principal emphasis of this report is on the distribution of the total volume of hospital services by pay status (insured, public charge, and so forth), type of accommodation, and hospital ownership (voluntary, municipal, and proprietary), and on the factors that influence such distribution. This emphasis governed the selection of data for inclusion in this chapter on the population of New

York City. The chapter consists of three parts: (1) demographic characteristics, (2) income, and (3) voluntary health insurance.

Demographic Characteristics

SIZE OF POPULATION

The United States Bureau of the Census reported the population of New York City in 1960 as 7,782,000—a decline of 110,000 since 1950.

This is the first time that the decennial census recorded a loss of population in New York City. The largest numerical gains in the City's population took place between 1900 and 1910 and between 1920 and 1930, but even the 1930s and the 1940s showed increases of the order of one-half million. By the 1930s the up-

Table 1.1. POPULATION, NEW YORK CITY, 1900–60

Census Year	Number	Change from Preceding Decade	
		Amount	Percent
1900	3,437,202	+ 929,788	+ 37.1
1910	4,766,883	+ 1,329,681	+ 38.7
1920	5,620,048	+ 853,165	+ 17.9
1930	6,930,446	+ 1,310,398	+ 23.3
1940	7,454,995	+ 524,549	+ 7.6
1950	7,891,957	+ 436,962	+ 5.9
1960	7,781,984	− 109,973	− 1.4

SOURCE: U.S. Bureau of the Census.

ward trend in the city's population had slowed down considerably; and between the 1940s and 1950s the direction of the curve was reversed.

A decline in population was first reported in 1957. This caused surprise. The decline could be reconciled with the large increase in dwelling units (one quarter of a million homes or apartments for the decade, all occupied) only on the assumption that a sizable decline in the average size of household had occurred. The ratio of persons to households was 3.52 in 1940, 3.20 in 1950, 3.07 in 1957,[1] and probably fell below 3.00 in 1960. The decline in household size is, in turn, attributable to the sharp increase in one- and two-person households in the city, owing to the disproportionate out-migration of families with children and an increased life expectancy for the aged.

New York City is not unique in having lost population in the 1950s. Its loss of 1.4 percent is smaller than that incurred by many large cities in the eastern and midwestern regions of the United States. For half a century or longer suburban counties grew at a higher rate than the central cities of their metropolitan areas. In the 1950s, while the suburbs continued to gain in population, many cities incurred losses.[2]

In the New York area the neighboring suburban counties have continued their rapid population growth. Illustrative are the increases in the four New York State counties that are part of the metropolitan area. Although the rates of increase in the 1940s

Table 1.2. POPULATION, FOUR SUBURBAN NEW YORK COUNTIES, 1940–60

County	Number			Percent Increase	
	1940	1950	1960	1940–50	1950–60
Total	1,251,922	1,663,986	2,912,649	32.9	75.0
Nassau	406,748	672,765	1,300,171	65.5	93.4
Suffolk	197,355	276,129	666,784	40.0	141.8
Westchester	573,558	625,816	808,891	9.1	29.3
Rockland	74,261	89,276	136,803	20.2	53.2

SOURCES: Regional Plan Association, *Population 1954–1975* (Bulletin No. 85; New York, 1954), p. 7, and U.S. Bureau of the Census, *Advanced Reports, 1960 Census of Population, Population Counts for New York State*, PC (A1)-34 (Washington, D.C., 1960).

were substantial, they were still higher in the 1950s.

NET MIGRATION

Closer analysis of population trends indicates that in New York City the 1950s represented a continuation, and perhaps acceleration, of past tendencies, rather than a reversal. Among the persistent tendencies is a decline in the average size of household noted above. Other factors are net out-migration, numerical and relative increases in the Puerto Rican and nonwhite population groups and decreases in the non-Puerto Rican white group, increases in the number of children and aged (65 years and over), and redistribution of population among the five boroughs.

It is helpful to analyze population changes in terms of two
components: natural increase and net migration. Natural increase is the difference between the number of births and the
number of deaths. Net migration is the balance between the
number of persons moving into an area and the number leaving it.

In most civilized countries today natural increase is positive,
that is, the number of births exceeds the number of deaths. Since
deaths are the relatively more stable factor, it is the number of
births that largely determines the direction and size of natural increase. In the 1930s the birth rate in New York City was low. The
birth rate rose substantially in the 1940s and has remained at the
new level (19 live births per 1,000 population) in the 1950s, with
small fluctuations from year to year.

In the 1930s net migration to New York City was positive;
the number of persons coming into New York exceeded the
number leaving it by 237,000.[3] In the 1940s, for the first time,
New York City lost more persons through out-migration than it
gained through in-migration, so that the increase in population
was entirely due to natural increase. Over-all net migration in the
1940s amounted to 139,000,[4] but net out-migration for the non-
Puerto Rican white population was approximately 500,000.[5] The
tendency toward net out-migration became accentuated in the
1950s.

During the period 1950–57 over-all net out-migration amounted
to 621,000, and for the non-Puerto Rican white population alone
it amounted to 970,000. If these figures were applicable to the full
decade 1950–60, net out-migration for the entire population
would approach 900,000 and for the non-Puerto Rican white
population alone, 1,250,000. It should be noted that some of the
difference in the rate of out-migration between the 1940s and
1950s is more apparent than real. A large share of the out-migration in the 1940s occurred in the second half of the decade, after
World War II.

Much of the out-migration from New York City has flowed
to suburban counties. The fact that some of the new residents of
these counties formerly lived in New York City has implications
for the use of the city's hospitals. Persons who continue to work

in New York City are likely to retain some association with hospitals here, whether as patients, financial contributors, members of the medical staff, or trustees. Even those who leave the city for the suburbs and do not commute to work here may retain ties with hospitals in New York City, at least during a transitional period, pending the development of new ties with physicians and the expansion of hospital facilities in the suburbs.

In time, however, residents of the suburbs build hospitals near their homes. In relocating hospitals in relation to major geographic shifts in population, planning on an area-wide basis becomes necesary in order to avoid constructing numerous small hospitals in the suburbs, wasting existing suitable and efficient hospital plants in the city, and weakening the educational and research potential of established medical centers in the city. It is significant that the Hospital Survey for New York, which was instrumental in establishing the Hospital Council of Greater New York, was conducted in New York City and in eight neighboring counties in New York State, New Jersey, and Connecticut.

The Hospital Council is now reviewing the geographic scope of its planning mission, with a view to extending both the area of study and the area of planning for hospital care beyond the confines of the five boroughs.

NEGRO AND PUERTO RICAN GROUPS

The particular problem of the Puerto Rican and nonwhite population groups lies in their being predominantly newcomers to the community and in their being handicapped educationally and in job opportunities. Some of their characteristics are as follows: they tend to occupy positions at the bottom of the economic ladder [6] and to earn low incomes; their ability to pay for hospital care is impaired by a relatively low rate of enrollment in voluntary insurance; and, to a greater extent than do other groups in similar financial circumstances, they receive hospital care in the ward and, especially, in municipal hospitals (see Chapter 3).

Moreover, the needs of the Puerto Ricans and nonwhites for certain types of medical and hospital services may exceed those of other groups, as, for example, in the field of tuberculosis and in maternal and child health. In 1957 they constituted 7 and 12 percent, respectively, of the city's population. In the same year they contributed 13 and 31 percent, respectively, of all new cases of active tuberculosis [7] (and of tuberculosis inpatients) and 12 and 18 percent, respectively, of all live births in New York City (as compared with 13 and 19 percent of all live births to residents). Indicative of greater need, perhaps as well as of greater neglect, is the fact that they contributed 15 and 29 percent, respectively, of total perinatal mortality (defined as infant deaths under seven days plus stillbirths of 20 or more weeks of gestation).[8]

On the other hand, Puerto Ricans and nonwhites need relatively fewer facilities for the aged at this time. In 1957, when 13 percent of the non-Puerto Rican white adult population was 65 years old and over, the corresponding proportion of Puerto Rican adults was 3 percent and of nonwhite adults, 7 percent.[9]

Negroes have been moving north and settling in large cities since World War I, and Puerto Ricans have been arriving in sizable numbers in the United States, especially in New York City, since World War II. As a result, the combined nonwhite and Puerto Rican component of the city's population has increased from 2 percent in 1910 to 7 percent in 1940 and to 13 percent in 1950.[10]

For April, 1957, the date of the special United States census, the Department of City Planning estimated the ethnic composition of the population of New York City. (The Census counted the population as white and nonwhite. To have a Puerto Rican component, it had to be estimated. The estimates prepared by the Department of City Planning tend to be lower than some other estimates, because they allow for the departure of Puerto Ricans from New York City to other cities on the mainland.) The categories in Table 1.3 are mutually exclusive, so that the "nonwhite" group is really "nonwhites other than Puerto Rican" and the "other whites" group is "whites other than Puerto Rican."

The United States census of 1950 reflected for the first time the large influx of Puerto Ricans into New York City. On the basis of what was then known about migration from Puerto Rico to the mainland, the Department of City Planning made certain projections in 1954 of the probable ethnic composition of the

Table 1.3. DISTRIBUTION OF POPULATION BY ETHNIC GROUP, NEW YORK CITY, 1957

Ethnic Group	Number	Percent
Total	7,795,471	100.0
Puerto Rican	566,000	7.3
Nonwhite	938,651	12.0
Other white	6,290,820	80.7

SOURCE: New York City Department of City Planning, unpublished data.

population of New York City in 1960.[11] These are not inconsistent with the figures presented in Table 1.3 for the Puerto Rican and nonwhite groups but are too high for the non-Puerto Rican white population. The last signifies that a larger out-migration has occurred than was expected.

Seventy percent of the increase in the city's Puerto Rican population in the 1950s came from in-migration. During the decade a pronounced shift took place in the sources of increase: in 1950 natural increase contributed 20 percent of that year's population growth and in-migration 80 percent; in 1959, it is estimated, the two sources were approximately equal.[12]

It may be that the peak of the Puerto Rican migration to New York City has passed. Although net migration from the Island fluctuates with employment opportunities on the mainland, there were 10,000 fewer migrants a year in the second half of the 1950s than in the first half.[13] In addition, the proportion of Puerto Rican migrants settling in New York City is believed to have declined from 85 percent in 1950 to 60 percent in 1958.[14]

One aspect of the Puerto Rican migration that may have escaped adequate notice is its two-way, or even three-way, character. Migrants leave the Island, but some also return. For fiscal year 1959 net migration from the Island to the United States is estimated at 37,000, but the number of new migrants leaving the Island is estimated to have been at least 10,000 higher and possibly 35,000 higher.[15] The Puerto Rican study of school children has similarly reported a substantial reciprocal flow between New York City and Puerto Rico.[16] In addition, as previously noted, some of the Puerto Ricans who leave New York City relocate elsewhere on the mainland.

Much of the increase in the nonwhite population in New

York City during the 1950s (two thirds) was the result of natural increase. At the same time there was some out-migration to the suburbs, in which the numbers of nonwhites have increased at the same high rate as the total population (see Table 1.2). In 1957, though, nonwhites still were fewer than 5 percent of the total population of these areas.[17]

CHILDREN AND AGED

Children tend to use less hospital care than the rest of the population, whereas the aged use more. Children tend to have the same rate of enrollment under voluntary health insurance as the rest of the population, whereas the aged have a lower rate. Both children and aged persons are relatively large users of ward accommodations in New York City (see Chapter 3).

Children increased both in number and in proportion to the city's total population in the 1940s and 1950s. Simultaneously, the number and proportion of aged persons (65 years and over) also increased. A substantial decline has occurred in the number and proportion of persons in age class 15 to 44.

Table 1.4. DISTRIBUTION OF POPULATION BY AGE GROUP, NEW YORK CITY, 1940, 1950, AND 1960

	1940		1950		1960	
Age Group	Number	Percent	Number	Percent	Number	Percent
Total	7,454,995	100.0	7,891,957	100.0	7,781,984	100.0
0–14 years	1,465,558	19.7	1,644,527	20.8	1,857,885	23.9
15–44	3,942,410	52.8	3,680,187	46.6	3,097,118	39.8
45–64	1,632,608	21.9	1,962,008	24.9	2,013,154	25.9
65 years and over	414,419	5.6	605,235	7.7	813,827	10.4

SOURCE: U.S. Bureau of the Census.

A major difference between the period 1940–50 and 1950–60 is in the behavior of age class 45 to 64. This group increased by 33,000 a year, on the average, in the former period and only by 5,000 in the latter.

REDISTRIBUTION OF POPULATION AMONG THE BOROUGHS

The geographic distribution of the population is an important consideration in locating and relocating hospitals. In New York City the boroughs of Queens and Richmond (Staten Island) have been gaining in population in recent years at the expense of Manhattan, the Bronx, and Brooklyn, which were settled at much earlier dates.

Manhattan reached its peak population in 1910, when it contained almost one half of the city's population. It lost population between 1910 and 1920 and between 1920 and 1930 but gained in the 1930s and 1940s. Each of the other four boroughs continued to gain in population through the United States census of 1950. The special census of 1957 reported losses for the first time for the Bronx and Brooklyn, and again for Manhattan. The census of 1960 seems to confirm the findings of 1957 and points to continuing gains for Queens and Richmond. Table 1.5 shows the distribution of the city's population among the boroughs in 1940, 1950 and 1960. The major shift among the boroughs has occurred between Manhattan and Queens, the former losing and the latter gaining.

Table 1.5. DISTRIBUTION OF POPULATION BY BOROUGH, NEW YORK CITY, 1940, 1950, AND 1960

	1940		*1950*		*1960*	
Borough	*Number*	*Percent*	*Number*	*Percent*	*Number*	*Percent*
New York City	7,454,995	100.0	7,891,957	100.0	7,781,984	100.0
Bronx	1,394,711	18.7	1,451,277	18.4	1,424,815	18.3
Brooklyn	2,698,285	36.2	2,738,175	34.7	2,627,319	33.8
Manhattan	1,889,924	25.4	1,960,101	24.8	1,698,281	21.8
Queens	1,297,634	17.4	1,550,849	19.7	1,809,578	23.3
Richmond	174,441	2.3	191,555	2.4	221,991	2.8

SOURCE: U.S. Bureau of the Census.

Another important development is the dispersal of the nonwhite and Puerto Rican populations among the four major boroughs. This is shown in Table 1.6.

In 1940 Mahattan contained 70 percent of the city's Puerto Ricans. Its proportion declined to 56 percent in 1950 and 46 percent in 1957.

The nonwhite population has also been extending to the other boroughs. Mahattan's share of the city's nonwhite population has declined from almost two thirds in 1940 to two fifths in 1957. Indeed, between 1950 and 1957 the number of nonwhites in Manhattan declined.

Table 1.6. DISTRIBUTION OF PUERTO RICAN AND NONWHITE
POPULATION BY BOROUGH, NEW YORK CITY,
1940 AND 1957

	Puerto Rican				Nonwhite			
	1940		1957		1940		1957	
Borough	Num-ber	Per-cent	Num-ber	Per-cent	Num-ber	Per-cent	Num-ber	Per-cent
New York City	76,800	100.0	566,000	100.0	469,811	100.0	936,000	100.0
Bronx	10,100	13.1	145,000	25.6	23,892	5.1	126,000	13.5
Brooklyn	11,200	14.6	150,000	26.5	108,834	23.2	300,000	32.0
Manhattan	54,000	70.3	260,000	45.9	307,299	65.4	382,000	40.8
Queens	1,300	1.7	10,000	1.8	26,803	5.7	120,000	12.8
Richmond	200	0.3	1,000	0.2	2,983	0.6	8,000	0.9

SOURCE: New York City Department of City Planning, unpublished data.

In 1957 Brooklyn had approximately one third of the city's
nonwhites and one quarter of the Puerto Ricans. The Bronx had
almost as large a number of Puerto Ricans as Brooklyn, but fewer
than one half as many nonwhites. By contrast, Queens had almost as many nonwhites as the Bronx, but relatively few Puerto
Ricans.

Despite the dispersal of nonwhites among the boroughs, their
basic pattern of settlement is still one of concentration in Harlem
and in several other neighborhoods, such as the Bedford-Stuy-
vesant district in Brooklyn and the South Jamaica–St. Albans
district in Queens.[18] Almost from the outset the Puerto Rican
population has been more widely scattered throughout the city's
many neighborhoods.

PROJECTIONS OF POPULATION

In 1954 the Regional Plan Association projected that the population of New York City would be 8,700,000 in 1975.[19] This
was broadly consistent with the estimate of 8,570,000 then projected by the City's Department of City Planning for the year
1970, but the distribution by borough was not.[20] In 1957 the
Regional Plan Association reduced its population estimates for
1975 to 8,400,000 mainly because of a lower estimate for Richmond.[21] The projected population for 1975 that is associated with
zoning revision is 8,340,000.[22] The major differences between this
projection and the 1957 projection by the Regional Plan Associa-

tion are a further reduction in the estimate for Richmond from 500,000 to 315,000 and an increase in the estimate for Queens from 1,900,000 to 2,200,000.

All of these projections of population may be on the high side. Vacant land is scarce, and the old settled areas of the city are likely to experience declines in population as result of redevelopment at lower rates of density, changes in land use from residential to nonresidential, and a further reduction in the average number of persons per household.[23]

Projection of the ethnic composition of the population cannot be divorced from the projection of the total. This is a necessary qualification to the most recent projection of the city's population in 1975 by ethnic status: [24]

Total number: 8,315,000	Percent
Puerto Rican	13.2
Nonwhite	14.6
Other white	72.2
	100.0

In the suburbs the outlook is for further population growth, probably at a reduced rate. In the four counties listed in Table 1.2, the Regional Plan Association projects a total population of 3.5 million in 1975,[25] an increase of 20 percent from 1960.

Individual and Family Income

Income is the best single measure of the ability of a community or group to pay for goods and services, including hospital care. This section examines the income of the residents of New York City, compares income trends in the city with income trends in other parts of the country, and describes differences among the three ethic groups.

TRENDS IN INCOME, NEW YORK CITY AND ELSEWHERE

The Metropolitan Region Study developed estimates of per capita income for each of the constituent counties for three years. Table 1.7 compares per capita income in New York City, the New York metropolitan region, New York State, and the United States.

In 1939 and 1947 New York City's per capita income was

Table 1.7. PER CAPITA INCOME (IN DOLLARS), NEW YORK CITY
AND SELECTED AREAS, 1939, 1947, AND 1956

Area	1939	1947	1956
New York City	997	1,892	2,562
New York metropolitan region	912	1,789	2,592
New York State	825	1,715	2,428
United States	556	1,316	1,979

SOURCES: Robert E. Graham, Jr., "General Rise in State Income in 1959," *Survey of Current Business*, XL, No. 8 (August, 1960), 17; Charles F. Schwartz and Robert E. Graham, Jr., *Personal Income by State, Supplement to Survey of Current Business* (Washington, D.C., 1956), pp. 142–43; and Harvey H. Segal, "Personal Income of the New York Metropolitan Region" (New York Metropolitan Region Study; New York, 1958; mimeographed), p. 49.

higher than in the entire metropolitan region, the state, or the nation. In 1956 the city's per capita income was slightly lower than in the metropolitan region, but higher than in the state or nation.

Clearly, per capita income has increased more slowly in New York City than in the Metropolitan Region. It has also increased more slowly in New York City than in the state or nation. Indeed, per capita income has increased more slowly in the New York metropolitan region and in New York State than in the United States as a whole. The explanation lies in part in a general tendency toward equalization of income between poorer states and richer states,[26] among sections of the country, and between metropolitan and nonmetropolitan areas within sections.[27] These developments reflect certain broad economic forces, which are sometimes reinforced by local influences, such as the growth of the Puerto Rican and nonwhite population in New York City.

In 1956 per capita income in New York City exceeded the nation-wide average by 30 percent and the New York State average by 5 percent. Although other sources present somewhat different figures, trend data indicate that these relationships have not changed materially since 1956.[28]

Higher per capita income is likely to be associated with a relatively larger proportion of income recipients in the upper brackets and fewer recipients in the lower brackets. Table 1.8 compares the percentage distribution of families by income in New York City, New York State, and the United States.

Compared with the United States as a whole, New York City

Table 1.8. PERCENTAGE DISTRIBUTION OF FAMILIES BY INCOME,
NEW YORK CITY, NEW YORK STATE, AND
UNITED STATES, 1949 AND 1956

	1949			1956		
Annual Income	New York City	New York State	United States	New York City	New York State	United States
Under $2,000	19.3	19.6	29.3	7.0	7.1	15.4
$ 2,000– 3,999	38.8	39.7	38.5	19.8	19.1	22.7
4,000– 5,999	24.1	23.6	19.9	31.6	31.6	28.6
6,000– 9,999	12.8	12.1	9.2	30.0	31.0	25.4
10,000 and over	5.0	4.8	3.1	11.6	11.2	7.9
Total	100.0	100.0 *	100.0	100.0	100.0	100.0
Median Income	$3,526	$3,487	$3,073	$5,478	$5,523	$4,783

* Due to rounding, does not add to 100 percent.
SOURCE: New York State Interdepartmental Committee on Low Incomes, Family Income in New York State, 1956 (Bulletin No. 1, Pt. 1; New York, 1958), Tables 1, 12, and 13.

has had—and still has—a large proportion of families with income of $6,000 or more and a smaller proportion of families with low income. Between New York City and New York State differences in the distribution of income are small.

The above distributions are based on information collected through household surveys. It is recognized that these do not account for all the income received by respondents [29] and that more complete data would increase the number of families with income of $6,000 or more.

Increases in income overstate improvement in economic welfare to the extent that prices of goods and services have risen. When allowance is made for the rise in the Consumer Price Index between 1949 and 1956, median family income is found to have increased in New York City by 38 percent, compared with 55 percent without such an allowance; and the proportion of families with annual income of $6,000 or more is found to have increased to 42 percent in 1956 from 24 percent in 1949, rather than from 18 percent, as shown in Table 1.8.[30]

The Metropolitan Region Study also developed estimates of per capita income in each of the city's five boroughs.

Manhattan, which has relatively more low-income recipients as well as high-income recipients than the other boroughs, has

Table 1.9. PER CAPITA INCOME (IN DOLLARS) BY BOROUGH,
          NEW YORK CITY, 1939, 1947, AND 1956

Borough	1939	1947	1956
Bronx	768	1,658	2,318
Brooklyn	917	1,622	2,317
Manhattan	1,489	2,662	2,964
Queens	723	1,656	2,749
Richmond	733	1,489	2,250

SOURCE: Harvey H. Segal, *Personal Income of the New York Metropolitan Region* (New York Metropolitan Region Study; New York, 1958; mimeographed), p. 49.

always led in per capita income, and still does. However, its lead is diminishing. Between 1939 and 1956 there was considerable shifting about in the ranks of the three other major boroughs. The rise of Queens from last place to second is noteworthy.

If the boroughs are ranked by cash income per household (exclusive of certain types of noncash income as well as institutional income that does not accrue to households) rather than by per capita income (as defined by the United States Department of Commerce), the borough of Queens assumes top rank, with Richmond joining Manhattan in the second rank.[31] This is pertinent to another finding, namely, that the residents of Richmond (Staten Island) have a relatively low proportion of ward to total hospital admissions (see Chapter 4).

INCOME OF PUERTO RICANS AND NONWHITES

Income data for each of the ethnic groups in New York City are available from the United States Bureau of the Census for the year 1949.

In the spring of 1957, the State Interdepartmental Committee on Low Incomes sponsored a sample survey of households in New York State, including New York City. From this survey, separate income data were derived for whites and nonwhites. A supplementary survey, conducted in New York City, was designed to yield information on Puerto Ricans and augmented information on nonwhites. Although the findings of the supplementary survey have not yet been published, they were kindly made available by the Division of Research and Statistics of the New York State Department of Labor.

Comparisons among Puerto Ricans, Nonwhites, and Other Whites. Data are available for the three ethnic groups on the median income of earners in 1949 and 1956. The incomes of all groups have risen but not at equal rates. Relationships among the ethnic groups have, therefore, changed somewhat. The median income of nonwhites relative to whites has improved slightly. Because of sampling variation, this may not be statistically significant. The median income of Puerto Ricans relative to whites has declined. Here, too, sampling variation is involved. Moreover, not enough is known of the forces at play, such as possible changes in the sex composition of income recipients and in the importance of part-time workers.

Table 1.10. MEDIAN MONEY EARNINGS (IN DOLLARS) OF PERSONS FOURTEEN YEARS OLD AND OVER BY ETHNIC GROUP, NEW YORK CITY, 1949 AND 1956

	1949		1956	
Ethnic Group	Amount	Percent of White Income	Amount	Percent of White Income
Puerto Rican	n.a.	n.a.	2,505	56.5
White	1,657	65.9	n.a.	n.a.
Nonwhite	1,513	60.3	n.a.	n.a.
Other nonwhite	1,707	68.0	3,069	69.5
Other white	2,517	100.0	4,430	100.0

SOURCE: U.S. Bureau of the Census and New York State Department of Labor, Division of Research and Statistics, unpublished tabulations.

For 1956 income distributions of families are available for each ethnic group.

Table 1.11. PERCENTAGE DISTRIBUTION OF WHITE, NONWHITE, AND PUERTO RICAN FAMILIES BY INCOME, NEW YORK CITY, 1956

Annual Income	All Families	White	Nonwhite	Puerto Rican
Under $2,000	2.5	1.7	8.2	11.8
$ 2,000– 3,999	17.9	13.8	41.6	46.2
4,000– 5,999	33.8	33.8	30.3	27.6
6,000– 9,999	32.9	35.7	18.9	13.1
10,000 and over	12.8	14.9	1.1	1.1
Total *	100.0 *	100.0 *	100.0 *	100.0 *
Median Income	$5,752	$6,050	$4,016	$3,510

* Due to rounding, does not add to 100 percent.
SOURCE: New York State Department of Labor, Division of Research and Statistics, unpublished tabulations.

The median income of nonwhite families in 1956 was 66 percent of the median income of white families and that of Puerto

Rican families was 58 percent. The incomes of all families shown here are higher than the corresponding figures for New York City families shown in Table 1.8. The difference between the two medians is $275, or five percent of the lower one. The relationship between the income distributions of white and nonwhite families is, however, consistent with the findings of the New York State interdepartmental Committee on Low Incomes.[32]

One half of all white families earn above $6,000. By contrast, one half of the nonwhite families earn under $4,000 and one half of the Puerto Rican families earn under $3,500. The figure of $6,000 is exceeded by 20 percent of the nonwhite families and by 14 percent of the Puerto Rican families.

Comparisons between Nonwhites and Whites

Data on the income of whites and nonwhites, without a separate breakdown for Puerto Ricans, are more plentiful for New York City and also for other areas. It is possible, for example, to compare trends in the median income of white and nonwhite income recipients in New York City by sex.

Table 1.12. MEDIAN INCOME (IN DOLLARS) OF WHITE AND NONWHITE INCOME RECIPIENTS BY SEX, NEW YORK CITY, 1949 AND 1956

			Increase 1949–56	
Color and Sex	*1949*	*1956*	*Amount*	*Percent*
All income recipients	2,410	3,035	625	25.9
White	2,517	3,210	693	27.5
Nonwhite	1,707	2,362	655	38.4
Total men	2,907	4,036	1,129	38.8
White	3,017	4,216	1,199	39.7
Nonwhite	2,099	3,015	916	43.6
Total women	1,758	2,037	279	15.9
White	1,844	2,084	240	13.0
Nonwhite	1,339	1,848	509	38.0

SOURCE: New York State Interdepartmental Committee on Low Incomes, *Income of Persons by Sex and Color, New York State* (Bulletin No. 3, Pt. 1; New York, 1958), Tables D, 1, and 2; and Gladys Engel Lang, *Minority Groups and Economic Status in New York State* and *Working Tables*, prepared for the New York State Commission against Discrimination (New York, 1958; mimeographed), Table 28.

In relative terms, the median income of nonwhites has shown slightly more improvement than that of whites in the case of men and much more improvement in the case of women. In terms of dollar amounts, the larger increase in median income has been shown by whites in the case of men and by nonwhites in the case of women. The data on white women should be interpreted with care, because they reflect a large increase in part-time employment.[33] The improvement shown by nonwhite women is, however, a real one. As for the income position of men, any conclusion concerning the relative progress of whites and nonwhites depends on whether changes in dollar amounts or in percentages are considered the more appropriate criterion.

There is no doubt whatever that the income position of nonwhites relative to whites is better in New York City than in the country as a whole. For both men and women the difference in income between whites and nonwhites, whether expressed as an amount or as a percentage, is smaller in New York City than in the United States as a whole or in the urban areas of the United States.

Table 1.13. MEDIAN INCOME (IN DOLLARS) OF WHITE AND NON-WHITE INCOME RECIPIENTS BY SEX, NEW YORK CITY, UNITED STATES TOTAL, AND UNITED STATES URBAN, 1956

	Men			*Women*		
Area	*White*	*Non-white*	*Percent Nonwhite to White*	*White*	*Non-white*	*Percent Nonwhite to White*
New York City	4,216	3,015	71.4	2,084	1,848	88.5
United States Total	3,827	2,000	52.2	1,267	727	57.5
United States Urban	4,165	2,624	63.0	1,486	994	66.8

SOURCE: New York State Interdepartmental Committee on Low Incomes, *Income of Persons by Sex and Color, New York State* (Bulletin No. 3, Pt. 1; New York, 1958), Tables A, D, 1, and 2.

DISCUSSION AND IMPLICATIONS

The data show that although nonwhites in New York City are better off than nonwhites elsewhere, the average income of nonwhites in New York City is substantially below that of whites. The disparity between Puerto Ricans and other whites is even greater.

Incomes of nonwhites and of Puerto Ricans in New York City have increased. Because of variation due to sampling size, it is not certain that the ratio of Puerto Rican income to that of other whites has declined. The relative change in the income position of nonwhites cannot be interpreted without ambiguity.

A study of the 1949 income statistics for New York City found that a much larger proportion of nonwhites than of whites had low income (as defined in the study), but that the large majority of families with low incomes—85 percent of the total—were white. The key factor to the lower income of nonwhites was found to be unequal job opportunity.[34]

Less is known about the factors affecting the income of Puerto Ricans. The outlook for the future is complicated by the two-way and perhaps three-way flow of population. It is conceivable that the average income of Puerto Ricans in New York City might be depressed by a continuing stream of new immigrants starting anew at the bottom of the economic ladder, despite improvement in the income position of long-term Puerto Rican residents.[35] The number and proportion of long-term residents is likely to increase, however.

Voluntary Health Insurance Enrollment

Today membership in health insurance plans may be, or is becoming, a better index than personal income of consumer ability to pay for hospital care. From the inception of the voluntary health insurance movement in this country the emphasis has been on covering employee groups. More recently, health insurance premiums are increasingly being paid for, in full or in part, by employer contributions to welfare funds, and enrollment of the individual worker is influenced more by his participation in the labor force than by his earnings.

In May, 1958, a household survey found that 71 percent of the residents of New York City had insurance for hospital care.[36] This is approximately the same proportion as for the nation as a whole.[37] An outstanding difference between New York City and the United States is that the former has a much higher proportion of Blue Cross enrollment (see Chapter 17).

In the spring of 1952 a household survey conducted by a special committee under the auspices of the Health Insurance Plan of Greater New York found that 56 percent of the population of New York City had some type of voluntary health insurance.[38] At that time the nation-wide proportion was also 56 percent. The 1952 finding was consistent with more selective data compiled by the United States Bureau of Labor Statistics for 1950, which showed that the proportion of the population with voluntary health insurance was significantly lower in New York City than in other large cities of the north.[39]

Contributing in part to the relative lag of health insurance enrollment in New York City has been the increase in the Puerto Rican and nonwhite population. It is estimated that enrollment among these groups is one half or less of the rate for the non-Puerto Rican white population.[40] In addition to lower income, higher rates of unemployment are undoubtedly one factor, and the distribution of members of the labor force by industry is another.

Growth in the proportion of the population of New York City with insurance is hampered by a lag in employer participation in the payment of voluntary health insurance premiums. The proportion of insured persons with some employer contribution to premiums was no higher in New York City in 1958 than in the nation in 1955.[41]

It should be noted that for one half of the employees in New York City whose premiums are paid, in full or in part, by their employers the contributions are directed to multiemployer union funds (those that receive contributions from two or more employers in an industry). This is a much higher frequency than in upstate New York, where employer contributions accrue to multiemployer union funds for one sixth of the employees involved and to single employer funds for five sixths.[42] Altogether, multiemployer union funds are encountered more frequently in New York State than in the country as a whole.[43] By pooling premium payments on behalf of employees in two or more firms, the multiemployer union fund increases the flexibility with which a given amount of money can be spent and enhances the leverage that can be applied.

In 1958, 63 percent of New York City's population had some type of insurance for doctors' bills.[44] This is approximately the same as the proportion of the population of the United States with surgical care insurance.[45] The comparison is not entirely valid, however, because a good many of the persons with medical care insurance in New York City have coverage for more than surgical care in the hospital. Coverage for many extends also beyond medical expense insurance in the hospital, as in the case of all subscribers to the Health Insurance Plan of Greater New York (HIP), one third or more of the subscribers to Group Health Insurance (GHI), and 7 percent of the subscribers to United Medical Service (Blue Shield).

On the other hand, New York City lags in enrollment under major medical insurance. (Major medical insurance is characterized by its broad scope, a deductible feature, and a coinsurance factor, as in fire insurance. Most often it supplements the benefits of regular health insurance.) In New York City 11 percent of all group subscribers to health insurance had major medical insurance in 1958, compared with 17 percent in the rest of New York State [46] and also in the nation.[47]

New York City has an unusually high proportion of the population enrolled under prepaid group practice plans—28 percent of the nation-wide total.[48] Included are the one-half million and more subscribers to HIP and approximately one-half million persons, employees and dependents, who are eligible for care in union health centers.

With one exception, union health centers in New York City are relatively new. Mostly they serve members of the union who are employees of a given industry, but frequently dependents are also eligible for care. Typically, they offer diagnostic and treatment services or diagnostic services only for ambulatory patients. Only one center provides services in the hospital as well.

Table 1.14 shows the estimated distribution of persons eligible for care in union health centers in New York City by type of service. Of 13 centers included in the above data, 12 were established after 1947 and 9 after 1950. Every center established after 1952 is limited by state statute to the provision of diagnostic services only.

Of some importance for hospitals in New York City are the estimated 370,000 persons who work but do not reside here.[49] The Roper Survey found that, in 1958, 85 percent of commuters carried hospital care insurance, compared with 83 percent for

Table 1.14. PERCENTAGE DISTRIBUTION OF PERSONS
ELIGIBLE FOR CARE IN UNION HEALTH
CENTERS BY TYPE OF SERVICE,
NEW YORK CITY, 1957

Type of Service	Eligible Persons Percent
Total number: 511,000	
Diagnosis and treatment for ambulatory patients plus inpatients	7.1
Diagnosis and treatment for ambulatory patients	53.5
Diagnosis only	39.4
	100.0

SOURCE: Margaret C. Klem, *Care Provided for Nervous and Mental Diseases at Union Health Centers in New York City, 1957*, paper delivered before Community Council of Greater New York, April 11, 1958 (mimeographed).

other residents of the suburbs, and 71 percent for the residents of New York City.[50] To the extent that commuters make use of hospitals in the city, they increase the demand for private and semiprivate accommodations and reduce the demand for ward accommodations.

Summary

1. The population of New York City declined for the first time in the 1950s, dropping to 7,780,000 in 1960.

2. The loss of 1.4 percent during the decade was smaller than that incurred by many large cities in the nation. The suburban counties of the metropolitan region gained in population here, as they did elsewhere. This points to the need for planning hospital care for an area larger than the city.

3. The decline in New York City's population reflected a continuing decline in average household size and accelerated out-migration of non-Puerto Rican whites.

4. Puerto Ricans and nonwhites increased in number during the 1950's. Both groups tend to occupy positions at the bottom of the economic ladder and have greater need for certain types of health service than the rest of the population.

5. The number and proportion of children and of aged (65 years and over) have increased in New York City.

6. The city's population has been redistributed among the five

boroughs, with Queens being the chief gainer and Manhattan the chief loser. Simultaneously, there has been some dispersal of Puerto Ricans and nonwhites from Manhattan to the other major boroughs. The nonwhite population continues to show evidence of concentration in certain neighborhoods.

7. The most recent projection of population for New York City envisages a population of 8,340,000 in 1975. This figure may prove to be on the high side. Puerto Ricans and nonwhites, it is projected, will constitute 28 percent of the total.

8. Per capita income of the residents of New York City has always exceeded that of the population of the United States and of New York State. Until recently, per capita income in New York City has also exceeded that of the New York metropolitan region.

9. The median income of the Puerto Rican and nonwhite earner in New York City is approximately three fifths and two thirds, respectively, of the median income of the non-Puerto Rican white earner.

10. The proportion of families with low income is larger for Puerto Ricans and nonwhites than for non-Puerto Rican whites, and the proportion of families with higher income is considerably smaller for Puerto Ricans and nonwhites than for non-Puerto Rican whites. Nevertheless, one fifth of nonwhite families in New York had income of $6,000 or more in 1956.

11. The ratio of income of nonwhite earners to that of white earners is much higher in New York City than in the United States as a whole or in urban sections of the United States.

12. Between 1949 and 1956 the ratio of the median income of nonwhite women in New York City to that of white women increased. The trend in income of Negro men relative to that of white men is more ambiguous.

13. Between 1949 and 1956 the median income of all familes in New York City increased 55 percent in money terms and 38 percent in real terms, after allowance for the rise in prices.

14. The ranks of the boroughs with respect to per capita income have changed. Although Manhattan is still in the lead, its margin is narrower than in the past. The other boroughs have shifted ranks, with the greatest gain occurring in Queens. The borough of Richmond ranks fifth when income is measured per

capita, but second when income is measured as cash income per household.

15. Seventy-one percent of the population of New York City is enrolled in hospital care insurance, the same proportion as in the country as a whole. The rate of enrollment in the suburbs is higher—83 percent. The major difference between New York City and the rest of the nation is the larger role played here by Blue Cross relative to commercial insurance.

16. Health insurance enrollment has lagged in New York City relative to other large cities in the north. This may be attributable, in part, to the increase in New York City's Puerto Rican and nonwhite population, whose rate of enrollment is only one half that of the rest of the population. In part, it may be attributable to a lower degree of employer participation in paying health insurance premiums.

17. A larger proportion of employer contributions than elsewhere is directed in New York City to multiemployer union funds. This enhances the leverage that welfare funds can apply.

18. In comparison with the rest of New York State and the United States as a whole, New York City is further distinguished by a lower proportion of the population enrolled under major medical insurance, a higher proportion of the population with insurance for doctors' services outside the hospital, and a high proportion of the population eligible for services in union health centers.

19. The last decade has witnessed a substantial expansion of union health centers. Every center chartered after 1952 is authorized to provide diagnostic services only.

2   PATTERNS OF HOSPITAL USE

This chapter deals with the services rendered by hospitals in New York City. Its primary aim is to assess the changing relative importance of the two major hospital systems, voluntary and municipal. Since proprietary hospitals also play a significant role in New York City, they are included in the data.

It is important to be clear about the terms employed. A voluntary hospital is operated by a nonprofit corporation; a municipal hospital is operated by the Department of Hospitals of the City of New York; and a proprietary hospital is operated by its owners for profit. There is a traditional division of patients by financial status among the three hospital systems. Briefly, municipal hospitals are by law intended primarily for the sick poor; proprietary hospitals care for patients able to pay; and voluntary hospitals typically care for all segments of the population. In turn, the classification of patients by pay status is associated with their classification by type of hospital accommodation—private, semi-private, and ward.

Hospital Services in 1958

The most recent year for which complete data were available is 1958. There were then 151 voluntary, municipal, and proprietary hospitals in New York City, with approximately 50,000 beds. Serving both residents of the city and patients from other areas, they admitted 1,050,000 inpatients and provided 14,435,000 days of care, an average daily census of almost 40,000. These hospitals also carried an average of 2,240 patients a day on home care, received 7,265,000 visits during the year in their outpatient and emergency departments, and responded to 345,000 calls with their emergency ambulances.

Excluded from the above are the following categories of hospitals and related facilities:

1. All federal hospitals in the city. Of particular importance are the three Veterans Administration general hospitals with 3,600 beds. Almost 85 percent of their patients are residents of New York City.[1]

2. All state hospitals. In New York City the four state hospitals are exclusively devoted to the care of psychiatric patients. Although 98 percent of their patients come from New York City, these hospitals, in turn, care for only 22 percent of all New York residents in the state mental hospital system. State hospitals with large numbers of patients from New York City are located in suburban Suffolk and Rockland counties, and with smaller numbers of New York City residents in Broome, Dutchess, and Orange counties.[2]

3. Most related facilities. All nursing homes or infirmaries apart from hospitals are excluded from the data. Included are those infirmary and nursing-home units that are integral parts of hospitals.

DISTRIBUTION OF SERVICES BY OWNERSHIP

The tables in this chapter present data on beds as well as on services, but the former serve mainly as bases for computing measures of hospital use. The focus of this chapter is on hospital services. Facilities as such are dealt with in Chapter 8.

Table 2.1 shows the volumes of services rendered by hospitals in New York City in 1958 and distributes the total for each type of service among the three hospital systems. Absent from the compilation are figures on services rendered to private ambulatory patients for which existing reporting fails to yield reliable information (see pages 57–58).

In 1958 voluntary hospitals provided one half or more of all inpatient and outpatient department services in New York City. Municipal hospitals provided one quarter to two fifths of inpatient services (depending on the criterion employed) and one half or more of all home-care patient days, emergency department

Table 2.1. DISTRIBUTION OF ALL HOSPITAL FACILITIES
BY OWNERSHIP, NEW YORK CITY, 1958

		Percent			
Facility or Service	Number, All Hospitals	All Hospitals	Volun- tary Hospitals	Munici- pal Hospitals	Proprie- tary Hospitals
Bed capacity	49,959	100.0	50.8	39.7	9.5
Bed complement	48,672	100.0	51.2	39.1	9.7
Discharges, inpatients	1,050,570	100.0	59.2	24.7	16.1
Patient days, inpatients	14,435,675	100.0	50.9	40.2	8.9
Patient days, home care	817,431	100.0	5.3	94.7	0
Visits, outpatient departments	5,445,709	100.0	51.4	48.6	0
Visits, emergency departments	1,820,844	100.0	46.3	53.1	0.6
Calls, emergency ambulance service	345,911	100.0	41.3	58.7	0

SOURCE: Hospital Council of Greater New York, annual inventory.

visits, and emergency ambulance calls. Proprietary hospitals provided 9 to 16 percent of inpatient services and a negligible fraction, or none, of the other types of service.

COMPARISON WITH SHORT-TERM HOSPITALS IN UNITED STATES

It is not practical to compare New York City and the nation
in total hospital services, because the residents of New York City
receive so large a proportion of their mental hospital services
outside the city. The obvious solution would be to exclude state
mental hospitals from the comparison. This cannot be done, because the nation-wide data combine the figures for state and local
government hospitals. It was, therefore, decided to limit the comparison to short-term hospitals, in which state hospitals usually
play a small part.

Data are available to compare New York City and the nation
in five categories of hospital beds and services, as shown in Tables
2.2 and 2.3. The comparison is made in two stages: (1) a percentage distribution of a given total by hospital ownership; and (2) a
ratio of beds or services per 1,000 population.

For this comparison municipal hospital centers, such as Bellevue, are treated as single institutions and classified as short-term
hospitals, inasmuch as this is the way the institution and its

counterparts report to the American Hospital Association and appear in the annual "Guide Issue" of the magazine *Hospitals*. Under this scheme of classification certain large facilities for long-term patients are parts of short-term hospitals, affecting the computed measures of hospital use, especially the average duration of patients' stay.

Table 2.2. DISTRIBUTION OF SHORT-TERM HOSPITAL FACILITIES
AND SERVICES BY OWNERSHIP, NEW YORK CITY
AND UNITED STATES, 1958

		Percent			
	Number, *		*Volun-*	*Govern-*	*Proprie-*
	All	*All*	*tary*	*ment*	*tary*
Facility or Service	*Hospitals*	*Hospitals*	*Hospitals*	*Hospitals*	*Hospitals*
Bed complement					
New York City	40,308	100.0	54.3	34.7	11.0
United States	609,732	100.0	69.5	24.6	5.9
Admissions or discharges, inpatients					
New York City	1,036	100.0	59.6	24.4	16.0
United States	21,684	100.0	73.0	19.9	7.1
Patient days, inpatients					
New York City	11,785	100.0	54.0	35.7	10.3
United States	164,668	100.0	71.4	23.4	5.2
Visits, outpatient departments					
New York City	5,407	100.0	51.3	48.7	0
United States	34,276	100.0	55.2	39.2	5.6
Visits, emergency departments					
New York City	1,819	100.0	46.2	53.2	0.6
United States	17,094	100.0	65.8	31.7	2.5

* In thousands, except for beds.
SOURCE: American Hospital Association, *Hospitals*, XXXIII, No. 15 (August 1, 1959), Pt. 2 (Guide Issue), and Hospital Council of Greater New York, annual inventory.

Distribution by Ownership. Because short-term government hospitals in the United States include some state hospitals, the table understates the actual difference between New York City and the nation in the relative importance of municipal hospitals. Even so, municipal hospitals play a larger role here than in the nation for every category of service compared. Conversely, voluntary hospitals play a smaller role here.

Services in Relation to Population. In 1958 New York City had 4.5 percent of the population of the United States. Table 2.3

shows the percentages of beds and of each type of service in New York City to the nation-wide total and compares the ratios of beds and services per 1,000 population in the two areas. The

Table 2.3. PERCENTAGE OF FACILITIES AND SERVICES IN SHORT-
TERM HOSPITALS IN NEW YORK CITY TO THOSE
IN UNITED STATES, AND RATIOS PER 1,000
POPULATION, 1958

Facility or Service	Percent New York City to United States	Ratios per 1,000 Population	
		New York City	United States
Bed complement	6.6	5.2	3.5
Admissions or discharges	4.8	133	125
Patient days	7.1	1,510	947
Visits, outpatient departments	15.8	693	197
Visits, emergency departments	10.6	233	98

SOURCE: Table 2.2 and U.S. Bureau of the Census, Statistical Abstract of the United States.

proportion of New York City's services to the nation's has a wide range—5 to 16 percent. It is lowest in inpatient services and highest in outpatient services.

Two factors that affect the comparisons in Table 2.3 deserve elaboration: (1) the proportion of all medical services rendered in hospitals; and (2) the proportion of hospital services in New York City rendered to nonresidents.

Outpatient departments of hospitals offer medical services to the sick poor. According to Table 2.3, they are used 3.5 times more often in New York City than in the nation. This ratio would rise if cognizance were taken of the large volume of services rendered to the sick in New York City by nonhospital clinics, including those operated by the Department of Health and by independent dispensaries (see page 53). There is apparently a real difference between New York City and the nation in the manner of providing medical care to ambulatory patients who are indigent or medically indigent. This difference is consistent with the higher proportion of inpatients in New York City who receive care in the ward (see Chapter 4).

A significant proportion of inpatient services rendered by short-term hospitals in New York City—almost one-tenth (see Chapter 3)—is received by nonresidents. In turn, some of the residents of New York City receive hospital care elsewhere. The net result is an annual rate of admission of 125 per 1,000 population, the same as in the nation (see below).

The comparison of patient days in Table 2.3 is also invalid, because the municipal hospital centers in New York City include a much larger volume of beds and services for long-term patients than do short-term hospitals in the nation at large. To anticipate the findings of a later section on general care facilities and services, average length of patient stay in New York City exceeds that in the nation by one third or more. With rates of admission identical, hospital use is higher in New York City than in the nation by the same one third or more—1,310 patient days per 1,000 population per year compared with 950.

Table 2.3 also shows that the use of emergency department services is two-and-one-third times greater in New York City than in the nation. The 1958 difference is smaller than in the past.[3]

It is known, although an exact quantitative comparison is not possible, that New York City uses more emergency ambulance services than do other large cities in the nation.[4]

Trends in Total Hospital Services, 1930–58

The situation in New York City in 1958 represents the culmination of developments over the years. Moreover, the total for all hospitals is the sum of the several types of hospital program.

The remainder of this chapter traces the trend in total hospital beds and services as far back as it was possible to go to develop reliable figures for each hospital system. This order of discussion is followed: (1) total hospital services for inpatients; (2) services for inpatients in general-care facilities; (3) services for ambulatory patients and in the home; (4) services for inpatients in non-general-care facilities.

For total hospital facilities and services it was possible to compile decennial data beginning in 1930, and for facilities only, beginning in 1920. For individual programs, however, data are usually presented beginning in 1940, except when they first became available at a later date.

Table 2.4 shows beds, discharges, and patient days by hospital ownership in 1930, 1940, 1950, and 1958.

Table 2.4. DISTRIBUTION OF FACILITIES AND SERVICES BY
HOSPITAL OWNERSHIP, NEW YORK CITY,
1930, 1940, 1950, AND 1958

Facility or Service	1930		1940		1950		1958	
	Num-ber*	Per-cent	Num-ber*	Per-cent	Num-ber*	Per-cent	Num-ber*	Per-cent
Bed complement								
All hospitals	36,575	100.0	41,160	100.0	43,493	100.0	48,672	100.0
Voluntary	19,466	53.2	22,017	53.5	22,559	51.9	24,883	51.2
Municipal	13,614	37.2	15,609	37.9	16,735	38.5	19,059	39.1
Proprietary	3,495	9.6	3,534	8.6	4,199	9.6	4,730	9.7
Discharges								
All hospitals	627	100.0	756	100.0	921	100.0	1,051	100.0
Voluntary	384	61.2	427	56.5	525	57.0	622	59.2
Municipal	176	28.1	253	33.5	251	27.3	259	24.7
Proprietary	67	10.7	76	10.0	145	15.7	170	16.1
Patient days								
All hospitals	10,218	100.0	12,637	100.0	13,743	100.0	14,436	100.0
Voluntary	5,062	49.6	6,116	48.4	6,525	47.5	7,350	50.9
Municipal	4,448	43.5	5,785	45.8	6,095	44.3	5,796	40.2
Proprietary	708	6.9	736	5.8	1,123	8.2	1,290	8.9

* In thousands, except for beds.
SOURCE: For 1930—Hospital Survey for New York, II (New York, 1937), pp. 116, 142,
and Eli Ginzberg, A Pattern for Hospital Care (New York, 1949), p. 151; for 1940—
see Appendix 2.A; for 1950 and 1958—Hospital Council of Greater New York, annual inventory.

The estimated bed figures for 1920 follow:[5]

Hospital Ownership	Number	Percent
All hospitals	30,231	100.0
Voluntary	16,636	55.0
Municipal	12,299	40.7
Proprietary	1,296	4.3

It is clear that the use of hospitals in New York City has been
rising. This was true even in the 1950s, after the resident population had ceased to grow (see Chapter 1). Although changes in the
proportion of beds, discharges, and patient days held by each hospital system have not always tended in the same direction, it may
be generalized that (1) in the past 40 years the relative importance
of proprietary hospitals has increased, with much of the increase
taking place in the 1920s and again in the 1940s; (2) the relative
importance of municipal hospitals in the provision of inpatient
services has declined since World War II, and (3) the relative

importance of voluntary hospitals has been reasonably constant over the long run, with some interim fluctuations.

In both beds and patient days, if proprietary hospitals received a weight of 1 in 1958, the weight of voluntary hospitals would be 5 and that of municipal hospitals 4. In discharges the corresponding weights would be 1.5, 6.0, and 2.5, respectively. These differences in relative weights between discharges, on the one hand, and patient days and beds, on the other, signify that municipal hospitals have by far the longest duration of patient stay. This reflects in part the longer stay of general-care patients in municipal hospitals than in other hospitals and in part the larger proportion of municipal hospital facilities devoted to non-general-care patients.

Services for General-Care Inpatients

For an analysis of trends in hospital use in New York City, without reference to other geographic areas, a more refined set of distinctions is available than that between short-term and long-term hospitals. One may classify facilities and services in terms of organized nursing units within a hospital by employing the classification scheme developed in the Hospital Council's *Master Plan for Hospitals and Related Facilities for New York City*,[6] as modified by subsequent usage.

Broadly, inpatient facilities are classified into (1) general care and (2) all other, with the latter further subdivided among psychiatric, tuberculosis, chronic, rehabilitation, and nursing home. General care has come to include acute communicable diseases.

A general-care facility is usually housed in a general or allied special hospital, such as maternity or children's. Since a general hospital may also contain units for patients with tuberculosis or psychiatric illness, the total number of beds and services reported by a general hospital may exceed the number of its general-care beds and services. In 1958, for example, the general care (general and allied special) hospitals in New York City had 40,300 beds in complement, 1,036,000 discharges, and 11,785,000 patient days (Table 2.2). The corresponding figures for general-care facilities were lower—35,700, 993,000, and 10,200,000, respectively (Table 2.5, below).

Data on general-care beds, discharges, and patient days by hospital ownership for the years 1940, 1950, and 1958 are shown in Table 2.5.

Table 2.5. DISTRIBUTION OF GENERAL-CARE FACILITIES
AND SERVICES BY HOSPITAL OWNERSHIP,
NEW YORK CITY, 1940, 1950, AND 1958

Facility or	1940		1950		1958	
Service	Number*	Percent	Number*	Percent	Number*	Percent
Bed complement						
All hospitals	32,542	100.0	32,584	100.0	35,670	100.0
Voluntary	19,005	58.4	19,180	58.9	21,220	59.5
Municipal	10,238	31.5	9,816	30.1	10,245	28.7
Proprietary	3,299	10.1	3,588	11.0	4,205	11.8
Discharges						
All hospitals	707	100.0	870	100.0	993	100.0
Voluntary	422	59.7	520	59.8	612	61.6
Municipal	210	29.7	209	24.0	216	21.7
Proprietary	75	10.6	141	16.2	165	16.7
Patient days						
All hospitals	9,387	100.0	9,785	100.0	10,217	100.0
Voluntary	5,070	54.0	5,411	55.3	6,102	59.7
Municipal	3,638	38.8	3,437	35.1	2,976	29.1
Proprietary	679	7.2	937	9.6	1,139	11.2

* In thousands, except for beds.
SOURCE: For 1940—see Appendix 2.A; for 1950 and 1958—Hospital Council of Greater New York, annual inventory.

General-care beds remained constant in the 1940s but increased 10 percent between 1950 and 1958, while the city's population declined slightly. Two thirds of the bed increase occurred in voluntary hospitals.

General-care discharges increased by 163,000 in the 1940s and by 123,000 between 1950 and 1958. Voluntary hospitals reported a substantial increase in each time interval, while proprietary hospitals had a substantial increase in the first interval and a moderate one in the second. Municipal hospitals had no appreciable change in either period.

Patient days increased by 400,000 in the 1940s and by more than 400,000 between 1950 and 1958. Voluntary and proprietary hospitals had substantial increases in both time intervals. Municipal hospitals had a decline of 200,000 in the first interval and a much larger one in the second.

If the number of general-care beds in proprietary hospitals were given a weight of 1, the respective weights of the voluntary and municipal systems would be roughly 6 and 3 (compared with weights of 1, 5, and 4 for total beds). Over the years the proportion of all general-care beds in voluntary hospitals has increased slightly, that in proprietary hospitals has increased somewhat, and that in municipal hospitals has declined.

In 1958 the percentage distribution of general-care patient days by hospital ownership was similar to that of beds. This had not been true in earlier years, when the municipal system's share of patient days exceeded its share of beds. The shift signifies that today the rate of occupancy in municipal hospitals is close to that in the other hospital systems and not much higher, as in the past.

Proprietary hospitals have always had a larger share of discharges than of patient days, whereas the converse is true of municipal hospitals. These relationships signify that the average duration of patient stay is longer in municipal than in proprietary hospitals. Since the difference between each hospital system's proportion of discharges and of patient days was smaller in 1958 than in 1950, the decade must have witnessed a narrowing of differences among the three hospital systems in average length of patient stay (see below for computed measures of hospital use).

In 1940 the percentage distribution of general-care discharges was similar to the distribution of beds. This is no longer true. In 1958 voluntary hospitals had approximately the same share of discharges as of beds. Municipal hospitals, however, had a lower proportion of discharges than of beds, while proprietary hospitals had a higher proportion of discharges than of beds. These shifts bear on changes in the average rate of bed turnover (the number of patients served by a bed during a specified period of time). They signify that the largest gains have occurred in proprietary hospitals and the smallest gains, if any, in municipal hospitals.

COMPUTED MEASURES OF HOSPITAL USE

The numerical values of the changes in rate of occupancy, length of stay, and rate of bed turnover in each hospital system can only be determined by computation. For present purposes the figures need not be exact. Much effort has been obviated by computing rate of occupancy on bed complement at the end of the year, rather than on the average number of beds in operation during the year. Length of stay was computed in the usual manner by relating discharges to total patient days for the year; this short cut yields acceptable results when applied to short-term hospitals.

It should be pointed out that the three measures of hospital use are interrelated mathematically, with the rate of bed turnover directly proportional to length of stay. The equation is this (see Appendix 2.B for its derivation):

$$\text{Average Annual Rate of Bed Turnover} = \frac{365 \times \text{Rate of Occupancy}}{\text{Length of Stay}}$$

The measures of hospital use are shown in Table 2.6.

Table 2.6. COMPUTED MEASURES OF HOSPITAL USE IN GENERAL-CARE FACILITIES BY OWNERSHIP, NEW YORK CITY, 1940, 1950, AND 1958

Measure of Hospital Use	1940	1950	1958
Rate of occupancy (percent)			
All hospitals	79.0	82.5	78.5
Voluntary	73.2	77.4	78.8
Municipal	97.4	96.0	79.8
Proprietary	56.4	72.1	74.3
Length of stay (days)			
All hospitals	13.3	11.2	10.3
Voluntary	12.0	10.4	10.0
Municipal	17.3	16.4	13.8
Proprietary	9.1	6.7	6.9
Annual rate of bed turnover (ratio)			
All hospitals	21.7	26.8	27.8
Voluntary	22.2	27.1	28.8
Municipal	20.5	21.3	21.1
Proprietary	22.7	39.3	39.2

SOURCE: Table 2.5.

Rate of Occupancy. For the three hospital systems combined the rate of occupancy of general-care beds in 1958 was about the same as in 1940 but lower than in 1950. The reason is that in the 1950s beds increased at a faster rate than patient days.

Formerly municipal hospitals were overcrowded, operating at an annual rate of occupancy of 95 to 100 percent. It is recognized that a short-term hospital cannot be operated efficiently at so high an average occupancy for the year. Too many factors militate against this, including random fluctuations in patient load; seasonal variations in the incidence of illness; vacation on the part of patients, physicians, or hospital personnel; weekend lulls; segregation of patients by pay status, sex, and clinical department; and maintenance of stand by facilities for emergency admissions. An annual rate of occupancy of 95 or 100 percent signifies the presence of patients in beds in the corridors of patients' rooms and in hallways on many days in the year.

At a rate of occupancy of 80 percent, municipal hospitals are operating at a level that was once regarded as optimum.[7] Today it is believed that general-care facilities can be effectively operated at a higher annual rate of occupancy, perhaps 85 percent or more. What the optimum rate of occupancy is for an individual institution depends on (1) the relative size of its obstetrical service, which tends to operate at a lower rate of occupancy than other clinical departments; (2) the extent to which physical plant lends itself to flexible use and the extent to which administration takes advantage of the plant's capabilities; and perhaps also (3) the average length of patient stay, with a longer stay being conducive to a higher rate of occupancy. In any event, with a complement of 10,200 general-care beds in the municipal system, improved occupancy may be expected to reduce the number of vacant beds by no more than 500 to 800.

The rate of occupancy in voluntary hospitals has steadily improved, but it is still slightly lower than in municipal hospitals. Rate of occupancy in voluntary hospitals by type of accommodation is discussed in the next section.

Occupancy in proprietary hospitals improved strikingly in the 1940s and continued to improve, more slowly, in the 1950s. The rate of occupancy in proprietary hospitals is still lowest but is now within four to five percentage points of the rate in the other two systems.

Length of Patient Stay. The average length of stay of general-care patients in all hospitals in New York City declined in the 1940s and also in the 1950s. However, the rate of decline in the second interval was only one half that in the first. In the voluntary and proprietary systems all or most of the decline in patient stay occurred in the 1940s. There was hardly any change in the 1950s. The experience of municipal hospitals was reversed. Here length of stay declined by one day in the 1940s and by two and one half days in the 1950s.

Immediately after World War II municipal hospitals were crowded, and bottlenecks in diagnostic facilities prolonged the period of examination and evaluation prior to treatment. In addition, overflow of patients from tuberculosis facilities raised the average length of patient stay in general-care units.

Toward the end of the 1940s the Department of Hospitals engaged in a concerted drive to expand ancillary services and eliminate diagnostic bottlenecks. Crowding was also eased by the adoption of more rigorous criteria for the admission of patients. The average period of initial evaluation therefore declined. Duration of stay was shortened in 1949 by the establishment of home-care programs and more effectively in 1952 by the initiation of a campaign to transfer patients to proprietary nursing homes and public-home infirmaries when definitive hospital care was completed. Finally, the composition of patients changed, as the proportion of obstetrical patients, who remain in the hospital only a few days, increased and as several municipal hospitals—new ones as well as existing ones that were relocated from Welfare Island to populated neighborhoods—became active institutions with more rapid turnover of patients.

Rate of Bed Turnover. The rate of turnover of general-care beds—a measure of the over-all effectiveness with which hospital beds are used—increased five times as rapidly in the 1940s as in the 1950s. The large increase in the first period reflects the confluence of two tendencies: increased occupancy and shortened patient stay. In the second interval the reduction in stay was partly offset by a decline in rate of occupancy.

Proprietary hospitals had a large increase in the rate of bed turnover during the period 1940–58, voluntary hospitals a moderate increase, and municipal hospitals only a slight increase. The entire gain in the proprietary system was confined to the 1940s. In the voluntary system a moderate gain occurred in the 1940s and a small one in the 1950s. In the municipal system the decline in rate of occupancy from a very high level served to offset a reduction in patient stay.

DISTRIBUTION BY TYPE OF ACCOMMODATION

Reference has been made to the association between patients' pay status and type of hospital accommodation—private, semiprivate, and ward. For example, all public-charge patients are in the ward, whereas most insured patients are semiprivate. Both private and semiprivate patients in the hospital receive care from their own physicians; the difference between them is that the former occupies a single-bed room while the latter occupies a multiple-bed room (usually containing two or four beds). If the number of beds in the multiple-bed room is large, say eight, the accommodation may be designated as private ward, a subclass under semiprivate. What is usually called the ward service is, more precisely, the general ward. More and more this designation has come to mean provision of medical care by one of the organized clinical departments of the hospital and the absence of a private physician rather than a large number of beds in the patient's room. In newly built or modernized hospitals designed for the flexible use of facilities, there are few, if any, patients' rooms with more than four beds: rooms with two, three, or four beds may be used interchangeably for semiprivate and ward patients, as needed.

All general-care patients in proprietary hospitals are either private or semiprivate, and all patients in municipal hospitals are general ward patients. (The single exception in the municipal system is Sydenham Hospital, which was allowed to maintain its private and semiprivate services when acquired by the City of New York in 1949.) Voluntary hospitals have both private (including semiprivate) and ward patients.

Private and Ward Services of Voluntary Hospitals. Most voluntary hospitals have all three types of accommodation. It is, therefore, necessary to distribute the facilities and services of the voluntary system by type of accommodation as a prerequisite to preparing such a distribution for all hospitals. Table 2.7 divides beds, discharges, and patient days in voluntary hospitals between private (including semiprivate) and ward services. Private and semiprivate patients are combined because (1) for many purposes, including the teaching role of hospitals, the important distinction is between them, on the one hand, and ward patients, on the other; (2) they must ultimately be combined in any analysis that includes proprietary hospitals in New York City, since most of the latter do not report separate statistics for private and semiprivate patients; and (3) the presentation and analysis of data are facilitated.

Table 2.7. GENERAL-CARE FACILITIES AND SERVICES IN VOLUN-
TARY HOSPITALS BY TYPE OF ACCOMMODATION,
NEW YORK CITY, 1940, 1950, AND 1958

Facility or Service	1940		1950		1958	
	Number*	Per-cent	Number*	Per-cent	Number*	Per-cent
Bed complement						
All accommodations	19,005	100.0	19,180	100.0	21,220	100.0
Private and semiprivate	8,001	42.1	9,958	52.0	13,004	61.3
Ward	11,004	57.8	9,222	48.0	8,216	38.7
Discharges						
All accommodations	422	100.0	520	100.0	612	100.0
Private and semiprivate	168	39.8	309	59.5	422	69.0
Ward	254	60.2	211	40.5	190	31.0
Patient days						
All accommodations	5,070	100.0	5,411	100.0	6,102	100.0
Private and semiprivate	1,918	37.8	2,942	54.4	3,851	63.1
Ward	3,152	62.2	2,469	45.6	2,251	36.9

* In thousands, except for beds.
SOURCE: See Table 2.5.

Between 1940 and 1958 general-care ward beds in voluntary hospitals declined by 2,800, whereas the number of private and semiprivate beds increased by 5,000. The increase in private and semiprivate beds in voluntary hospitals was achieved in part by expanding plant by 2,200 beds and in part by transferring ward facilities to semiprivate use (with or without physical conversion). Private beds declined by 400 between 1940 and 1958, and private ward beds (classified under semiprivate) declined by 800.[8] Only semiprivate beds increased—by 6,200.

The ward service of voluntary hospitals declined in discharges and patient days as well as in beds. At the same time, total general-care discharges and patient days in the voluntary system increased, so that the gains of the private (including semiprivate) service must have exceeded the losses of the ward service. The relative importance of the ward has, therefore, declined. The greatest decline has occurred in the proportion of ward to total discharges and the smallest in the proportion of ward to total beds, with the proportion of ward to total patient days in between. These shifts signify certain changes in the measures of hospital use, and these can be examined directly.

Table 2.8. COMPUTED MEASURES OF HOSPITAL USE IN GENERAL-CARE FACILITIES OF VOLUNTARY HOSPITALS BY TYPE OF ACCOMMODATION, NEW YORK CITY, 1940, 1950, AND 1958

Measure of Hospital Use	1940	1950	1958
Rate of occupancy (percent)			
All accommodations	73.0	77.4	78.8
Private and semiprivate	65.7	81.0	81.1
Ward	78.5	73.5	75.0
Length of stay (days)			
All accommodations	12.0	10.4	10.0
Private and semiprivate	11.4	9.5	9.1
Ward	12.5	11.7	11.8
Annual rate of bed turnover (ratio)			
All accommodations	22.1	27.1	28.8
Private and semiprivate	21.0	31.0	32.5
Ward	23.0	22.9	23.1

SOURCE: Table 2.7.

Whereas the rate of bed turnover in the private (including semiprivate) service rose strikingly in the 1940s and modestly in the 1950s, it remained unchanged in the ward in both periods. In the 1940s a reduction in average length of patient stay in the ward was offset by a decline in rate of occupancy, and in the 1950s a slight improvement in occupancy was offset by a small prolongation of stay. It will be recalled that the rate of bed turnover in municipal hospitals behaved in similar fashion, although the timing of the changes in rate of occupancy and length of stay differed.

Computing Rates of Occupancy in Two Types of Accommodation. Since World War II the rate of occupancy in the private (including semiprivate) service of voluntary hospitals has consistently exceeded that in the ward. The rate of occupancy in the semiprivate service alone is, however, higher than shown in the table, and that in the private service is much lower. In 1958 the rates of occupancy in the private, semiprivate, and ward general-care services were, respectively, 68, 85, and 75 percent.

Many voluntary hospitals report a rate of occupancy in the high 80s or 90s for their semiprivate service, and in the 60s or low 70s for their ward. At first glance it would seem that such hospitals must have large numbers of vacant ward beds. In fact, this is true only in hospitals in which semiprivate and ward facilities are segregated and not used interchangeably. It is not true in a hospital where a patient applying for a semiprivate bed is admitted to the ward in the absence of a vacant semiprivate bed. Although physically located in the ward, such a patient, who is under the care of his own physician, is classified as semiprivate. Under this procedure the rate of occupancy of the semiprivate service is overstated and that of the ward understated.

The situation described above is particularly common in hospitals which report services for private ward patients but do not designate any private ward beds. In 1957 a special analysis of the Hospital Council's inventory data found that 82,000 private ward patient days (equivalent to an average daily census of 224) were reported by six voluntary hospitals that reported no private ward beds. These hospitals computed rates of occupancy of 54 percent in the ward and of 101 percent in semiprivate accommodations. When the physical location of patients was taken into account, the result was a rise in ward rate of occupancy to 75 percent and a reduction in semiprivate occupancy to 80 percent.

For hospitals that use their beds flexibly for both semiprivate and ward patients there are no firm bases on which to compute the rate of occupancy of each type of accommodation. Reported rates of occupancy should be viewed with caution. It may be sensible to compute a rate of occupancy for all multiple-bed rooms combined, rather than separately for semiprivate and ward accommodations.

Trends in Private and Ward Services. It is now possible to analyze trends in private (including semiprivate) and ward facilities and services for general-care patients in all hospitals, before examining the respective roles of the three hospital systems.

Table 2.9. GENERAL-CARE FACILITIES AND SERVICES IN ALL
HOSPITALS BY TYPE OF ACCOMMODATION,
NEW YORK CITY, 1940, 1950, AND 1958

	1940		1950		1958	
Facility or Service	Number*	Percent	Number*	Percent	Number*	Percent
Bed complement						
All accommodations	32,542	100.0	32,584	100.0	35,670	100.0
Private and semiprivate	11,300	34.7	13,619	41.8	17,270	48.4
Ward	21,242	65.3	18,965	58.2	18,400	51.6
Discharges						
All accommodations	707	100.0	870	100.0	993	100.0
Private and semiprivate	243	34.4	452	52.0	589	59.4
Ward	464	65.6	418	48.0	404	40.6
Patient days						
All accommodations	9,387	100.0	9,785	100.0	10,217	100.0
Private and semiprivate	2,597	27.7	3,895	39.8	5,006	49.0
Ward	6,790	72.3	5,890	60.2	5,211	51.0

* In thousands, except for beds.
SOURCE: See Table 2.5.

In each item—beds, discharges, and patient days—the ward service has declined, and the private (including semiprivate) service has gained by an even greater amount. The proportion of ward to total general-care facilities and services has, therefore, declined.

Notwithstanding, general-care ward patients, who constitute two fifths of all discharges in New York City, still receive more than one half of patient days. Some of the factors underlying this relatively high use of the ward in New York City are explored in Chapter 4.

Since the proportion of ward to total has declined much faster for discharges than for beds, the rate of bed turnover in ward facilities has lagged behind that in the private (including semiprivate) service. Indeed, the computed measures show no change for the former, compared with a large increase for the latter.

	Rate of Bed Turnover		
Accommodation	1940	1958	Difference
Private and semiprivate	21.5	34.1	+ 12.5
Ward	21.8	21.7	− 0.1

Trends in Private Service by Hospital Ownership. Table 2.10 shows the respective roles of the three hospital systems in caring for private (including semiprivate) patients in 1940, 1950, and 1958. The role of municipal hospitals is negligible, being limited to Sydenham Hospital.

Table 2.10. PRIVATE (INCLUDING SEMIPRIVATE) GENERAL-CARE FACILITIES AND SERVICES BY HOSPITAL OWNERSHIP, NEW YORK CITY, 1940, 1950, AND 1958

Facility or Service	1940		1950		1958	
	Number*	Percent	Number*	Percent	Number*	Percent
Bed complement						
All hospitals	11,300	100.0	13,619	100.0	17,270	100.0
Voluntary	8,001	70.8	9,958	73.1	13,004	75.4
Municipal	0	0	73	0.5	61	0.3
Proprietary	3,299	29.2	3,588	26.4	4,205	24.3
Discharges						
All hospitals	243	100.0	452	100.0	589	100.0
Voluntary	168	69.2	309	68.5	422	71.6
Municipal	0	0	2	0.4	2	0.3
Proprietary	75	30.8	141	31.1	165	28.1
Patient days						
All hospitals	2,597	100.0	3,895	100.0	5,006	100.0
Voluntary	1,918	73.8	2,942	75.6	3,851	76.9
Municipal	0	0	16	0.4	16	0.3
Proprietary	679	26.2	937	24.0	1,139	22.8

* In thousands, except for beds.
SOURCE: See Table 2.5.

Voluntary hospitals have had a rising share of private (including semiprivate) beds, discharges, and patient days. Although proprietary hospitals have experienced sizable growth in numerical terms, their rate of expansion has been below that of the private service of voluntary hospitals.

Proprietary hospitals have a higher proportion of discharges than of patient days. This is consistent with their below-average patient stay. As previously shown, length of stay in proprietary hospitals is 7 days, compared with 9 days in the private (including semiprivate) service of voluntary hospitals.

Rate of occupancy in proprietary hospitals is 74 percent, compared with a reported rate of 81 percent in the private (including semiprivate) service of voluntary hospitals.

Trends in Ward Service by Hospital Ownership. Table 2.11 shows the roles of voluntary and municipal hospitals in caring for ward patients in 1940, 1950, and 1958.

Table 2.11. WARD GENERAL-CARE FACILITIES AND SERVICES
BY HOSPITAL OWNERSHIP, NEW YORK CITY,
1940, 1950, AND 1958

Facility or Service	1940		1950		1958	
	Number*	Percent	Number*	Percent	Number*	Percent
Bed complement						
All hospitals	21,242	100.0	18,965	100.0	18,400	100.0
Voluntary	11,004	51.8	9,222	48.6	8,216	44.6
Municipal	10,238	48.2	9,743	51.6	10,184	55.4
Discharges						
All hospitals	464	100.0	418	100.0	404	100.0
Voluntary	254	54.6	211	50.4	190	47.1
Municipal	210	45.4	207	49.6	214	52.9
Patient days						
All hospitals	6,790	100.0	5,890	100.0	5,211	100.0
Voluntary	3,152	46.5	2,469	42.0	2,251	43.2
Municipal	3,638	53.5	3,421	58.0	2,960	56.8

* In thousands, except for beds.
SOURCE: See Table 2.5.

The ward service in voluntary hospitals has definitely declined, whatever the criterion. In municipal hospitals ward beds
and ward discharges have each increased slightly, whereas patient
days have declined appreciably. As a result, the share of voluntary
hospitals in the general-care ward service has declined and that of
municipal hospitals increased. In 1940 municipal hospitals had
more than one half of all ward patient days, but less than one
half of beds and of discharges; by 1950 they also had more than
one half of ward beds; and by 1958 they had, in addition, more
than one half of all ward discharges.

Between 1940 and 1958 the proportions of ward beds, discharges, and patient days held by each system converged. As a
result, the differences between the two hospital systems in ward
rate of occupancy, length of stay, and rate of bed turnover have
narrowed.

Hospital Use (Computed measure)	1940			1958		
	Voluntary Ward	Munici-pal	Differ-ence	Voluntary Ward	Munici-pal	Differ-ence
Rate of occupancy (percent)	78.5	97.4	+ 18.9	75.0	79.8	+ 4.8
Length of stay (days)	12.5	17.3	+ 4.8	11.8	13.8	+ 2.0
Turnover rate (ratio)	23.0	20.5	− 2.5	23.1	21.1	− 2.0

It may be that one of the factors leading to convergence is the increased proportion of public-charge patients in the wards of voluntary hospitals (see Chapter 14).

Services for Ambulatory Patients and in the Home

Traditionally, a short-term voluntary or municipal hospital in New York City has operated an outpatient department for the sick poor. A more recent development—a postwar phenomenon in its present size—is the emergency department, which frequently started in the outpatient department and in some instances still cannot be separated from it. Organized home-care programs radiating from hospitals have old antecedents but in New York City they represent a postwar revival and growth. Also discussed in this section are the emergency ambulance service and, more briefly, services to private ambulatory patients, including those furnished by diagnostic clinics in hospitals.

OUTPATIENT DEPARTMENT

The number of visits to outpatient departments of voluntary and municipal hospitals in New York City has fluctuated considerably. Data for selected years are shown in Table 2.12. The volume of outpatient department visits in both hospital systems in 1958 was almost the same as in 1930 or 1950 but substantially below that in 1940—at the end of a decade of depression. Compared with more recent years, the volume of visits in 1958 was the same as in 1951 but 400,000 higher than in 1955.

Table 2.12. OUTPATIENT DEPARTMENT VISITS BY HOSPITAL OWNERSHIP, NEW YORK CITY, 1925–58

| Year | Number (in Thousands) | | | Percent | |
	Total	Voluntary	Municipal	Voluntary	Municipal
1925	3,596	2,798	798	77.8	22.2
1930	5,623	4,275	1,348	76.0	24.0
1940	7,720	4,805	2,915	62.2	37.8
1950	5,577	3,436	2,141	61.6	38.4
1958	5,446	2,801	2,644	51.4	48.6

SOURCE: For 1925, 1930, and 1940—United Hospital Fund of New York, Out-Patient Service Statistics Relating to Hospitals and Independent Dispensaries in New York City (New York, 1926–41); for 1950 and 1958—Hospital Council of Greater New York, annual inventory.

In voluntary hospitals the volume of visits in 1958 was the same as in 1925 but well below the volume in the intervening years shown in the table. Conversely, the 1958 volume of visits in municipal hospitals was four times that in 1925, double that in 1930, and only 10 percent below that in 1940. All of the increase in total visits between 1955 and 1958 occurred in municipal hospitals. The postwar tendency toward more visits in municipal hospitals and fewer visits in voluntary hospitals was arrested in 1959, when the effects of the new payment policy by government first became felt.

In September, 1958, the City of New York undertook to pay voluntary hospitals $5 per outpatient department visit by recipients of public assistance, provided certain criteria were met. At the same time, the State of New York agreed to reimburse the City $2.50 per visit by recipients of public assistance in municipal and voluntary hospitals.

Visits in outpatient departments of voluntary hospitals have declined from three fourths of the total in 1930 to five eighths in 1940 and 1950 and to approximately one half in 1958. Future trends in outpatient department services will depend on a number of factors. One is the growth of health insurance for medical services outside the hospital. It is perhaps surprising in the face of both rising per capita income and health insurance enrollment in New York City that the volume of outpatient department visits rose in the second half of the 1950s. This was accompanied by an even more rapid increase in emergency department visits (see below).

There have been no compensatory declines in similar or possibly substitute services. Visits by ambulatory patients in Department of Health clinics and independent dispensaries under voluntary control amounted to 2.5 million in 1958, the same as in 1950. Here, too, the tendency in recent years has been for the volume of services in governmental clinics to increase and in voluntary clinics to decline.

It is fair to note that during the postwar period the number of clinic visits for dental care, for which there is little voluntary health insurance coverage, has increased faster than for any other type of service. Between 1947 and 1956 visits to dental clinics of hospitals, Health Department, and independent dispensaries rose by more than 400,000. During this period there was also a large increase in visits to pediatric clinics—more than 300,000. The largest single reduction—more than 400,000 visits—occurred in syphilis clinics, as a result of changes in medical practice.[9]

Examination of changes in the number of visits to the outpatient department and emergency department of hospitals operting both services fails to reveal a shift from the former to the latter. The relationship between the two types of service is complex, and under certain conditions one department may be expected to gain simultaneously with the other. Under other conditions one gains at the expense of the other.[10]

Analysis of data for individual voluntary hospitals shows that there is an inverse relationship between changes in average income per visit and in number of visits to outpatient departments. In general, the larger the increase in income, the larger is the reduction in volume of visits. In specific instances, however, increases in outpatient department charges, if unaccompanied by other steps, may serve to raise the proportion of free visits, rather than to reduce the total volume. The greatest reductions in outpatient department load have occurred in clinics in which rigid adherence to district lines or to formal eligibility criteria was introduced or became more firmly enforced.

The decline in outpatient visits in voluntary hospitals is consistent with the decline in their ward services. In 1940, when voluntary hospitals had 55 percent of all general-care ward patients, they had 62 percent of all outpatient department visits. In 1950, the voluntary hospitals' proportions were 50 and 62 percent, respectively, and by 1958, 47 and 51 percent, respectively. However, in individual hospitals there is no uniform relationship between the volumes of the two services. As reported by one survey, the proportion of ward patients referred by, or originating in, the outpatient department varies greatly, from 15 percent in one hospital to 65 percent or more in another.[11] Some of the variation has to do with differences in the diagnostic composition of referred patients, but much of it is not yet understood.

Municipal hospitals in New York City do not charge for outpatient department services. For several years a proposal has been pending to charge outpatients one dollar a visit, with suitable adjustment downward for persons who cannot afford the fee. The major stated objective of the proposal is to reduce overcrowding in the outpatient departments of municipal hospitals and thereby permit available physicians' time to be concentrated on fewer patients. This is expected to improve the quality of care.

In support of the proposal it is argued that persons who do not require the services of a physician should not be encouraged to come to the outpatient department, add to its crowded condition, and consume scarce services. It is also pointed out that inpatients who can afford it are required to pay, so that there is no reason why the same requirement should not in principle apply to ambulatory patients. An arrangement to reduce or waive the fee for those unable to pay would provide protection against denial of needed services.[12]

In opposition it has been argued that a charge may operate indiscriminately, effecting a reduction in visits by patients who need the services of a physician as well as by patients who do not. It is also observed that certain patients, particularly among the aged, do not like a means test and prefer to forego necessary medical care rather than submit to one. Similarly, it has been argued that other groups of dependents, such as children and pregnant women, may be deprived of needed services if a charge is levied. Finally, it has been suggested that direct efforts to improve the quality of care—an objective that enlists general support —may prove to be more fruitful.

EMERGENCY DEPARTMENT

The year 1948 is the first for which data on hospital emergency departments could be obtained for both voluntary and municipal hospitals. Because the volume of services rendered by proprietary hospitals is so small—10,500 visits in 1958—it has not been compiled routinely and is omitted from Table 2.13.

Considerable variation exists among hospitals in the role assigned to the emergency department and in the manner of counting its services. One large teaching hospital in New York City still does not report any emergency department visits but assigns them all to the outpatient department. Although detailed comparisons

Table 2.13. EMERGENCY DEPARTMENT VISITS BY HOSPITAL
OWNERSHIP, NEW YORK CITY,
1948, 1950, AND 1958

	Number (in Thousands)			Percent	
Year	Total	Voluntary	Municipal	Voluntary	Municipal
1948	880	539	341	61.3	38.7
1950	1,052	579	473	55.0	45.0
1958	1,811	842	969	46.5	53.5

SOURCE: For 1948—New York State Department of Social Welfare, unpublished information, and United Hospital Fund of New York, unpublished information; for 1950
and 1958—Hospital Council of Greater New York, annual inventory.

may be unwise without thorough study of the programs involved,
there is no doubt that the sharp upward trend in the reported
figures on visits to hospital emergency departments is real.

Within a decade the volume of emergency department visits
in New York City has doubled. The annual rate of increase for
the decade was 7 percent, but in the most recent four years it
averaged 10 percent. Emergency department visits increased in
both hospital systems. Between 1948 and 1958 they increased by
more than one half in voluntary hospitals and increased more
than threefold in municipal hospitals. As a result, the municipal
system's share of the total has increased from 39 to 54 percent,
exceeding 50 percent for the first time in 1957.

The increase in emergency department visits is a significant
development in the use of hospitals after World War II. Indeed,
the rate of expansion in other parts of the country has frequently
exceeded that in New York City. In an analysis of available data,
the Hospital Council found that trends in injuries, changes in the
use of the emergency ambulance service, shifts of patients from
the outpatient department, and increases in the number of visits
paid for by Blue Cross cannot account for more than a small fraction of the increase in emergency department visits in New York
City.[13]

Other factors have been offered in explanation, including the
relative unavailability of physicians at certain hours of the day
and on certain days of the week, increasing acceptance of the
hospital as a community health center, and changes in the ethnic
composition of the city's population. It would be worth while to
ascertain the relative importance of these factors in New York

City, as well as of others that might emerge in the course of study. The factors responsible for the increased use of hospital emergency departments influence the characteristics of patients served and their needs for services. These, in turn, are the proper bases for staffing and equipping hospital emergency departments.

SERVICES FOR PRIVATE AMBULATORY PATIENTS

The Hospital Council's hospital inventory for the year 1958 shows 222,000 visits by private ambulatory patients to the 37 voluntary hospitals that reported such visits. Projected to the 62 voluntary hospitals that report offering services to private ambulatory patients, the resulting estimate is 350,000 to 425,000 visits by 200,000 persons. In addition to being incomplete, the reported figures are probably not very reliable, in view of the evident lack of uniform criteria among hospitals in answering this question.

The United Hospital Fund reports an increase of 30 percent between 1955 and 1959 in the number of private ambulatory patients cared for in its member hospitals. A large part of the increase may be attributed to more complete reporting. Most of the services reported are diagnostic x-ray and laboratory tests.

In its annual inventory the Hospital Council also inquires about special diagnostic centers offering a medical examination and complete evaluation. Under this program physicians on the attending staff make use of the hospital's diagnostic tools and equipment.[14] At the end of 1958, six voluntary hospitals reported diagnostic centers.

The year 1958 marked the closing of the pioneer diagnostic center in New York City, namely, the Mount Sinai Hospital's consultation service for persons of moderate means, which was established in 1931. This service accepted patients only on referral by physicians and assured their return to the latter for treatment. The reason for closing the clinic was insufficient demand for this service by physicians, relative to that for other hospital services. Among the factors advanced as accounting for the insufficient demand were the following: the growth of union health centers and their concentration on diagnostic services (see Chapter 1); the provision of similar services by some of the centers affiliated with the Health Insurance Plan of Greater New York; and the rise in Mount Sinai's flat fee from $35 to $80 in the course of a decade. It was observed at the time that the Hospital's cancer detection clinic, which does not require the patient's referral by a physician, was gaining in popularity while the diagnostic clinic was losing.[15] Also noteworthy is termination of community service during 1959 at the diagnostic clinic operated by the Department of Health.

Eight municipal general hospitals have diagnostic clinics. These do not admit patients referred by physicians but serve in effect as coordinating mechanisms for screening and evaluating patients already accepted by the outpatient department.

EMERGENCY AMBULANCE SERVICE

The emergency ambulance service may be viewed as a transportation service, first-aid medical service, and means of distributing inpatients among participating hospitals. It is obviously important in the first two roles, but its third role also deserves attention. The ability of a hospital to redirect and transfer to another hospital patients brought by its own ambulance permits the former to be selective in admitting patients and leads to some of the prevailing differences among hospitals and hospital systems in patient composition.

Table 2.14 shows the number of emergency ambulance service calls in voluntary and municipal hospitals since 1930. Proprietary hospitals do not participate in this service, which is operated in municipal hospitals or subsidized by the City of New York in voluntary hospitals.

Table 2.14. EMERGENCY AMBULANCE CALLS BY HOSPITAL
OWNERSHIP, NEW YORK CITY,
1930, 1940, 1950, AND 1958

	Number (in Thousands)			*Percent*	
Year	*Total*	*Voluntary*	*Municipal*	*Voluntary*	*Municipal*
1930	193	109	84	56.5	43.5
1940	494	293	201	59.3	40.7
1950	344	178	166	51.8	48.2
1958	346	143	203	41.3	58.7

SOURCE: New York City Department of Hospitals, *Number and Disposition of Ambulance Calls* (New York, 1931–59; mimeographed).

The total number of emergency ambulance calls in 1958 was the same as in 1950, but the municipal system's share increased during the eight-year interval, whereas that of the voluntary system declined. The rise in the proportion of calls made by municipal hospitals is even greater if 1940 is taken as the base year. Although the number of calls in municipal hospitals was the same in 1958 as in 1940, there had been a sharp decline during World War II and an almost uninterrupted rise afterward. In voluntary hospitals the number of calls declined by one half between 1940 and 1958, as a sharp drop during World War II was followed first by a small rise and then by another decline.

Today 26 of 71 voluntary general hospitals in New York City operate an emergency ambulance service, while 14 of 15 municipal general hospitals do so. During the 1950s eight voluntary hospitals, all in Brooklyn, relinquished their emergency ambulance service whereas only two new voluntary hospitals, one in the Bronx and one in Queens, established it. Since the assigned emergency ambulance zones in the aggregate cover the total area of New York City, without overlap and without gaps, hospitals that continue the service have had to assume responsibility for additional territory and sometimes for changed territory. The fact that an ambulance district radiates from a hospital that agrees to participate in the service means that, regardless of the initial plan, after some hospitals join and others abandon the service, districts are inevitably unequal in size and different in shape.

Underlying the decisions by some voluntary hospitals to abandon the emergency ambulance service were a number of factors, long run and immediate. Chief among the long-run factors was recognition that the emergency ambulance service is properly a transportation service, not a medical service.[16] Some hospitals also believed that the emergency ambulance service is a liability to a hospital's public relations; this adverse effect became aggravated with the removal of physicians from routine ambulance duty. An immediate factor was the large financial loss incurred prior to the sizable increase in the City's payment per ambulance in 1953.

Only hospitals that participate in the emergency ambulance service ordinarily care for patients picked up by ambulance. There are two circumstances under which a hospital that does not participate may receive ambulance patients: (1) by special arrangement with a participating hospital for the referral of certain types of patient, usually to complete its teaching program; and (2) at the request of the individual patient. The result is that many voluntary hospitals, including several of the major teaching centers, do not care for emergency ambulance patients.

Whereas municipal hospitals keep most of their ambulance patients who require hospital admission, voluntary hospital ambulances take many of their patients to other hospitals, especially to municipal hospitals. Patients are more likely to be redirected to another hospital at night than during the day, indicating that some hospitals are not so well prepared to care for emergency inpatients at night. Redirection of patients to other hospitals is in compliance with ambulance rules and regulations.[17]

A decade ago the Hospital Council discussed the practices of voluntary hospitals in redirecting ambulance patients in these words:

Part of this movement [of patients] is accounted for by the policy of voluntary teaching hospitals to select for admission certain types of cases. The low reimbursement rate traditionally paid by the City to the voluntary hospitals for the care of public charges has undoubtedly contributed to this tendency. The most important factor, however, is the fact that the voluntary hospitals with emergency ambulance service have only one third the ward capacity of the municipal hospitals in which to accommodate ambulance patients.[18]

Today the corresponding ratio is one fourth, although voluntary hospital ambulances respond to more than two fifths of all calls.

As emergency departments of hospitals continue to expand, it may become more practicable for hospitals that do not participate in the emergency ambulance service to join in caring for patients picked up by ambulance. It may be desirable to consider delineating ambulance districts around receiving hospitals rather than around the smaller number of hospitals that operate ambulances.

ORGANIZED HOME CARE

In 1947 Montefiore Hospital instituted its program of home care, by which the hospital organization makes available certain hospital personnel, facilities, and services to the patient at home.

In many instances the result is care that is more appropriate to the patient's needs than can be provided in the hospital, as well as cheaper care. The attitude of the patient and his family toward home care is an important factor in the program's success.

Among voluntary hospitals in New York City home care has failed to secure a large measure of acceptance. Only four such programs are reported, two of which are small ones financed by a special fund for cancer patients and one is primarily designed for teaching medical students.

In 1949 the New York City Department of Hospitals established home care in its hospitals, in order to provide more appropriate care to the sick poor and, more urgently, to help relieve severe overcrowding of beds. Today every municipal general hospital but one and both municipal hospitals for the chronically ill have home care programs. Since the Hospital Council's comprehensive study of home care was completed in 1956,[19] two programs operated by municipal tuberculosis hospitals have been terminated. One ceased when the parent hospital closed. In the other the conclusion was reached that under modern methods of treatment a tuberculosis patient who has been discharged from the hospital can travel to an outpatient department or clinic for further medical care.

The year 1949 was the first in which both hospital systems operated organized home-care programs. The volume of services rendered, as expressed in patient days, has been stable in recent years.

Table 2.15. PATIENT DAYS REPORTED FOR PATIENTS ON HOME CARE BY HOSPITAL OWNERSHIP, NEW YORK CITY, 1949, 1950, AND 1958

	Number (in Thousands)			Percent	
Year	Total	Voluntary	Municipal	Voluntary	Municipal
1949	216	27	189	12.5	87.5
1950	531	34	497	6.4	93.6
1958	817	43	775	5.3	94.7

SOURCE: Hospital Council of Greater New York, annual inventory.

Comparison of Cost. Average daily census on home care increased from 590 in 1949 to 1,450 in 1950 and 2,240 in 1958. Although it cannot be assumed that all these patients would occupy hospital beds in the absence of a home-care program, some would. In New York City the saving in hospital beds attributable to home care has been estimated at roughly one fourth of the number of patients on home care,[20] after allowance for the retransfer of patients from home to hospital for medical reasons. For the year 1958 a saving of 660 beds is thus indicated, on the assumption that a rate of occupancy of 85 percent could have been attained. In New York City most of the saving—95 percent—is achieved in municipal hospitals.

Higher estimates of bed saving have been made. If as many as three fourths of the patients on home care were to be hospitalized in the absence of a home-care program,[21] the saving in New York City would amount to 2,000 beds.

In comparing the cost of caring for a patient on home care and in the hospital, the estimate of bed saving is important from the standpoint of both capital expenditures and operating expenditures. Existing knowledge is insufficient to permit a choice between the two extreme fractions cited above. It is recognized, however, that a valid comparison of cost would take account of the additional expenditures incurred by the patient's family due to his presence at home.

During interviews with hospital administrators the staff of the Hospital Council learned that some voluntary hospitals consider lack of money as the chief obstacle to establishing a home-care program. Even if this program were accepted as an economical device from the community's standpoint, it would still entail expenditures to the individual hospital for which there are no obvious sources of income.

Broadening of Program. Several administrators also reported difficulty in finding in their hospitals a sufficient number of patients likely to benefit from home care. They are more pessimistic than the findings of surveys cited in the Hospital Council's study of home care [22] or the findings of more recent studies by Associated Hospital Service of New York (AHS).[23]

Currently in negotiation between AHS and some of its member hospitals is a program of early hospital discharge of Blue Cross subscribers, with subsequent visits to patients' homes by Visiting Nurse Service. AHS will pay the bill. A pilot project found that this program could save money for Blue Cross, and recent State legislation authorized its incorporation as a benefit in subscribers' contracts. Since most AHS subscribers are private or semiprivate patients and all existing home-care programs in New York City are for ward patients, the new program represents a significant departure from traditional practice. It may be expected that patients will be younger than in existing home-care programs, that a significant proportion of them will be short-term, convalescent patients, and that the individual private physician will make some of the decisions that have hitherto been made by the home-care team. The organization of home-care services will, therefore, require adaptation to the needs of a new group of patients. Elsewhere some home-care programs have successfully served private and semiprivate patients.[24]

It cannot be assumed that hospitals have the necessary personnel required to staff an organized home-care program. The Hospital Council's study of programs found great variation in staffing and in frequency of home visits by physicians, nurses, social workers, and physical therapists. The range of variation was wide even among hospitals in the municipal system. It may be that an extramural program is more vulnerable to reduction in staff and deterioration in quality of care than a program operated within the confines of a hospital.

All of the existing home-care programs in New York City, voluntary and municipal, care for patients discharged from the hospital. Home care can be provided to persons prior to, or without, their admission to the hospital, if they are properly evaluated. One voluntary hospital for long-term patients in New York City has recently undertaken to demonstrate this on a pilot basis, with provision for research and evaluation.

Services in Non-General-Care Facilities

The data in Table 2.4 pertain to all hospital facilities in New York City under voluntary, municipal, and proprietary ownership. Hospitals under federal and state ownership are excluded. Although certain nursing-home facilities are included in the data, most are omitted. When the data on general care facilities and services (Table 2.5) are subtracted from the corresponding figures in Table 2.4, the differences represent figures for non-general-care facilities (Table 2.16). These include facilities for patients with tuberculosis and mental illness and also for patients in rehabilitation and in receipt of long-term care. The last is further subdivided between beds in hospitals for the chronically ill and nursing-home beds.

The data in Table 2.4 include only those nursing-home units that are integral parts of hospitals which admit persons directly from the community. Excluded, therefore, are nursing-home facilities that are located separately, at homes for the aged, or at institutions that offer hospital services only to their own inpatients. The excluded facilities and their services are discussed in the last section of this chapter.

Table 2.16. DISTRIBUTION OF FACILITIES AND SERVICES FOR
NON-GENERAL-CARE PATIENTS BY HOSPITAL OWNER-
SHIP, NEW YORK CITY, 1940, 1950, AND 1958

Facility or Service	*1940*		*1950*		*1958*	
	*Number**	*Percent*	*Number**	*Percent*	*Number**	*Percent*
Bed complement						
All hospitals	*8,618*	*100.0*	*10,909*	*100.0*	*13,002*	*100.0*
Voluntary	3,012	34.9	3,379	31.0	3,663	28.2
Municipal	5,371	62.4	6,919	63.4	8,814	67.8
Proprietary	235	2.7	611	5.6	525	4.0
Discharges						
All hospitals	*49*	*100.0*	*51*	*100.0*	*58*	*100.0*
Voluntary	5	10.2	5	9.8	10	17.3
Municipal	43	87.8	42	82.4	43	74.1
Proprietary	1	2.0	4	7.8	5	8.6
Patient days						
All hospitals	*3,250*	*100.0*	*3,958*	*100.0*	*4,219*	*100.0*
Voluntary	1,046	32.2	1,114	28.1	1,248	29.6
Municipal	2,147	66.0	2,658	67.2	2,820	66.8
Proprietary	57	1.8	186	4.7	151	3.6

* In thousands, except for beds.
SOURCE: See Table 2.5.

In 1958 municipal hospitals reported two thirds of the beds and patient days in non-general-care facilities, and voluntary hospitals reported most of the remaining one third. The same year municipal hospitals reported three fourths of all discharges from these facilities, a marked decline from their share in 1940 and 1950. Since municipal hospitals have retained a constant proportion of patient days, they must have experienced a prolongation of patient stay relative to voluntary and proprietary hospitals. Part of the prolongation is attributable to the development of public-home infirmary units in the municipal system.

So far totals have been distributed by hospital ownership. It is helpful also to view the role of non-general-care facilities within each ownership group. Table 2.17, therefore, shows the amounts in Table 2.16 as percentages of the corresponding amounts in Table 2.4.

Table 2.17. PROPORTION OF FACILITIES AND SERVICES FOR NON-GENERAL-CARE PATIENTS TO TOTAL BY HOSPITAL OWNERSHIP, NEW YORK CITY, 1940, 1950, AND 1958

Facility or Service	Percent of Total		
	1940	1950	1958
Bed complement			
All hospitals	20.6	25.1	26.7
Voluntary	13.7	15.0	14.8
Municipal	34.4	41.3	46.3
Proprietary	6.7	14.6	11.1
Discharges			
All hospitals	6.5	5.5	5.5
Voluntary	1.2	1.0	1.6
Municipal	17.0	16.8	16.6
Proprietary	1.3	2.8	2.9
Patient days			
All hospitals	25.7	28.8	29.3
Voluntary	17.1	17.1	17.0
Municipal	37.1	43.6	48.6
Proprietary	7.9	16.5	11.7

SOURCE: Tables 2.4 and 2.16.

Because non-general-care patients include a large number of long-stay patients, they account for a much higher proportion of total patient days than of discharges—29 percent compared with 6 percent. In the municipal system the proportion of patient days by non-general-care patients has been rising and approached one half in 1958. In the voluntary system this proportion has remained constant, at 17 percent. In the proprietary system, it has fluctuated a great deal—between 8 and 16 percent—primarily because of changing arrangements in the care of patients with tuberculosis.

The proportions shown for beds are close to the corresponding proportions for patient days, but always lower. This means that non-general-care facilities tend to operate at higher rates of occupancy than general-care facilities.

Between 1940 and 1958 the entire increase in beds in the municipal system was assigned to non-general-care facilities. By

Table 2.18. DISTRIBUTION BETWEEN GENERAL CARE AND
OTHER CARE OF INCREASE IN BED COMPLEMENT,
BY HOSPITAL OWNERSHIP, NEW YORK CITY, 1940–58

Hospital Ownership	Number			Percent	
	Total	General Care	Other	General Care	Other
All hospitals	7,512	3,128	4,384	41.6	58.4
Voluntary	2,866	2,215	651	77.3	22.7
Municipal	3,450	7	3,443	0.2	99.8
Proprietary	1,196	906	290	75.8	24.2

SOURCE: Tables 2.5 and 2.16.

contrast, in the other two hospital systems between three fourths and four fifths of the increase in total beds was devoted to general-care facilities and between one fifth and one fourth to non-general-care facilities.

This contrast is even more striking for patient days than for beds. In voluntary and proprietary hospitals non-general-care

Table 2.19. DISTRIBUTION BETWEEN GENERAL CARE AND
OTHER CARE OF INCREASE IN PATIENT DAYS,
BY HOSPITAL OWNERSHIP, NEW YORK CITY, 1940–58

Hospital Ownership	Number (in Thousands)			Percent	
	Total	General Care	Other	General Care	Other
All hospitals	1,799	830	969	46.1	53.9
Voluntary	1,234	1,032	202	83.7	16.3
Municipal	11	– 662	673	– 6,019.0	6,119.0
Proprietary	554	460	94	83.0	17.0

SOURCE: Tables 2.5 and 2.16.

facilities accounted for one sixth of the increase in total patient days between 1940 and 1958. In municipal hospitals total patient days remained virtually unchanged, so that the increase in non-general-care facilities offset a substantial decline in general care.

The non-general-care facilities of hospitals comprise a hetero-
geneous group. Table 2.20 shows the distribution of beds and
services by type of program. As usual, the percentage distribution

Table 2.20. DISTRIBUTION OF NON-GENERAL-CARE BEDS
           AND SERVICES BY TYPE OF PROGRAM,
           NEW YORK CITY, 1958

Type of Program	Beds		Discharges		Patient Days	
	Number*	Percent	Number*	Percent	Number*	Percent
Total	13,002	100.0	58	100.0	4,219	100.0
Psychiatry	2,111	16.2	37	63.8	730	17.3
Tuberculosis	4,622	35.6	10	17.3	1,364	32.4
Physical medicine and rehabilitation	725	5.6	2	3.4	177	4.2
Hospital for chronically ill	3,641	28.0	7	12.1	1,286	30.4
Nursing home or pub-lic-home infirmary	1,903	14.6	2	3.4	662	15.7

* In thousands, except for beds.
SOURCE: Hospital Council of Greater New York, annual inventory.

of patient days is similar to that of beds, and the distribution of
discharges differs from the other two. Only in physical medicine
and rehabilitation is the proportion of discharges close to the
proportion of patient days. In psychiatry and in nursing-home
facilities the two percentages display the widest divergence, with
the former having the much higher proportion of discharges and
the latter the higher proportion of patient days. These relationships mean that among non-general-care patients psychiatric patients have the shortest duration of stay and nursing-home patients
the longest.

Trends and developments will next be considered by type of
program, as follows: (1) psychiatric facilities; (2) tuberculosis
facilities; (3) long-term facilities—(a) rehabilitation, (b) hospitals
for chronically ill, (c) nursing homes serving as integral parts of
hospitals, (d) other types of nursing homes. Before this is done, it
is appropriate to introduce a brief analysis for one year of the distribution of non-general-care facilities by type of accommodation.

In 1955 almost 94 percent of all such beds were assigned to
the ward service and only 6 percent to private and semiprivate

services. In the municipal system all non-general-care beds were classified as ward, whereas in the proprietary system all such beds were classified as private or semiprivate, except for the tuberculosis unit in one hospital, which was used under a special arrangement with the City of New York. In the voluntary system the proportion of ward beds to total varied by program, ranging from a low of 64 percent in psychiatry, to 80 percent in hospital beds for chronically ill, 94 percent in tuberculosis, and 100 percent in physical medicine and rehabilitation; 83 percent of the non-general-care beds in voluntary hospitals were assigned to the ward.

In part the high proportion of ward care reflects the manner in which these programs are paid for, but in part it also reflects decisions to provide physicians' services through the clinical departments of hospitals rather than through the private physicians of patients.

Psychiatric Services

In this country most hospital services to psychiatric inpatients are furnished in state hospitals. In recent years the patient census in these hospitals has declined. Reversal of the long-term upward trend in 1955 came about because a speeding-up in the rate and number of discharges overtook the continuing increase in the rate and number of admissions.[25]

At the same time psychiatric facilities and services in community general hospitals have increased in the United States. Beds set aside for psychiatric patients increased from 10,600 in 1954 to 14,400 in 1958 and admissions increased from 202,400 to 257,300, respectively. The latter figure was substantially higher than the number of admissions to public mental hospitals, 210,000.[26]

Psychiatric facilities in general hospitals play a more important role in hospital admissions than in patient days. This means that their average patient stay is shorter than in state mental hospitals.

In New York City in 1958 psychiatric units of general hospitals reported 32,000 admissions and 530,000 patient days. In 1957 New York City residents were responsible for 12,000 admissions to state mental hospitals and 15.8 million patient days. Although the state hospitals reported only 27 percent of the combined admissions, they reported 97 percent of the combined patient days.

Table 2.21 shows the data on all psychiatric facilities in New York City under voluntary, municipal, and proprietary ownership. Excluded are state hospitals and psychiatric facilities in federal hospitals. Both beds and patient days doubled in volume

Table 2.21. DISTRIBUTION OF FACILITIES AND SERVICES FOR
PSYCHIATRIC INPATIENTS BY HOSPITAL OWNERSHIP,
NEW YORK CITY, 1940, 1950, AND 1958

Facility or Service	1940		1950		1958	
	Number*	Percent	Number*	Percent	Number*	Percent
Bed complement						
All hospitals	1,028	100.0	1,561	100.0	2,111	100.0
Voluntary	88	8.6	308	19.7	485	23.0
Municipal	705	68.5	979	62.7	1,338	63.4
Proprietary	235	22.9	274	17.6	288	13.6
Discharges						
All hospitals	34	100.0	35	100.0	37	100.0
Voluntary	†	†	1	2.8	2	5.6
Municipal	33	97.1	31	88.6	31	83.9
Proprietary	1	2.9	3	8.6	4	10.5
Patient days						
All hospitals	360	100.0	583	100.0	730	100.0
Voluntary	25	7.0	95	16.3	161	22.0
Municipal	278	77.2	402	69.0	495	67.9
Proprietary	57	15.8	86	14.7	74	10.1

* In thousands, except for beds.
† Less than 500.
SOURCE: See Table 2.5.

between 1940 and 1958, whereas discharges increased less than 10 percent. More than two thirds of the increase in patient days took place in the first interval, between 1940 and 1950, whereas the increase in beds was evenly divided between the two intervals.

New York City's municipal hospitals continue to play a preponderant role in caring for psychiatric inpatients in the community. Their relative importance is declining, however, and that of voluntary hospitals is rising.

Unlike general-care facilities, psychiatric facilities report the shortest duration of patient stay in municipal hospitals and the longest stay in voluntary hospitals. The computed data for 1958 follow:

	Average Length of Patient Stay (Days)
All hospitals	19.9
Voluntary	78.0
Municipal	16.0
Proprietary	19.2

When separate psychiatric hospitals are eliminated from the comparison, length of stay in psychiatric units of general hospitals is 52.2 days in the voluntary system and 14.8 days in the municipal system. This difference reflects the fact that psychiatric units in municipal hospitals are heavily oriented toward diagnostic and screening services, whereas psychiatric units in voluntary hospitals tend to emphasize treatment for a short term—up to three months.

In the 1940s there was a modest increase in the number of visits to psychiatric clinics of hospitals, and in the 1950s the increase was large. During the same period visits to psychiatric clinics of independent dispensaries under voluntary ownership declined from 51,000 in 1940 to 30,000 in 1950 and 300 in 1958. Psychiatric services in family and other social service agencies are omitted from these counts.

Table 2.22. VISITS TO PSYCHIATRIC CLINICS OF OUTPATIENT DEPARTMENTS BY HOSPITAL OWNERSHIP, NEW YORK CITY, 1940, 1950, AND 1958

	Number (in Thousands)			Percent	
Year	Total	Voluntary	Municipal	Voluntary	Municipal
1940	48	22	26	45.8	54.2
1950	68	28	40	41.2	58.8
1958	178	63	115	35.4	64.6

SOURCE: United Hospital Fund of New York, *Outpatient Service Statistics Relating to Hospitals and Independent Dispensaries in New York City* (New York, 1941–59), and unpublished information.

Visits to psychiatric clinics of voluntary hospitals increased slightly in the 1940s and more than doubled in the 1950s, but in each decade their rate of increase was lower than in municipal hospitals. In the latter, visits increased one half in the 1940s and almost tripled again in the 1950s. As a result, the municipal hospitals' proportion of psychiatric visits to outpatient departments rose from 54 to 65 percent. Although trends for inpatients and for outpatients have run in opposite directions—with voluntary hospitals reporting an increasing proportion of the former and a declining proportion of the latter—the share of voluntary hospitals in outpatient services is still well above that for inpatient services, 35 percent compared with 22 percent. (The latter figure is the voluntary hospitals' share of patient days; their share of discharges is only 6 percent, because of a relatively longer patient stay.)

A significant factor in the expansion of services in psychiatric clinics of hospitals has been financial support received through the New York City Community Mental Health Board, whose budget is augmented by State funds. In the voluntary system contracts with individual hospitals subsidize expansion of services. In effect, the City pays 50 percent of expeditures for psychiatric clinics as long as services are increased, provided that the amount paid does not exceed the increase in expenditures occasioned by the expansion of services.

In its *Master Plan* the Hospital Council stated that "the care of psychiatric patients should be an important function of general hospitals." [27] Subsequently, the Hospital Council elaborated:

The additional psychiatric units in general hospitals will provide needed care promptly when the patient is most likely to benefit from it. In the units of the voluntary hospitals psychiatrists will be able to care for their private patients. The organization of a psychiatric staff in a general hospital will also serve to extend knowledge of the emotional factors of illness to other services of the hospital.[28]

Despite an initial reluctance by voluntary hospitals to establish psychiatric units, a conjuncture of circumstances, including the development of tranquilizer drugs and increased financial support from government, have recently enabled them to move in the desired direction. Since 1954 the number of patients in psychiatric units of voluntary general hospitals in New York City has doubled. In 1958 seven voluntary general hospitals in New York City had psychiatric units, and another five, without designated beds, were listed as admitting psychiatric patients in emergencies, for treatment, or both.[29] Of those with psychiatric units six are located in Manhattan and one in the Bronx. An additional psychiatric unit opened in the Bronx in 1959.

In the municipal system two newly built general hospitals have established psychiatric units in recent years. Plans have been initiated to establish psychiatric facilities in a fifth and a sixth municipal hospital, with the simultaneous aim of reducing the size of, and eliminating overcrowding in, the psychiatric service at Bellevue Hospital Center. If these additional facilities materialize, there will be psychiatric units in three municipal general hospitals in Manhattan and in one each in the Bronx, Brooklyn, and Queens.

Tuberculosis Facilities

In the summer of 1953 the upward trend in tuberculosis patients in hospitals in New York City was reversed for the first time. Since then there has been an uninterrupted decline.

The downturn was sharp, apparently reflecting the introduction in 1952 of a new set of drugs. The hydrozides of nicotinic acid, used separately or in combination with other drugs, have resulted in a substantial reduction in patient stay. Table 2.23 gives data on tuberculosis patients in hospitals in New York City in 1940, 1950, and 1958.

Between 1940 and 1950 there was a sizable decline in tuberculosis beds in voluntary hospitals. This reflects mostly the inability of one hospital to continue under voluntary ownership and its sale to the City of New York. The increase in municipal hospital beds between 1940 and 1950 reflects the City's acquisition of this hospital and also the opening of a tuberculosis facility in Queens. In addition, to meet the demand for beds, tuberculosis units in existing hospitals were expanded to the utmost and beds for acute communicable diseases were diverted to tuberculosis patients. Total tuberculosis facilities were further augmented in 1949 when a proprietary hospital agreed to assign several hundred beds to this purpose, under a special arrangement with the Department of Hospitals.

Between 1950 and 1958 tuberculosis beds declined in each hospital system, as did discharges. Most striking is the decline in patient days (and, equivalently, average daily census).

Table 2.23. DISTRIBUTION OF FACILITIES AND SERVICES FOR
PATIENTS WITH TUBERCULOSIS BY HOSPITAL
OWNERSHIP, NEW YORK CITY,
1940, 1950, AND 1958

Facility or Service	1940		1950		1958	
	Number*	Percent	Number*	Percent	Number*	Percent
Bed complement						
All hospitals	4,754	100.0	5,506	100.0	4,622	100.0
Voluntary	1,588	33.4	962	17.4	700	15.1
Municipal	3,166	66.6	4,207	76.5	3,685	79.8
Proprietary	0	0	337	6.1	237	5.1
Discharges						
All hospitals	11	100.0	11	100.0	10	100.0
Voluntary	3	27.3	1	9.1	1	10.0
Municipal	8	72.7	9	81.8	8	80.0
Proprietary	0	0	1	9.1	1	10.0
Patient days						
All hospitals	1,901	100.0	2,010	100.0	1,364	100.0
Voluntary	574	30.2	333	16.6	240	17.6
Municipal	1,327	69.8	1,577	78.4	1,047	76.8
Proprietary	0	0	100	5.0	77	5.6

* In thousands, except for beds.
SOURCE: See Table 2.5.

It should be noted that the total number of tuberculosis inpatients reported by hospitals is consistently lower than the number reported by the Tuberculosis Register, a perpetual inventory
of persons with active tuberculosis. A comparison of the estimated
number of persons in tuberculosis facilities at the end of 1950 and
1958, as reported by hospitals and by the Register, follows:

Source of Data	1950	1958	Decline 1950–58
Hospitals	5,860	3,427	– 2,433
Register	6,714	4,378	– 2,336
Difference	+ 854	+ 951	– 97

The two sources report approximately the same size of decline in tuberculosis patients between 1950 and 1958—2,350 to
2,450. The number reported by the Register at a given time is,
however, 850 to 950 higher. The direction of the difference is
surprising, since logically the Register should deal with the
smaller number of patients: (1) it lists active tuberculosis cases
only, whereas a hospital unit may be caring for some arrested
cases; and (2) it lists tuberculosis cases only, whereas a hospital

unit may also be caring for patients with nontuberculous conditions of the chest.

After analysis of data and consultation with experts, it was concluded that for the purpose of tracing the use of tuberculosis hospitals and units over time the data from hospitals are probably more reliable than those from the Register.

The relative importance of voluntary hospitals in tuberculosis care has declined: from one third in 1940 to 15 percent in 1958, as measured by beds; and from 27 to 10 percent, as measured by discharges. Conversely, the relative importance of municipal hospitals has increased. This trend remains substantially unchanged when hospitals located outside the city that serve primarily New York City residents are included in the data. In 1950 there were almost 900 such beds. The number was well in excess of 1,000, if beds in State hospitals used by New York City residents, though not specifically allocated to them, are also counted. The complete data on tuberculosis facilities and services for residents of New York City, including those located outside the city are shown in Table 2.24; these show larger volumes of services than in Table 2.23 above, and raise the relative importance of voluntary hospitals in past years. Since the year 1958 is not affected, the result is to continue the decline in the relative importance of voluntary hospitals into the 1950s.

By 1958 the net decline from peak in all hospitals serving New York City residents was of the order of 2,150 beds, or 31 percent. The decline in patient days from peak was 1,080,000 or 43 percent (see Table 2.24). The rate of occupancy in tuberculosis facilities declined from 96 percent in 1952 to 81 percent in 1958. In municipal hospitals the decline was from 99 to 78 percent, paving the way for a sizable reduction in bed complement in 1959.

In the modern treatment of tuberculosis it is feasible to perform a smaller part of the total care in the hospital than formerly.[30] Visits to tuberculosis clinics of hospitals show an increase from 80,000 in 1950 to 108,000 in 1958, with the share of municipal hospitals rising from 72 to 86 percent. More striking is the relative gain of Department of Health clinics, which cared for 70 percent of all clinic cases with active tuberculosis in 1958, compared with 50 percent in 1950.[31]

Table 2.24. DISTRIBUTION OF FACILITIES AND SERVICES FOR
PATIENTS WITH TUBERCULOSIS BY HOSPITAL
OWNERSHIP, NEW YORK CITY AND
ENVIRONS, 1940, 1950, AND 1958

Facility or Service	1940		1950 †		1958	
	Number*	Percent	Number*	Percent	Number*	Percent
Bed complement						
All hospitals	5,579	100.0	6,381	100.0	4,622	100.0
Voluntary	2,013	36.0	1,417	22.2	700	15.1
Municipal	3.566	64.0	4,627	72.5	3,685	79.8
Proprietary	0	0	337	5.3	237	5.1
Discharges						
All hospitals	11,925	100.0	11,732	100.0	9,735	100.0
Voluntary	2,959	24.8	1,898	16.2	1,371	14.1
Municipal	8,966	75.2	9,388	80.0	7,943	81.6
Proprietary	0	0	446	3.8	421	4.3
Patient days						
All hospitals	2,180	100.0	2,286	100.0	1,364	100.0
Voluntary	712	32.7	461	20.1	240	17.6
Municipal	1,468	67.3	1,725	75.5	1,047	76.8
Proprietary	0	0	100	4.4	77	5.6

* In thousands, except for beds.
† Between 1950 and 1952 beds increased by 400, discharges by 850, and patient days
by 160,000.
NOTE: Approximately 200 New York City residents in state hospitals, with 43,000
patient days, are not included in this table.
SOURCE: See Table 2.5.

There is considerable overlap in role between tuberculosis
clinics operated by hospitals and chest clinics operated by the
Department of Health. One difference is that hospital outpatient
departments focus more on the follow-up of discharged inpatients,
while Department of Health clinics focus more on the care of
newly diagnosed patients and on supervising patients' families.

Although the tuberculosis patient load is declining, eradica-
tion of the disease is not yet in sight.[32] There remains a need for
sound planning to provide adequate facilities for the care of
tuberculosis patients. Appropriate roles for general hospitals, particularly teaching hospitals, and provision for a reasonable geographic distribution of facilities are dealt with elsewhere (see
Chapter 11).

Reporting early in 1959, the Committee on the Tuberculosis
Survey expressed satisfaction with the length of patient stay in
tuberculosis hospitals and units in New York City and concluded

that the existing supply of beds was ample. True, 5 percent of all newly reported active cases of tuberculosis fail to accept hospitalization (even though it is fully paid for by government in New York State), but this proportion is probably not reducible.[33]

Of special concern is provision of care for long-term patients with tuberculosis, who frequently have associated medical conditions. They require well organized programs, with adequate personnel and equipment.

Management of tuberculosis patients is dispersed among various types of facility, and care of the individual patient may be fragmented. With total treatment of a patient seldom lasting less than two years and subsequent supervision taking much longer, extra effort and ingenuity must be exerted to coordinate services for a mobile population.[34]

Facilities for Long-Term Patients

As previously listed, facilities for long-term patients comprise units for rehabilitation; hospital beds for the chronically ill; and nursing-home or infirmary beds. In this report the last group is divided into facilities attached to hospitals (and included in the data presented in this chapter) and those that are not.

REHABILITATION FACILITIES

Since World War II the public and the medical profession have become aware of the potential contribution of rehabilitation services to the welfare of all types of patient, whether on the way to full recovery or undergoing adjustment to a permanent impairment. Since a regimen of intensive rehabilitation begins early in the patient's hospital stay, it should be instituted in the general hospital while the patient is receiving medical or surgical care.

In the community general hospital the rehabilitation service is essentially a clinical department under the direction of the chief of physical medicine, and as such it seldom requires a special assignment of beds for the patients it serves. To be distinguished from the department of physical medicine of a general hospital is the so-called rehabilitation facility or center. Under the definition employed by the Hill-Burton program, a rehabilitation facility is expected to provide integrated diagnostic evaluation and treatment services, including medical, psychiatric, social, and vocational. These services are provided through the team approach, and this calls for the participation of many different medical specialists and auxiliary personnel. A rehabilitation facility may serve both inpatients and ambulatory patients, depending on the availability of beds. Under the Hill-Burton program grants for beds are treated separately from grants for the rehabilitation facility itself.

An inventory of rehabilitation facilities and services conducted in 1955 by the State Hill-Burton agency, then called the New York State Joint Hospital Survey and Planning Commission, listed 25 hospitals in New York City, 19 voluntary and 6 municipal. Ten hospitals—5 voluntary and 5 municipal—assigned beds to rehabilitation patients. Most voluntary hospitals that admitted and cared for rehabilitation inpatients did not assign a specific number of beds to the service. There were, in addition, 5 rehabilitation facilities outside hospitals, all under voluntary ownership, with four for outpatients only and one for inpatients only. Every hospital reported that it served outpatients as well as inpatients.

The Hospital Council's annual inventory reported 107 beds for patients in rehabilitation in 1950, all in municipal hospitals, but did not report any service statistics for them. For the year 1958, 14 hospitals—5 voluntary and 9 municipal—reported data on beds, discharges, and patient days.

Table 2.25. DISTRIBUTION OF REHABILITATION FACILITIES AND SERVICES FOR INPATIENTS BY HOSPITAL OWNERSHIP, NEW YORK CITY, 1958

Facility or Service	Number*	Percent
Bed complement		
All hospitals	725	100.0
Voluntary	222	30.6
Municipal	503	69.4
Discharges		
All hospitals	2	100.0
Voluntary	1	50.0
Municipal	1	50.0
Patient days		
All hospitals	177	100.0
Voluntary	36	20.4
Municipal	141	79.6

* In thousands, except for beds.
SOURCE: Hospital Council of Greater New York, annual inventory.

The municipal system reports four fifths of the patient days received by rehabilitation patients. In fact this is an understatement, for in one municipal hospital with 240 beds assigned to rehabilitation, discharges and patient days are not separated from services to other long-term patients.

HOSPITAL FACILITIES FOR THE CHRONICALLY ILL

Hospital facilities for the chronically ill are intended for long-term patients in need of active medical or surgical care. Counting these facilities is not a simple matter, since it is sometimes difficult to separate and distinguish them from general-care facilities, on the one hand, and nursing-home or infirmary facilities, on the other hand.

Specifically, the New York State Plan for administering the Hill-Burton program draws certain distinctions between hospital and nursing-home care of the chronically ill. The hospital for the chronically ill is defined as "a place for the patient needing active around-the-clock medical and professional nursing care and observation. Hospital care is necessary when difficult diagnostic procedures are indicated, when the severity of illness requires constant medical observation, and when highly skilled nursing techniques must be applied." [35] The role of the nursing home is outlined below.

Hospital facilities for the chronically ill, as counted in this report, are a residual group. For the year 1940 they include all beds other than those designated for general care, psychiatry, and tuberculosis. For 1950 rehabilitation beds are also deducted, though their services are not reported separately. By 1958 nursing-home and infirmary beds are separated and deducted. Because of the frequency with which facilities for long-term patients may be reclassified from one category to another, as well as differences among authorities in classifying a given facility and the high degree of uncertainty that surrounds the classification of certain facilities, the data on hospital facilities for the chronically ill and their services must be interpreted with caution.

Subject to these reservations, data on hospital facilities for the chronically ill are presented in Table 2.26 for the years 1940, 1950, and 1958.

Table 2.26. DISTRIBUTION OF HOSPITAL FACILITIES AND
SERVICES FOR CHRONICALLY ILL BY HOSPITAL
OWNERSHIP, NEW YORK CITY, 1940, 1950, AND 1958

Facility or Service	1940		1950		1958	
	Number*	Percent	Number*	Percent	Number*	Percent
Bed complement						
All hospitals	2,836	100.0	3,735	100.0	3,641	100.0
Voluntary	1,336	47.1	2,109	56.4	1,741	47.8
Municipal	1,500	52.9	1,626	43.6	1,900	52.2
Discharges						
All hospitals	4	100.0	5	100.0	7	100.0
Voluntary	2	50.0	3	60.0	5	71.4
Municipal	2	50.0	2	40.0	2	28.6
Patient days						
All hospitals	989	100.0	1,365	100.0	1,286	100.0
Voluntary	447	45.3	686	50.3	630	49.0
Municipal	542	54.7	679	49.7	656	51.0

* In thousands, exept for beds.
SOURCE: See Table 2.5.

In this field the two hospital systems play approximately equal roles in beds and patient days but not in discharges. One hospital reports more than one half of all discharges from the voluntary system, though it has only 15 percent of the beds. Perhaps all or part of this facility should be considered for reclassification to general care, as a result of continuing changes in the types of patient cared for.

It should be recognized, of course, that general care units of hospitals treat some long-term patients, and properly so. To limit their role to caring for the acutely ill would be to deprive the long-term patients of the benefits of medical progress. At times of diagnostic evaluation, surgery, or exacerbations of illness, long-term patients do not differ from acutely ill patients in the degree or types of active care required. Indeed, in certain areas, such as physical therapy or radiation therapy, long-term patients may require more personnel and more complex facilities than short-term patients. Nor is it likely that other institutions can provide as adequate a level of care for these long-term patients as can the general-care hospital.

Existing information on the use of general-care hospitals in New York City by long-stay patients is scanty. It is insufficient to support any conclusions regarding the propriety of such use.

NURSING-HOME FACILITIES IN HOSPITALS

There are other long-term patients who do not need active hospital care but need skilled nursing care and related services in an institution, under medical direction. Such a facility, as described by the Hill-Burton Act, is a nursing home that admits patients solely because they are sick but offers them a home-like atmosphere and security during their prolonged stay. It is not a custodial institution or boarding home.[36]

Data on nursing-home facilities that are integral parts of hospitals are presented for the year 1958 in Table 2.27. It is possible that the facilities so classified today performed the same function in 1950 or even in 1940, when they were classified as hospital beds for the chronically ill. Over the years classification of facilities has become more refined because of two parallel developments: (1) increasing complexity of medical care and, therefore, increasing specialization of personnel and facilities providing the care; and (2) increasing availability of funds from a variety of sources, which eventually calls for a finer adjustment of rates of payment to services rendered. Of particular importance in the financial realm are amendments to the public assistance provisions of the Social Security Act, because these have raised Federal participation in support of long-term patients in institutions. In some parts of the country voluntary health insurance plans offer subscribers limited benefits for care in nursing homes.

Table 2.27. DISTRIBUTION OF NURSING-HOME BEDS IN HOS-
PITALS BY OWNERSHIP, NEW YORK CITY, 1958

Facility or Service	Number*	Percent
Bed complement		
All hospitals	1,903	100.0
Voluntary	515	27.1
Municipal	1,388	72.9
Discharges		
All hospitals	2	100.0
Voluntary	1	50.0
Municipal	1	50.0
Patient days		
All hospitals	662	100.0
Voluntary	181	27.3
Municipal	481	72.7

* In thousands, exept for beds.
SOURCE: Hospital Council of Greater New York, annual inventory.

Municipal hospitals contribute almost three fourths of the beds and patient days in these facilities.

As will be seen in the next section, this proportion may be misleading, since only a small segment of nursing-home facilities are counted here. Indeed, municipal facilities of this type, officially designated as public-home infirmaries, have not expanded as projected. One reason is that some of the facilities that were built could not be staffed. Another important reason is the opposition of the medical staffs of university hospitals to establishing and operating such units. The recent decision by Bellevue Hospital Center to staff a public-home infirmary when the new plant is completed marks a significant break with this policy.

OTHER NURSING-HOME FACILITIES

Outside the hospital four categories of nursing-home facilities are recognized in New York City: the incorporated nursing home under voluntary ownership; the infirmary of a home for the aged, also under voluntary ownership; the infirmary of a public home; and the proprietary nursing home.

For lack of data it is not possible to prepare a table for nursing-home facilities outside hospitals that would go back to 1940 or even to 1950. For the year 1958, however, the data are complete and mesh with those developed for hospitals.

Not shown in this table are nonhospital facilities for shorter-term patients. In 1958 there were 250 beds in convalescent homes in New York City, which reported almost 3,000 discharges and 73,000 patient days. Outside the city there are certain convalescent homes that serve primarily residents of New York City. These had 1,050 beds in 1957,[37] after a generation in which convalescent homes had closed or reduced their capacity.[38]

Proprietary nursing homes play a major role in the care of long-term patients. This is a relatively new phenomenon, with their significant expansion dating back to the early 1950s. In 1950, for example, there were 2,400 beds in proprietary nursing homes and in 1952, 3,090, but in 1955, 5,400, and in 1958, 9,160.

The role of infirmaries of homes for the aged has also increased in recent years, but at a slow rate. Some additional infirmary facilities were created by converting facilities for domicili-

Table 2.28. DISTRIBUTION OF NURSING-HOME FACILITIES
OUTSIDE HOSPITALS AND THEIR SERVICES
BY OWNERSHIP, NEW YORK CITY, 1958

Facility or Service	Number*	Percent
Bed capacity		
All facilities	14,152	100.0
Voluntary	4,528	32.0
Nursing homes	1,062	7.5
Infirmaries, homes for aged	3,466	24.5
Municipal	468	3.3
Proprietary	9,156	64.7
Discharges		
All facilities	12	100.0
Voluntary	6	50.0
Nursing homes	1	8.3
Infirmaries, homes for aged	5	41.7
Municipal	†	†
Proprietary	6	50.0
Patient days		
All facilities	4,083	100.0
Voluntary	1,373	33.6
Nursing homes	284	6.9
Infirmaries, homes for aged	1,089	26.7
Municipal	184	4.5
Proprietary	2,526	61.9

* In thousands, except for beds.
† Less than 500.
SOURCE: Adapted from New York State Joint Hospital Survey and Planning Commission, Hospitals and Related Facilities in New York State (Albany, N. Y., 1960; typewritten).

ary patients, and others were newly built. In the latter effort, the Hill-Burton program has furnished some assistance.

The separate voluntary nursing homes have increased their capacity 50 percent since 1950, when the number of beds was 710.

There has been no formal change in the capacity of the infirmary section of the public home on Staten Island. However, the City Home on Welfare Island, with some facilities of this type, was closed in 1953.

The four categories of nursing homes share these characteristics: almost all of their patients need long-term care, and the majority are aged (65 years and over) and in receipt of Old Age Assistance. There are differences among the facilities, however, in the way in which patients are admitted, so that some differences arise in the degree and types of illness of patients and in their cultural and social characteristics.[39] These are described at length in another report.[40]

It is interesting that public-charge patients constitute a majority of patients in proprietary nursing homes. By contrast, proprietary general hospitals have no public charges.

A striking finding from Table 2.29 is that in 1958 the number of beds in nursing homes outside hospitals exceeded the total number of beds in hospitals for non-general-care patients (Table 2.16). If psychiatric and tuberculosis facilities are eliminated from the comparison, the relative importance of nursing-home facilities outside hospitals in caring for long-term patients is increased substantially.

Table 2.29. DISTRIBUTION OF FACILITIES AND SERVICES FOR LONG-TERM CARE BY OWNERSHIP AND BY LOCATION WITH RESPECT TO HOSPITALS, NEW YORK CITY, 1958

Facility or Service	Number*			Percent	
	Total	In Hospitals	Outside Hospitals	In Hospitals	Outside Hospitals
Bed capacity					
Total	20,421	6,269	14,152	30.7	69.3
Voluntary	7,006	2,478	4,528	35.4	64.6
Municipal	4,259	3,791	468	11.0	89.0
Proprietary	9,156	0	9,156	0	100.0
Discharges					
Total	23	11	12	47.8	52.2
Voluntary	13	7	6	53.8	46.2
Municipal	4	4	†	100.0	†
Proprietary	6	0	6	0	100.0
Patient days					
Total	6,208	2,125	4,083	34.2	65.8
Voluntary	2,220	847	1,373	38.2	61.8
Municipal	1,462	1,278	184	87.4	12.6
Proprietary	2,526	0	2,526	0	100.0

* In thousands, except for beds.
† Less than 500.
SOURCE: Tables 2.25–2.28.

(The bed figures in Table 2.29 represent capacity, rather than complement, because only the former were available for nursing homes outside hospitals. In this instance there is, however, no difference between bed capacity and bed complement for long-term facilities in hospitals.)

Over-all nursing home facilities outside hospitals represent 70 percent of all facilities for long-term care. They report more than one half of all discharges and two thirds of all patient days.

In the proprietary system all facilities for long-term care are located apart from hospitals and have no ties with them. In the municipal system the large majority of facilities are in hospitals and the outside unit is affiliated with a hospital for medical staffing. In the voluntary system the majority of facilities are outside hospitals, but some have ties of varying intensity with hospitals.

The percentage distribution by ownership is given in Table 2.30. When facilities for long-term care outside hospitals are taken

Table 2.30. PERCENTAGE DISTRIBUTION OF TOTAL FACILITIES AND SERVICES FOR LONG-TERM CARE BY OWNER-SHIP, NEW YORK CITY, 1958

Ownership	Bed Capacity	Discharges	Patient Days
Total	100.0	100.0	100.0
Voluntary	34.3	56.5	35.8
Municipal	20.9	17.4	23.5
Proprietary	44.8	26.1	40.7

SOURCE: Table 2.29.

into account, it is the proprietary system that looms largest and the municipal system smallest by far. These findings are the very opposite of those derived from studying only long term facilities in hospitals.

Summary

1. This chapter describes changes in the respective roles of voluntary, municipal, and proprietary hospitals in New York City in providing services to inpatients and to ambulatory patients. It was possible to trace back total beds to the year 1920 and total services to 1930. Almost every series on individual programs begins not later than 1940.

2. At the end of 1958 there were 151 hospitals with a capacity of almost 50,000 beds. During calendar year 1958 they cared for 1,050,000 inpatients and reported 14.4 million patient days. They also reported 0.8 million patient days on home care, 5.4 million visits to outpatient departments, 1.8 million visits to emergency departments, and roughly 0.4 million visits by private ambulatory

patients. Finally, they responded to 350,000 emergency ambulance calls.

3. Excluded from the above are the following:

(a) Federal hospitals in New York City, chiefly Veterans Administration hospitals. In 1958 the latter had 3,600 beds, and 85 percent of their occupants were residents of the city.

(b) State hospitals. The four institutions in New York City had 10,700 beds, and 98 percent of their occupants were from New York City. However, these hospitals accommodated only 22 percent of the city's residents in the state mental hospital system. The remaining 78 percent were cared for in hospitals located in neighboring counties in New York State.

(c) Nursing home facilities for long-term patients outside hospitals. These aggregated 14,200 beds in 1958, compared with fewer than 2,000 nursing-home beds that were integral parts of hospitals.

(d) Convalescent home facilities for shorter-term patients. The number of beds located in New York City was only 250, but the number of beds in the suburbs that served the city's residents amounted to 1,050.

4. A comparison between New York City's short-term hospitals and the nation's in 1958 shows the following:

(a) The admission rate to hospitals of the resident population was 125 per 1,000 in both instances.

(b) Average length of stay was higher by one third in New York City. Consequently, hospital use per person per year was higher by one third.

(c) Outpatient departments of hospitals were used 3.5 times as often in New York City.

(d) Emergency departments of hospitals were used 2.3 times as often in New York City.

(e) Municipal hospitals play a larger role here in every item that is compared, and voluntary hospitals a smaller one. Proprietary hospitals are relatively more important in New York City in inpatient care and less important in services for ambulatory patients.

5. There are two aspects to the summary of trends in facilities and services: the direction of the total and changes in the relative importance of the two major hospital systems.

6. Total bed complement in hospitals increased from 30,200 in 1920 to 36,600 in 1930, 41,200 in 1940, 43,500 in 1950, and 48,700 in 1958. The largest increase occurred in the 1950s and the smallest in the 1940s. Patient days show a smaller increase in the 1950s than in the 1940s or 1930s. The increase in discharges in the 1950s was the same as in the 1940s and larger than in the 1930s.

7. Beginning in 1940 the share of voluntary hospitals has increased in total discharges and patient days but decreased in beds. The share of municipal hospitals has changed in the opposite direction for each item. Proprietary hospitals registered both numerical and relative gains in the care of inpatients; they play scarcely any part in caring for ambulatory patients.

8. In 1958 general care beds constituted 73 percent of all hospital beds, but their discharges constituted 94 percent of all hospital discharges. On the whole, general care facilities and services increased in both the 1940s and 1950s. The share of voluntary hospitals continued to rise and that of municipal hospitals declined. Proprietary hospitals also reported a larger share of beds, discharges, and patient days.

9. The three computed measures of hospital use behaved differently:

(*a*) Rate of occupancy in general care facilities rose in the 1940s and declined in the 1950s.

(*b*) Length of stay declined by two days in the 1940s and by one day in the 1950s.

(*c*) Rate of bed turnover rose sharply in the 1940s and only slightly in the 1950s.

10. There has been an absolute, as well as a relative, decline in the ward service and an increase, both absolute and relative, in the private (especially semiprivate) service. Even so, the ward still reported 41 percent of all general care discharges in 1958 and 51 percent of all general care patient days.

11. The share of municipal hospitals in the ward service has steadily increased and that of voluntary hospitals decreased. In 1940 the former had more than one half of all general-care patient days, but less than one half of beds or discharges; by 1950 they also had more than one half of all ward beds; and by 1958, they had, in addition, more than one half of all ward discharges. Proprietary hospitals do not maintain a ward service.

12. In the private (including semiprivate) service the share of voluntary hospitals has increased and that of proprietary hospitals declined. The municipal system plays a negligible part.

13. Visits to outpatient departments of hospitals increased during the depression of the 1930s and declined during World War II and subsequently. There was little change in total volume during the 1950s.

14. The share of voluntary hospital outpatient departments has steadily declined. Their volume of visits has continued to fall, while that of municipal hospitals rose in the 1950s, after a drop in the 1940s. By 1958 the share of municipal hospitals was almost one half.

15. Between 1948 and 1958 visits to emergency departments of hospitals more than doubled. Volume of service increased in each hospital system, but at a much more rapid rate in municipal than in voluntary hospitals. The former reported more than one half of all emergency department visits for the first time in 1957.

16. Available data on services to private ambulatory patients are incomplete and not reliable. The number of visits to voluntary hospitals in 1958 is estimated between 350,000 and 425,000. A reported increase between 1955 and 1958 may be more apparent than real.

17. Diagnostic centers in hospitals have not expanded as anticipated. The year 1958 marked the closing of the pioneer consultation service in New York City for persons of moderate means.

18. The total number of calls answered by the emergency ambulance service in 1958 was the same as in 1950 but smaller than in 1940. The volume of services rendered by voluntary hospitals continued to decline, whereas that rendered by municipal hospitals rebounded from the sharp wartime drop. As a result, the share of voluntary hospitals declined from 59 percent in 1940 to 41 percent in 1958.

19. Home-care patient days rose rapidly between 1949 and 1950 and for several years thereafter. By 1955 a plateau was reached, with all but one municipal general hospital operating an organized home-care program and only four voluntary hospitals doing so. Among the latter two are very small, and one is primarily intended for teaching. Ninety-five percent of the average daily census on home care is reported by municipal hospitals.

20. Facilities and services in hospitals for non-general-care patients have also increased since 1940. Three fourths of the increase has occurred in the municipal system. By 1958, almost one half of all patient days in municipal hospitals were for nongeneral-care patients, compared with one sixth in voluntary hospitals and one eighth in proprietary hospitals.

21. Both beds and patient days in psychiatric services of voluntary, municipal, and proprietary hospitals have doubled since 1940, while discharges have increased but slightly. Although the municipal system remains predominant, the share of voluntary hospitals has increased.

22. Visits to psychiatric clinics of hospitals have expanded even more rapidly. Here, unlike the inpatient service, the share of voluntary hospitals has been contracting.

23. Tuberculosis facilities and services expanded through the summer of 1953, and then a long-term decline set in. Both major hospital systems have reduced facilities and services for inpatients, with voluntary hospitals proceeding at the faster rate. The share of municipal hospitals is four fifths of the total.

24. Outpatient services are of rising importance in tuberculosis care. The chest clinics of the Department of Health play a prominent role.

25. Many hospitals with a rehabilitation department do not assign any beds to it. In 1958 14 hospitals reported such assignments, which aggregated 725 beds. Most of the beds and services were in municipal hospitals, and the remainder in voluntary hospitals.

26. Hospital facilities for the chronically ill, as counted for this study, failed to increase in the 1950s. The share of each major system is close to one half of the total. All numbers should be interpreted with caution, however, because of difficulties in classifying and reclassifying facilities for long-term patients.

27. Nursing-home types of facility in hospitals have expanded less rapidly than anticipated. Municipal hospitals have almost three fourths of all such beds.

28. Nursing-home types of facility outside hospitals have expanded rapidly. Included are separate nursing homes, infirmaries of homes for the aged, and an infirmary of a public home. In 1958

proprietary nursing homes reported 65 percent of these beds and 62 percent of the patient days, compared with 32 and 34 percent, respectively, for the voluntary system and only 3 and 4 percent, respectively, for the municipal system.

29. If all facilities for long-term patients are combined, they amount to 20,400 beds in 1958, 70 percent of them outside hospitals and 30 percent inside. They reported only 23,000 discharges but 6.2 million patient days.

30. Of the total number of patient days reported by long-term facilities in New York City the proprietary system contributed two fifths, the voluntary system one third, and the municipal system less than one fourth.

31. Among a number of substantive and technical problems discussed are the following:

(a) Rates of occupancy by type of hospital accommodation— private, semiprivate, and ward—cannot be interpreted unequivocally.

(b) The rate of bed turnover is shown to be related mathematically to the two traditional computed measures of hospital use—rate of occupancy and length of stay.

(c) Changes in the outpatient department volume of visits are analyzed in relation to changes in charges and income. Potential effects on quality of care are cited.

(d) Future tendencies in hospital home-care programs are explored as Blue Cross extends benefits to this area and one hospital establishes a pilot program for patients who have not recently been in a hospital. Factors entering into a proper comparison of cost between home care and hospital care are enumerated.

(e) Problems raised by the present organization of the emergency ambulance service are considered in relation to the expanding role of the hospital emergency department.

Appendix 2.A

ESTIMATING NUMBERS OF BEDS, DISCHARGES, AND PATIENT DAYS FOR 1940

In general, the data on beds and services for inpatients in 1940 are based on the published data of the United Hospital Fund,[41] as adjusted.

Special problems were posed by the need to convert figures on patients treated into figures on discharges, that is, to estimate and subtract the number of patients in the hospital at the beginning of the year. These were handled by reference to relationships between the number of patients in a given type of accommodation in a given hospital at the beginning of the year and on the average during the year (average daily census), when both figures were available from the Hospital Council's annual inventory.

To obtain more complete counts than those published, several adjustments were made.

HOSPITAL SYSTEM TOTALS

Voluntary Hospitals. The psychiatric unit at New York Hospital was added from data in the Hospital Council's files. Doctors Hospital and The Hospital of the Rockefeller Institute were also added from data furnished by the hospitals.

Proprietary Hospitals. Two psychiatric hospitals licensed by the New York State Department of Mental Hygiene were added, which are not included in United Hospital Fund counts. The data were taken from the "Hospital Service" issue of the *Journal of the American Medical Association.*[42]

Municipal Hospitals. None.

TYPE OF CARE

Tuberculosis. Data were obtained from the annual compilation published by New York Tuberculosis and Health Association.[43]

Psychiatry. Data were obtained as follows:

(a) *Voluntary hospitals.* The New York Hospital unit, as above.

(b) *Municipal hospitals.* From the *Annual Report* of the New York City Department of Hospitals.[44]

(c) *Proprietary hospitals.* Two hospitals, as above, plus one hospital included in the United Hospital Fund count.[45]

Chronically Ill. Figures were calculated as follows:

(a) *Voluntary hospitals.* Total less tuberculosis (above) less psychiatry (above) and less general care (below).

(b) *Municipal hospitals.* United Hospital Fund, as given.

(c) *Proprietary hospitals.* Taken as zero.

General Care. Data were obtained as follows:

(a) *Voluntary hospitals.* General-care hospitals, as reported by United Hospital Fund, plus Doctors and Rockefeller Hospitals (as above) less tuberculosis in general hospitals.[46]

(b) *Municipal hospitals.* General-care hospitals (including acute communicable diseases) less tuberculosis in general-care hospitals [47] and less psychiatry.[48]

(c) *Proprietary hospitals.* United Hospital Fund total less one psychiatric hospital.[49]

Appendix 2.B

DERIVATION OF RELATIONSHIP AMONG RATE OF BED TURNOVER, RATE OF OCCUPANCY, AND LENGTH OF PATIENT STAY

The three terms are defined as follows:

$$\text{Rate of bed turnover} = \frac{\text{Admissions or Discharges (in a year)}}{\text{Beds}}$$

$$\text{Rate of occupancy} = \frac{\text{Average Daily Census}}{\text{Beds}}$$

$$\text{Length of stay} = \frac{\text{Patient Days}}{\text{Admissions or Discharges}}$$

These relationships hold true:

$$\text{Beds} = \text{Average Daily Census} \div \text{Rate of Occupancy}$$

$$\therefore \text{Beds} = \frac{\text{Patient Days}}{365 \times \text{Rate of Occupancy}}$$

$$\text{Admissions or Discharges} = \frac{\text{Patient Days}}{\text{Length of Stay}}$$

Substitute:

$$\text{Rate of bed turnover} = \frac{\text{Patient Days}}{\text{Length of Stay}} \div \frac{\text{Patient Days}}{365 \times \text{Rate of Occupancy}}$$

$$= \frac{\text{Patient Days}}{\text{Length of Stay}} \times \frac{365 \times \text{Rate of Occupancy}}{\text{Patient Days}}$$

$$= 365 \times \frac{\text{Rate of Occupancy}}{\text{Length of Stay}}$$

3   CHARACTERISTICS OF PATIENTS IN SHORT-TERM HOSPITALS

It is important to compare the three ownership groups (voluntary, municipal, and proprietary) and the two types of hospital service (private and ward) with respect to the characteristics of patients in short-term hospitals. Such information is a prerequisite to realistic planning for a more coordinated network of hospital facilities and services.

In view of the differences in mission assumed by the three hospital systems, it is not surprising that their patients differ in pay status (insured, public charge, and so forth). Other characteristics of persons, such as age, ethnic status, or residence, are associated with pay status but may play an independent role in distributing patients by hospital ownership and by accommodation.

This chapter discusses the following characteristics of patients in short-term hospitals in New York City: (1) pay status; (2) residence—in the city or outside; (3) ethnic status—Puerto Rican, non-white, or non–Puerto Rican white; (4) age; (5) length of stay; (6) diagnostic category; (7) need of hospital care.

For the purposes of this report the most important comparisons are between the wards of voluntary and municipal hospitals.

Pay Status

Differences in pay status of patients are much greater among the three hospital systems than between the ward services of voluntary and municipal hospitals. The latter are sizable, however.

To facilitate computation and to simplify presentation of data, all patients in municipal hospitals are treated in this chapter as if they were in the ward. This is not actually so, but the only private (including semiprivate) service (at Sydenham Hospital) is of modest size, serving fewer than 2,000 patients a year with 16,000 patient days.

Table 3.1 shows rates per 100 discharges and per 100 patient day for three categories of pay status. An AHS patient is paid for in full or in part by Associated Hospital Service of New York. A public charge in a voluntary hospital is someone for whom government assumes financial responsibility in full or in part. The concept of a public charge in a municipal hospital poses some difficulty; it was handled in this context by classifying as public charges all patients, except those with Blue Cross or Workmen's Compensation coverage and those who pay full rates. Public-charge patient days in municipal hospitals were computed from the ratio of tax funds to total income. Public assistance recipients in hospitals, included among public-charge patients, are easily defined but pose some difficulty in counting (see Appendix 3.A).

Altogether, 44 percent of the patients discharged from general-care hospitals in New York City in 1957 were Blue Cross subscribers and 27 percent were public charges. However, government paid for more patient days than Blue Cross, 39 percent compared to 37 percent. One fifth of the patient days paid for by government were for the indigent (recipients of public assistance) and four fifths were for the medically indigent (persons who normally pay their way but cannot afford to pay for hospital care).

Proprietary hospitals do not care for public charges, whether indigent or medically indigent, and neither does the private (including semiprivate) service of voluntary hospitals.

Comparison of the two ward services shows that voluntary hospitals have 2.5 times as many Blue Cross subscribers per 100 patients as municipal hospitals. There is a further difference between the Blue Cross subscribers in the two ward services, in that 42 percent of all AHS days in municipal hospitals are discount days compared with 30 percent in voluntary hospital wards. (A discount day is one for which AHS pays 50 percent of the full benefit and the subscriber pays 50 percent of regular charges.)

Municipal hospitals have approximately twice as many public charges and public assistance recipients per 100 patients as the

Table 3.1. RATE PER 100 DISCHARGES AND RATE PER 100 PATIENT
DAYS ACCORDING TO PAY STATUS OF PATIENTS IN
GENERAL-CARE HOSPITALS, BY HOSPITAL OWNER-
SHIP AND TYPE OF ACCOMMODATION,
NEW YORK CITY, 1957

| | | Voluntary | | | | |
Pay Status	All Hospitals	All Accommo- dations	Private and Semi- private	Ward	Munici- pal	Proprie- tary
Discharges						
Associated Hospital Service subscribers	44	51	67	23	9	64
Public charges	27	14	0	44	85	0
Public-assistance recipients	6.5	4	0	11.5	20	0
Patient days						
Associated Hospital Service subscribers	37	47	65	20	8	62
Public charges	39	20	0	50	91	0
Public-assistance recipients	8	4.5	0	11	17	0

SOURCES: United Hospital Fund of New York, Central Tabulating Service Bureau, unpublished tabulations for all subscribing hospitals in New York City; Appendix 3.A; and Table 17.4.

wards of voluntary hospitals. In both ward services public assistance recipients are responsible for a higher proportion of discharges than of patient days. This means that their hospital stay
is shorter than that of other ward patients, largely because maternity patients with a relatively short stay constitute a high proportion of hospitalized persons receiving assistance under the
program of Aid to Dependent Children.

The proportions of public charges and of Blue Cross subscribers in the wards of voluntary hospitals have been rising. In
1947 public charges received 31 percent of all ward days in voluntary general hospitals in New York City and Blue Cross subscribers, 9 percent; the corresponding figures in 1957 were 50
and 20 percent, respectively. The proportion of Blue Cross subscribers in municipal hospitals has increased to 9 percent from
3.5 percent in 1950.

The question arises whether the difference between the wards
of the two hospital systems in the proportion of public assistance
recipients is a true one or a reflection of the difference in the

ethnic composition of patients. For one group of public-assistance recipients the difference appears to be a true one. A higher proportion of Old Age Assistance recipients than of any other group of public-assistance recipients [1] receives care in municipal hospitals, despite the fact that the proportion of Puerto Ricans and nonwhites—who tend to concentrate in municipal hospitals—is lower among recipients of Old Age Assistance than among recipients of any other category of public assistance.[2]

Nonresidents

Closely associated with pay status is the patient's general area of residence. Hospitals in New York City are not likely to have many nonresident public charges or public-assistance recipients, because other local units of government will not pay for their care here. Conversely, patients able to pay for their care are free to travel to the hospital of their (or their physician's) choice.

Table 3.2 shows the percentage of nonresident discharges in the three hospital systems in New York City in 1933 and 1957, including a breakdown between the private (including semiprivate) and ward services for voluntary hospitals. Between 1933 and 1957 the proportion of nonresident discharges in New York City hospitals doubled. This came about not because the proportion of nonresident patients increased in each hospital system and type of accommodation, but rather because those hospitals and types of accommodation that have always had a sizable proportion of nonresident patients increased in relative importance.

Table 3.2. PROPORTION (PERCENT) OF NONRESIDENTS AMONG DISCHARGES FROM VOLUNTARY, MUNICIPAL, AND PROPRIETARY GENERAL-CARE HOSPITALS, NEW YORK CITY, 1933 AND 1957

Hospital Ownership	1933	1957
All hospitals	App. 4.5	9
Voluntary	6	11
Private and semiprivate	12	15
Ward	4	4
Municipal	1	1
Proprietary	n.a.	7

SOURCES: Neva R. Deardorff and Marta Fraenkel, *Hospital Discharge Study* (2 vols.; New York, 1942); Hospital Discharge Study, unpublished summary books in custody of Hospital Council of Greater New York; and Appendix 3.B.

Table 3.3 shows how nonresident patients were distributed in 1957. Almost three fourths of all nonresidents were discharged from voluntary hospitals and another one fourth from proprietary hospitals. Of the small number discharged from municipal hospitals, almost one third were accident cases.[3]

Table 3.3. DISTRIBUTION BY HOSPITAL OWNERSHIP OF NON-RESIDENT DISCHARGES FROM GENERAL-CARE HOSPITALS, NEW YORK CITY, 1957

Hospital Ownership	Number	Percent
All hospitals	91,000	100.0
Voluntary	67,000	73.6
Private and semiprivate	59,000	64.8
Ward	8,000	8.8
Municipal	2,000	2.2
Proprietary	22,000	24.2

SOURCE: See Table 3.2.

Nine tenths of all nonresidents were dischared from private (including semiprivate) accommodations. The proportion of private patients among New York City residents is, therefore, lower than among all patients hospitalized in New York City.

The ethnic composition of nonresident patients may be inferred from the data on live births. In the period September-November, 1956, Puerto Rican and nonwhites constituted only 2 percent of all live births to nonresidents in hospitals in New York City.[4]

There is some indication in the birth statistics that the number of suburban residents receiving care in New York City hospitals may be declining.[5] This is associated with the expansion of hospitals in the suburbs.

Ethnic Status

Complete, or nearly complete, information on the ethnic status of patients in hospitals in New York City became available for the first time from the Hospital Discharge Study of 1933. At that time Negroes constituted 14 percent of the patients discharged from municipal general hospitals and 3 percent of the patients discharged from voluntary general hospitals—less than 0.5 percent of those discharged from private and semiprivate services and 4 percent of those discharged from the ward.[6] Negroes then constituted approximately 5 percent of the population of New York City.[7]

Proprietary hospitals did not participate in the Hospital Discharge Study. For them there is no information on the ethnic composition of patients until the year 1951.

For the period between 1933 and 1951 there are no data on the ethnic composition of patients in voluntary hospitals. There is, however, an intervening estimate for municipal hospitals: in 1946 nonwhites constituted 31 percent of all discharges from municipal general care hospitals.[8]

THE YEAR 1951

For 1951 a sample of persons hospitalized in New York City has been tabulated by hospital ownership and by ethnic status. The data were obtained in the course of a household survey conducted in 1952 by a special committee of the Health Insurance Plan of Greater New York (HIP) and were made available to the Hospital Council.

Table 3.4. DISTRIBUTION BY HOSPITAL OWNERSHIP OF PUERTO RICAN, NONWHITE, AND OTHER WHITE RESIDENT ADMISSIONS, NEW YORK CITY, 1951

Hospital Ownership	Total	Puerto Rican	Nonwhite	Other White
Number in sample (all hospitals)	882	33	114	735
Percent				
Voluntary	58.0	30.4	22.8	64.6
Municipal	23.8	57.5	76.3	14.2
Proprietary	18.2	12.1	0.9	21.2
	100.0	100.0	100.0	100.0

SOURCE: Punch cards from Household Survey conducted by Health Insurance Plan of Greater New York.

The complete sample of hospitalized residents of New York City amounted to 939. Included are 2 percent who were admitted to Federal and State hospitals and 4 percent who were admitted to hospitals outside the city. The latter equals almost 40 percent of the number of nonresidents hospitalized in New York City.

Table 3.4 shows that in 1951 three fourths of the nonwhites admitted to hospitals in New York City received care in municipal hospitals and the remainder in voluntary hospitals. Puerto Ricans received more than one half of their care in municipal hospitals and most of the remainder in voluntary hospitals. (In view of the size of the sample, the distribution of Puerto Rican patients by hospital ownership may not be reliable.) Non–Puerto Rican whites received two thirds of their care in voluntary hospitals and another one fifth in proprietary hospitals.

What was the ethnic composition of resident patients in each hospital system in 1951? To answer this question percentages are distributed by ethnic group.

Table 3.5. DISTRIBUTION BY ETHNIC STATUS OF RESIDENT ADMISSIONS TO VOLUNTARY, MUNICIPAL, AND PRO-PRIETARY HOSPITALS, NEW YORK CITY, 1951

Hospital Ownership	Total		Percent		
	Number in Sample	Percent	Puerto Rican	Nonwhite	Other White
All hospitals	882	100.0	3.7	12.9	83.4
Voluntary	511	100.0	2.0	5.1	92.9
Municipal	210	100.0	9.1	41.4	49.5
Proprietary	161	100.0	2.5	0.6	96.9

SOURCE: See Table 3.4.

Puerto Rican patients constituted almost one tenth of the admissions to municipal hospitals and only 2 percent of the admissions to voluntary hospitals. Nonwhites were more than two fifths of the admissions to municipal hospitals and 5 percent of the admissions to voluntary hospitals. In combination, Puerto Rican and nonwhite patients are shown to have constituted in 1951 more than one half of the admissions to municipal hospitals; this may be an overstatement of the true facts (see Appendix 3.C).

An obvious shortcoming of the above data on hospital admissions, apart from the size of sample, is the lack of a breakdown between private (including semiprivate) and ward patients in voluntary hospitals.

THE YEAR 1957

This deficiency is remedied in the estimates developed for the year 1957. Admissions to general-care hospitals were distributed by ethnic status and by hospital ownership and type of accommodation on the basis of data and according to procedures described in Appendix 3.C.

Table 3.6. DISTRIBUTION OF PUERTO RICAN, NONWHITE, AND OTHER WHITE ADMISSIONS TO GENERAL-CARE HOSPITALS BY HOSPITAL OWNERSHIP AND TYPE OF ACCOMMODATION, NEW YORK CITY, 1957

Hospital Ownership	Total		Puerto Rican		Nonwhite		Other White	
	Num- ber	Per- cent	Num- ber	Per- cent	Num- ber	Per- cent	Num- ber	Per- cent
All hospitals	962,400	100.0	78,100	100.0	132,000	100.0	752,300	100.0
Voluntary	584,100	60.7	34,600	44.3	48,200	36.5	501,300	66.7
Private and semiprivate	392,600	40.8	5,900	7.6	11,800	8.9	374,900	49.9
Ward	191,500	19.9	28,700	36.7	36,400	27.6	126,400	16.8
Municipal	208,900	21.7	41,800	53.5	79,500	60.2	87,600	11.6
Proprietary	169,400	17.6	1,700	2.2	4,300	3.3	163,400	21.7

SOURCE: See Appendix 3.C.

In comparison with 1951, voluntary hospitals played a larger role in 1957 for each ethnic group, whereas the role of municipal hospitals was smaller. In part this is a true difference, and in part it reflects the inclusion of nonresidents in the 1957 data; nonresidents constitute a significant proportion of patients in voluntary hospitals and a negligible one in municipal hospitals. The differences between 1951 and 1957 shown for proprietary hospitals are probably not real but reflect the influence of large sampling variation in the 1951 data.

Municipal hospitals reported 22 percent of all admissions in 1957. Their relative importance to the ethnic groups varied from 12 percent for non–Puerto Rican white patients to more than 50 percent for Puerto Ricans and 60 percent for nonwhites. Conversely, proprietary hospitals, with 18 percent of all admissions, accounted for 22 percent of non–Puerto Rican white patients and for only 2 or 3 percent of Puerto Rican and nonwhite patients. Voluntary hospitals were of substantial importance to each ethnic group, ranging from as many as two thirds of non–Puerto Rican white admissions to just over one third of nonwhite admissions.

The breakdown in 1957 between the private (including semiprivate) and ward services in voluntary hospitals is new. Five sixths of Puerto Rican admissions to voluntary hospitals were ward patients, as were three fourths of nonwhite admissions. By contrast, only one fourth of non–Puerto Rican white admissions to voluntary hospitals were ward patients.

Admissions to the wards of voluntary hospitals were almost equal in number to admissions to municipal hospitals. The two ward systems were not, however, equally important to the three ethnic groups. Municipal hospitals cared for almost 70 percent of nonwhite ward patients, 60 percent of Puerto Rican ward patients, and 40 percent of non–Puerto Rican white ward patients.

Patients in the wards of both hospital systems comprise the following proportions of all patients in the three ethnic groups: Puerto Rican, 90 percent; nonwhite, 88 percent; other white, 28 percent.

In summary, the proportion of Puerto Rican patients receiving care in wards is approximately the same as for nonwhites but three times as high as for non–Puerto Rican whites. Among ward patients a majority of non–Puerto Rican whites (60 percent) use voluntary hospitals, and a majority of Puerto Ricans and of non-whites (60 percent or more) use municipal hospitals. The proportion of ward patients using municipal hospitals is higher for nonwhites than for Puerto Ricans.

What was the ethnic composition of patients admitted to each hospital system in 1957 and to each type of accommodation?

Table 3.7. DISTRIBUTION BY ETHNIC STATUS OF ADMISSIONS TO VOLUNTARY, MUNICIPAL, AND PROPRIETARY GENERAL-CARE HOSPITALS, NEW YORK CITY, 1957

Hospital Ownership	Total		Percent		
	Number	Percent	Puerto Rican	Nonwhite	Other White
All hospitals	962,400	100.0	8.0	14.0	78.0
Voluntary	584,100	100.0	6.0	8.0	86.0
Private and semiprivate	392,600	100.0	1.5	3.0	95.5
Ward	191,500	100.0	15.0	19.0	66.0
Municipal	208,900	100.0	20.0	38.0	42.0
Proprietary	169,400	100.0	1.0	2.5	96.5

SOURCE: Table 3.6.

Proprietary hospitals had relatively few Puerto Rican and non-white patients in 1957.

Together Puerto Rican and nonwhite patients constituted almost three fifths of the admissions to municipal general-care hospitals and 14 percent of the admissions to voluntary general-care hospitals. In the latter system Puerto Rican and nonwhite patients constituted fewer than 5 percent of private (including semiprivate) admissions and 34 percent of ward admissions.

Supplementary data for one group of voluntary general hospitals indicate that among public-charge patients, the combined proportion of Puerto Ricans and nonwhites to total is 40 percent.[9] This is a somewhat higher figure than for all ward patients in voluntary hospitals but much lower than for the patients in municipal hospitals—58 percent.

USE OF HOSPITALS BY NONWHITES

Nonwhites constituted 38 percent of the discharges from municipal hospitals in 1957, compared with 14 percent in 1933. This marks an increase of 170 percent. Their rate of increase in voluntary hospitals was approximately the same—from 3 percent of the total in 1933 to 8 percent in 1957. Their rate of increase in the wards of voluntary hospitals was much greater—from 4 percent of the total to 19 percent. Still, in 1957 the proportion of nonwhite patients was only one half as large in the wards of voluntary hospitals as in municipal hospitals.

Table 3.7 also shows that in 1957 nonwhites comprised 14 percent of all admissions to short-term hospitals in New York City. This is higher than their proportion in the population in 1957—12 percent. A high birth rate accounts for a significant fraction, perhaps one half, of the relative excess in hospital admissions. It has been suggested that some fraction of the excess may represent readmissions owing to adverse socioeconomic circumstances.[10]

The conclusion that nonwhites in New York City tend to use more hospital care than other groups in the population is confirmed by earlier studies on hospital admissions or discharges. In 1951, for example, as shown by Table 3.5, nonwhites constituted 13 percent of all resident admissions to voluntary, municipal, and

proprietary hospitals in the city. If other hospitals in and out of
the city are also considered, nonwhites constituted 12.5 percent of
all admissions by New York City residents. They constituted 9.5
percent of the city's population in 1950.[11]

In 1935–36 the National Health Survey measured morbidity
and the use of medical and hospital services by population groups.
Negroes in New York City were found to use 20 percent more
hospital care than whites.[12]

In 1933 nonwhites constituted 5 percent of the population of
New York City and accounted for 8 percent of the discharges from
voluntary and municipal general hospitals.[13] Had proprietary
hospitals been included, the proportion of nonwhite discharges
would have been under 8 percent but probably no less than 7
percent.

INFLUENCE OF ETHNIC STATUS IN DISTRIBUTING PATIENTS

Differences in ethnic composition of patients stem in part from
patients' differences in income and in health insurance enrollment, as discussed in Chapter 1. The question arises whether
ethnic status also exerts an influence of its own in the distribution
of patients among hospital systems and between types of accommodation. Several studies shed light on this question.

For example, one study of obstetrical care in New York City
found that Puerto Ricans and nonwhites make less use of private
physicians than do "other white" patients. In 1955, 83 percent of
non–Puerto Rican white live births were attended by private
physicians, compared with only 11 percent for nonwhite births
and 5 percent for Puerto Rican births. Moreover, a much higher
proportion of "other white" births with fathers in a low occupa-
tional status (laborers and others) had a private physician than did
Puerto Rican and nonwhite births with fathers in a high occupa-
tional status (professional, managerial, and technical).[14]

It is possible to isolate the ethnic factor to some degree by
holding income constant. This can be done by studying the distribution among hospitals and between accommodations of persons admitted to hospitals from low-income public housing
projects, in which tenants' income is uniformly low.

For a group of housing projects in the northern half of Manhattan these were the findings regarding the use of wards in the two hospital systems:

Ethnic Status	Proportion (Percent) Ward to Total Admissions	Proportion (Percent) Municipal to All Ward Admissions
Puerto Rican	90	40
Nonwhite	90	72
Other white	85	42

There was a small difference among the three ethnic groups in the extent to which they used ward accommodations. There was, however, a large difference between nonwhites and the others in the extent to which they used municipal hospitals.

In a similar study of hospital admissions from a poor neighborhood in which both voluntary and municipal hospitals are accessible, the Hospital Council found that the proportion of patients with Blue Cross insurance using the ward was about twice as high as in the city as a whole.[15] Furthermore, public housing tenants with Blue Cross insurance who use the ward are much more likely to go to a voluntary hospital than to a municipal hospital. The ratio was of the order of three to one.[16]

A study of patients in a group of nine voluntary general hospitals found wide variations among the three ethnic groups in the proportion of patients with Blue Cross insurance who use the ward. Among non–Puerto Rican white patients with Blue Cross 10 to 15 percent use the ward; among nonwhites the proportion exceeds 50 percent; and among Puerto Ricans, it reaches 70 percent.[17]

The tendency for nonwhite patients to make greater use of municipal hospitals than their white neighbors is not new. Analysis of unpublished data for 1933 yields the same result. At that time the tendency was perhaps even stronger than today.[18]

There is one further aspect of the use of municipal hospitals that merits attention. Because they are disproportionately used by nonwhites, who are a relatively younger population, municipal hospitals would be expected to have a higher proportion of nonwhite discharges in the younger ages than in the older ages. This effect is accentuated by the tendency of white patients in municipal hospitals to concentrate in the older ages. In consequence, age class 15–44 in municipal general hospitals contains more nonwhite than white discharges, but age class 65 and over contains six times as many white discharges as nonwhite.[19]

Age Composition

Aged persons (65 years and over) stay longer in the hospital than other patients. They are more likely to suffer from medical conditions that require prolonged treatment and to be without a suitable home. They may pose a discharge problem when definitive care in the hospital is completed. In consequence of their longer stay the aged constitute a higher proportion of the patient census of a hospital on a given day than of the patients admitted to, or discharged from, the hospital during a time interval. The two ways of looking at the age composition of patients are useful for different purposes, but they should be clearly distinguished. In this report the one will be designated "one-day patient census" and the other, "discharges or admissions."

DATA FOR EARLIER YEARS

Distributions of discharges by age class are available for the year 1933 for voluntary and municipal hospitals but not for proprietary hospitals. The 1933 data reflect the pattern of hospitalization at the depth of the depression. Little would be gained today from a detailed comparison of the age composition of patients in municipal and voluntary hospitals at that time. The 1933 distributions of discharges by age class are therefore presented in Appendix 3.D (see Table 3.18).

It was possible to develop distributions of hospital admissions by age for all three hospital systems for the year 1951. The data are taken from tabulations of punch cards furnished by HIP. Because of certain limitations inherent in household surveys (mostly, omission of the hospitalization experience of persons who died during the survey period), the distributions are clearly deficient in the older ages. Accordingly, these data are presented for the record in Appendix 3.D (see Table 3.19).

Distributions of a one-day patient census by age are available for the fall of 1953. Hospitals were requested to submit an age distribution of patients as of a given date to the American Medical

Association,[20] which furnished the Hospital Council with the machine tabulations for all hospitals in New York City that completed the questionnaire.

Table 3.8. PERCENTAGE DISTRIBUTION BY AGE GROUP OF ONE-DAY PATIENT CENSUS IN VOLUNTARY, MUNICIPAL, AND PROPRIETARY GENERAL-CARE HOSPITALS, NEW YORK CITY, 1953

Age Group (Years)	Voluntary	Municipal	Proprietary
0–14	11.1	12.8	6.6
15–44	36.1	29.7	45.2
45–64	33.0	29.1	36.4
65 and over	19.8	28.4	11.8
	100.0	100.0	100.0

SOURCE: American Medical Association, unpublished data for New York City hospitals collected through special questionnaire. See Frank G. Dickinson, *Age and Sex Distribution of Hospital Patients* (Bulletin 97; Chicago, Bureau of Medical Economic Research, American Medical Association, 1955).

In 1953 municipal hospitals had the highest proportion of aged patients and proprietary hospitals had the lowest, with voluntary hospitals in the intermediate position. Municipal hospitals also had the highest proportion of children, and proprietary hospitals again had the lowest proportion. In age class 15–44 proprietary hospitals had the highest proportion by far. This was in large part attributable to their high proportion of obstetrical patients at that time.

In the 1953 survey voluntary hospitals were not asked to distinguish between private and ward services. It is, therefore, not possible to compare the age composition of patients in municipal hospitals with that in wards of voluntary hospitals.

DATA FOR RECENT YEARS

For 1957 and 1958 it was possible to develop selected distributions by age class of a one-day patient census and of admissions (or discharges). Private and ward patients in voluntary hospitals are presented separately.

1. Admissions to voluntary general hospitals for the year 1958 and discharges from municipal hospitals for 1957. There is no comparable distribution for proprietary hospitals.

2. One-day patient census in voluntary, municipal, and pro-

prietary hospitals in 1958. These are estimates developed separately for each hospital system, as described in Appendix 3.D. (Appendix 3.D also contains Tables 3.20 and 3.21, with selected distributions of patients by age class for intervening years.)

Discharges from, or Admissions to, Hospitals. Table 3.9 shows admissions to voluntary hospitals in 1958 and discharges from municipal hospitals in 1957. Voluntary hospitals had a lower pro-

Table 3.9. PERCENTAGE DISTRIBUTION BY AGE GROUP OF ADMISSIONS TO VOLUNTARY GENERAL HOSPITALS BY TYPE OF ACCOMMODATION, AND OF DISCHARGES FROM MUNICIPAL GENERAL HOSPITALS, NEW YORK CITY, 1958 AND 1957

Age Group (Years)	Admissions, Voluntary Hospitals, 1958					Discharges, Municipal General Hospitals, 1957
	Total	Private	Semi-private	Private and Semiprivate	General Ward	
0–14 *	14.9	3.7	12.9	11.9	22.5	15.7
15–44 *	44.4	40.1	45.5	44.7	43.8	48.3
45–64	27.4	37.1	29.6	30.5	19.7	17.9
65 and over	13.3	19.1	12.0	12.9	14.0	18.1
	100.0	100.0	100.0	100.0	100.0	100.0

* In voluntary hospitals the age breakdown is 0–12 and 13–44.
SOURCES: United Hospital Fund of New York, Central Tabulating Service Bureau, unpublished tabulations for 33 subscriping general hospitals in New York City, 1958; and Hospital Morbidity Reporting, Joint Project of the New York City Departments of Health and Hospitals, *Bulletins*, 1–11, special reports, and tabulations, prepared by Marta Fraenkel (New York, 1957–58; mimeographed).

portion of aged and of children than municipal hospitals. The semiprivate service is chiefly responsible for the former and the private service for the latter. The proportion of aged patients in municipal hospitals was higher than in the wards of voluntary hospitals but lower than in the private service of voluntary hospitals.

It is now possible to compare trends in the population of New York City and in each hospital system with respect to the aged. Between 1933 and 1957 the proportion of aged in the population rose from approximately 4.5 percent (3.8 percent in 1930 and 5.6 percent in 1940) to 9 percent, that is, it doubled. During this period the proportion of aged to total discharges or admissions rose from 5 percent to 13 percent in voluntary general hospitals and from 6.5 percent to 18 percent in municipal general hospitals.

It is concluded that (1) the proportion of aged among hospital patients rose faster than in the population at large and (2) that the proportion of aged patients rose at the same rate in each hospital system.

One-Day Patient Census. Table 3.10 shows for the year 1958 the estimated age composition of a one-day patient census in each hospital system and type of accommodation. A more detailed breakdown of age class 65 and over is presented in another report.[21]

Table 3.10. DISTRIBUTION OF AGE GROUPS IN ONE-DAY PATIENT CENSUS IN GENERAL-CARE HOSPITALS BY HOSPITAL OWNERSHIP AND TYPE OF ACCOMMODATION, NEW YORK CITY, 1958

| | All Ages | | Age Group (Years) | | | | | | | |
| | | | 0–14 | | 15–44 | | 45–64 | | 65 and over | |
Hospital Ownership	Num- ber	Per- cent	Num- ber	Per- cent	Num- ber	Per- cent	Num- ber	Per- cent	Num- ber	Per- cent
All hospitals	29,275	100.0	2,948	100.0	9,444	100.0	9,873	100.0	7,010	100.0
Voluntary	17,098	58.3	1,682	57.1	5,562	58.9	6,049	61.3	3,805	54.3
Private and semi- private	10,353	35.3	570	19.3	3,471	36.8	4,093	41.5	2,219	31.7
Ward	6,745	23.0	1,112	37.8	2,091	22.1	1,956	19.8	1,586	22.6
Municipal	8,930	30.5	1,072	36.3	2,680	28.4	2,589	26.2	2,589	36.9
Proprietary	3,247	11.2	194	6.6	1,202	12.7	1,235	12.5	616	8.8

SOURCE: See Appendix 3.D.

In every age class voluntary hospitals had a majority of the patients, ranging from 54 percent in age class 65 and over to 61 percent in age class 45–64. Among ward patients municipal hospitals had a majority in three of the four age classes, children being the exception.

If patients in each age class are classified by type of accommodation, the highest proportion of ward patients is among children, not among the aged, as one might expect.

Age Class	Proportion (Percent) Ward to Total Patients
0–14 years	74.0
15–44	50.5
45–64	46.0
65 and over	59.5
All ages	53.5

One reason for the high proportion of ward patients among children is that most pediatric facilities in voluntary hospitals are classified as ward accommodations.

How were the patients in each hospital system and type of accommodation distributed by age? Municipal hospitals had a

Table 3.11. DISTRIBUTION BY AGE GROUP OF ONE-DAY PATIENT CENSUS IN VOLUNTARY, MUNICIPAL, AND PROPRIETARY GENERAL-CARE HOSPITALS, NEW YORK CITY, 1958

	All Ages		Percent in Age Group (Years)			
Hospital Ownership	Number	Percent	0–14	15–44	45–64	65 and over
All hospitals	29,275	100.0	10.0	32.3	33.7	24.0
Voluntary	17,098	100.0	9.8	32.5	35.4	22.3
Private and semiprivate	10,353	100.0	5.5	33.5	39.5	21.5
Ward	6,745	100.0	16.5	31.0	29.0	23.5
Municipal	8,930	100.0	12.0	30.0	29.0	29.0
Proprietary	3,247	100.0	6.0	38.0	37.0	19.0

SOURCE: Table 3.10.

higher proportion of aged and of children than did proprietary or voluntary hospitals. Proprietary hospitals had the lowest proportion of aged and, along with the private (including semiprivate) service of voluntary hospitals, had the lowest proportion of children.

It should be added that public-charge patients in voluntary hospitals have a higher proportion of aged than the other ward patients in voluntary hospitals but a lower proportion than patients in municipal hospitals.

Table 3.12. PERCENTAGE DISTRIBUTION BY AGE GROUP OF ONE-DAY PATIENT CENSUS IN WARDS OF VOLUNTARY AND MUNICIPAL GENERAL-CARE HOSPITALS, NEW YORK CITY, 1958

	Voluntary Hospital Wards		
Age Group (Years)	Other than Public Charges	Public Charges	Municipal Hospitals
0–14	17.3	15.9	12.0
15–44	31.1	30.7	30.0
45–64	31.6	27.5	29.0
65 and over	20.0	25.9	29.0
	100.0	100.0	100.0

SOURCES: See Appendix 3.D and Table 3.11.

It was possible to estimate the number and proportion of aged among patients in receipt of public assistance in each hospital system (see Appendix 3.A). The proportions are shown below both for discharges and for patient days:

	Proportion (Percent) of Aged among Public-Assistance Recipients in General-Care Hospitals	
Category	Voluntary	Municipal
Discharges	14	19
Patient days	30	44

In each hospital system the proportion of aged discharges among public-assistance recipients is approximately the same as the proportion of aged among all ward discharges (Table 3.9). However, the proportion of all patient days used by the aged is much higher for public-assistance recipients than for ward patients (see Table 3.11). It follows that the average duration of hospital stay of aged persons on public assistance is much longer than that of other aged patients in the ward.

Length of Patient Stay

One well-known difference among patients in voluntary, municipal, and proprietary hospitals is in the average length of patient stay. Similar, but smaller, differences also obtain between private (including semiprivate) and ward patients in voluntary hospitals.

In 1958 the average length of stay of general-care patients in New York City hospitals was as follows:

	Days
Voluntary hospitals, all services	10.0
Private and semiprivate service	9.1
Ward service	11.8
Municipal hospitals	13.8
Proprietary hospitals	6.9
All hospitals	10.3

The average length of stay of public-charge patients in voluntary hospitals was 13.2 days—1.4 days more than that of all patients in voluntary hospital wards. This difference, which reflects differences between public charges and other ward patients in almost every clinical service, has been constant for four years.[22] At the same time the difference in average length of stay between public-

charge patients in voluntary and municipal hospitals has been
steadily narrowing.

It has long been accepted that the diagnosic composition of
patients (the proportion of patients admitted for tonsillectomy or
obstetrics, on the one hand, and neurology or orthopedic surgery,
on the other hand) is an important cause of differences among
hospitals in average length of patient stay. Also important are the
socioeconomic circumstances of the patient and his family, for
these bear on the availability of a home to which the patient can
be discharged and on the likelihood of the patient's having received a prior diagnostic evaluation, so that he is ready for treatment upon admission.

Recently data have appeared that show persistent differences
among local hospital systems in the average length of stay of
patients with the same diagnostic condition.[23] The implications of
these findings are not clear, in the absence of information regarding possible differences among the hospital systems' patients in
the complexity of their diagnostic problems and in the presence of
associated medical conditions.

Only this year have data appeared that point to differences among the regions of this country in average length of stay
of patients with identical diagnostic condition and with membership in the same medical care plan.[24] Such geographic differences
in patient stay apparently reflect differences in medical practice,
about which relatively little can be said with assurance at this time.

Differences in average length of patient stay typically reflect
consistent differences in the distribution of discharged patients by
length of stay. For municipal hospitals distributions of patients
by length of stay have been available for several years, as a result
of the work of the Hospital Morbidity Reporting Project. Distributions for all three hospital system are available only for the year
1951 and are presented in Table 3.13. These distributions suffer
from the usual limitations of the household survey in reporting
hospital use.

Seventeen percent of the patients discharged from municipal
hospitals remained 21 days or longer; 12 percent of the patients
in voluntary hospitals and 2 percent of the patients in proprietary
hospitals stayed as long. Similarly, seven tenths of the patients dis-

Table 3.13. DISTRIBUTION BY LENGTH OF STAY OF DISCHARGES
FROM VOLUNTARY, MUNICIPAL, AND PROPRIETARY
HOSPITALS, NEW YORK CITY, 1951

Length of Stay	Total	Voluntary	Municipal	Proprietary
Number in sample				
(all discharges)	856	500	199	157
Percent				
1– 2 days	14.0	13.6	12.0	17.8
3– 6 days	30.3	27.6	31.7	37.0
7–13 days	34.8	37.0	27.2	37.6
14–20 days	9.5	9.6	12.0	5.7
21 days or more	11.4	12.2	17.1	1.9
	100.0	100.0	100.0	100.0
Average (mean) number				
of days	11.0	10.8	14.0	6.5

SOURCE: Punch cards from Household Survey conducted by Health Insurance Plan
of Greater New York.

charged from municipal hospitals left within 13 days; this compares with almost eight tenths for voluntary hospitals and more
than nine tenths for proprietary hospitals.

A distribution of patient days by the length of stay of discharged patients shows that long-stay patients, who constitute a
small proportion of all patients, account for a large proportion of
total patient days.

Table 3.14. DISTRIBUTION BY LENGTH OF STAY OF PATIENT
DAYS OF DISCHARGED PATIENTS, VOLUNTARY,
MUNICIPAL, AND PROPRIETARY HOSPITALS,
NEW YORK CITY, 1951

Length of Stay	Total	Voluntary	Municipal	Proprietary
Number of days in sample				
(all discharges)	9,434	5,442	2,940	1,052
Percent				
1– 2 days	1.6	1.5	1.1	3.3
3– 6 days	13.3	12.5	10.6	25.4
7–13 days	28.2	30.4	16.8	48.2
14–20 days	14.6	15.0	13.9	14.6
21 days or more	42.3	40.6	57.6	8.5
	100.0	100.0	100.0	100.0

SOURCE: See Table 3.13.

It is sometimes useful to separate the total stay of long-stay patients into two parts: the number of days incurred prior to a
specified length of stay and the number of days incurred after that.

In the above distributions patients who stayed 21 days or longer constituted 11 percent of all discharges and accounted for 42 percent of all patient days—21 percent prior to the twenty-first day and 21 percent afterward. This distinction is important in evaluating the possibilities of reducing hospital use, since a saving at the terminal end of a patient's stay is perhaps more likely than the elimination of his entire hospital stay. (See also comparisons of hospital admission rate and length of stay in New York City and United States in Chapter 2.)

For the year 1957 distributions of discharged patients by length of stay are available for patients in receipt of Old Age

Table 3.15. PERCENTAGE DISTRIBUTION BY LENGTH OF STAY OF
OLD AGE ASSISTANCE RECIPIENTS, GENERAL-CARE
VOLUNTARY AND MUNICIPAL HOSPITALS,
NEW YORK CITY, 1957

Length of Stay (Days)	Voluntary	Municipal
All discharges	100.0	100.0
0–14	48.1	44.0
15–19	12.4	9.3
20–29	14.9	13.7
30–59	16.6	20.4
60–89	4.4	6.6
90 and over	3.6	6.0

SOURCE: Sadie Zuchovitz and William Kaufman, *Hospital Utilization by Recipients in the Public Assistance Programs in New York City, 1957* (Special Research and Statistical Reports No. 15; Albany, N. Y., New York State Department of Social Welfare, 1960).

Assistance. In voluntary hospitals one fourth of all discharged Old Age Assistance recipients stayed 30 days or longer; in municipal hospitals one third did so.

Selected Diagnostic Categories

Detailed and current information on the diagnostic composition of patients is available only for municipal hospitals. For all hospital systems in New York City information is available for the year 1954 for selected diagnostic categories; these data were furnished the Hospital Council by the American Medical Association (AMA). Unfortunately, the questionnaire did not ask voluntary hospitals to distinguish between patients on private (including semiprivate) service and those on ward service.

Variations in the response rate may affect the reliability of the data. However, a comparison of the AMA data with those reported by the Hospital Morbidity Reporting Project for the municipal hospitals in the year 1956 shows no material differences, except for obstetrics. It is known that in recent years the number and proportion of obstetrical patients have increased in municipal hospitals and declined in proprietary hospitals.

In the instructions to hospitals the diagnostic categories were defined in terms of the codes of the *Standard Nomenclature of Diseases and Operations* and the *International Statistical Classification of Diseases, Injuries and Causes of Death*. For each patient only the primary diagnosis (the final diagnostic statement of the condition for which the patient was admitted to the hospital) was requested.[25]

Table 3.16 summarizes the data submitted to the American Medical Association by hospitals in New York City, expressing the number of discharges in each diagnostic category as a rate per 100 total discharges.

Table 3.16. RATE PER 100 DISCHARGED PATIENTS FOR SELECTED DIAGNOSTIC CATEGORIES IN VOLUNTARY, MUNICIPAL, AND PROPRIETARY GENERAL-CARE HOSPITALS, NEW YORK CITY, 1954

Diagnostic Category	Voluntary	Municipal	Proprietary
Tonsillectomies (including tonsils and adenoids)	5.5	1.5	8
Appendectomies	2.5	0.7	4.5
Malignant neoplastic disease	5	6	2.5
Cardiac disease	5	10	4
Fractures	3	6	2
Obstetrical (excluding Caesarean section)	20	17	23

SOURCE: American Medical Association, unpublished data for New York City hospitals collected through special questionnaire. See Frank G. Dickinson and James Raymond, *Some Categories of Patients Treated by Physicians in Hospitals* (Bulletin 102; Chicago, Bureau of Medical Economic Research, American Medical Association, 1956).

The smallest differences among the three hospital systems are in the proportion of obstetrical patients to total. These have been further reduced in the interim, as previously noted. The largest differences occur in tonsillectomies and in appendectomies. The rate in proprietary hospitals exceeds that in municipal hospitals five or six times. Smaller differences—ratios of two or three to one

—occur in cardiac disease, malignant neoplastic disease, and fractures. Here municipal hospitals have the highest rates and proprietary hospitals the lowest.

Data computed from a recent publication by Associated Hospital Service of New York also show a substantial difference between voluntary and proprietary hospitals in New York City in the proportion of tonsillectomies to total patients paid for by AHS—2.5 compared with 6 per 100.[26] Both rates are lower than those reported in 1954 for all hospital patients, regardless of pay status.

How Many Patients Do Not Belong in the Hospital?

On various occasions estimates have been given of the number of patients in the wards of voluntary hospitals and in municipal hospitals in New York City who do not require the services of a hospital and could, therefore, be discharged to another type of facility. Usually such estimates are not made simultaneously for both systems by the same person or team applying uniform criteria.

The Hospital Survey for New York, which was conducted in the middle 1930s, did examine patients in both hospital systems at the same time, but the sample was exceedingly small—admissions to selected services in four hospitals in the single month of November, 1935. On the basis of forms completed by the medical staff of each hospital, which are now in possession of the Hospital Council, it was concluded that 17 percent of the ward patients in voluntary hospitals and 6 percent of patients in municipal hospitals had been unnecessarily hospitalized from a medical standpoint. When home conditions were also taken into account, it was concluded that 5 and 3 percent, respectively, of the admissions had been unnecessary.[27]

In April, 1946, the New York City Department of Hospitals surveyed its patient load at the request of the Hospital Council. It found that 22.5 percent of the patients in its general hospitals and 20 percent of the patients in all municipal hospitals were chronically ill. The report on this survey does not furnish the criteria employed to classify patients as chronically ill, but a brief discussion in the Hospital Council's *Bulletin* at that time indicates that these were patients with long-term illnesses who occupied acute beds for lack of appropriate substitute facilities. The *Bulletin* adds, without amplification, that previous studies had shown that 20 percent of the general-care beds in voluntary hospitals were occupied by chronically ill patients.[28]

In March, 1954, the special staff of the Hospital Council's home-care study found that 20 percent of the patients in the ward of a large voluntary hospital were eligible for home care from a medical standpoint. The final report on this study also cites another survey, and this obtained the same results in the ward of another large voluntary hospital in New York City with similar admission policies. The Hospital Council staff also determined that two thirds of the medically eligible patients were socially eligible for home care, so that 13 percent of all ward patients might be expected to be suitable candidates for such a program.[29]

In 1955 a survey of patients in municipal hospitals concluded that 19 percent of the one-day patient census did not require hospital care. Two thirds of the almost 2,000 patients so classified were in the Department's long-term hospitals (Goldwater Memorial and Bird S. Coler), and another 12 percent were in Metropolitan and City Hospitals, then still located on Welfare Island and much less active than today. The other 13 active municipal general hospitals accounted for the remaining 20 percent of the patients in the system who no longer required hospital care.[30] By 1955 a number of measures had been instituted designed to reduce the number patients in municipal hospitals who could profit from other facilities and programs (see Chapter 2).

The important question of the use of the hospital by patients who do not require hospital services is difficult to resolve. From the beginning voluntary health insurance in this country has emphasized coverage of the costs of hospital care. It is likely that this emphasis may have contributed to the use of hospitals by private patients for purposes that are perhaps not essential. Absence of financial reasons to leave the hospital may unnecessarily prolong the stay of public-charge patients. This problem calls for constant attention at the medical and administrative levels.

To determine who does and who does not belong in the hospital, it is necessary to consider the existence of appropriate substitute facilities and programs of adequate quality, and also their cost in personnel, money, and organization. Furthermore, potential savings in hospital beds cannot be estimated reliably on the basis of an evaluation of patients on a single day but rather should take into account the trend of discharges in the immediate period thereafter. The recent survey of tuberculosis patients in hospitals in New York City did conduct such a follow-up, with the result that the estimate of the number of patients in the hospital classified as unnecessarily hospitalized was substantially reduced.[31]

There is good reason why surveys performed at various times and for various purposes yield different conclusions. The past surveys are of value, however, in providing useful leads for future research in this area. A survey of patients in hospitals to determine which ones belong there and which do not and, among the latter, which require substitute facilities and which do not, is a necessary step in any attempt to develop a long-range plan for facilities for the care of the sick in New York City.

Summary and Discussion

The following trends in patient composition are described:

1. The proportions of Blue Cross and public-charge patients and patient days have increased in each hospital system since the late 1940s.

2. The proportion of nonresident patients in New York City hospitals approximately doubled between 1933 and 1957. A downturn may now be under way. It is roughly estimated that the number of residents of New York City who seek care outside is 40 percent of the number of nonresidents cared for in hospitals in New York City (all figures are exclusive of Federal and State hospitals).

3. Between 1933 and 1957 the proportion of nonwhite patients increased at the same rate in both hospital systems but at a faster rate in the wards of voluntary hospitals. However, the proportion of nonwhite to total ward patients in voluntary hospitals is only one half that in municipal hospitals.

4. Since 1933 the proportion of aged (65 and over) has increased faster in hospitals than in the population at large but at approximately the same rate in voluntary and municipal hospitals.

Apart from the comparisons between patients in voluntary hospital wards and municipal hospitals that are shown in Table 3.17, the following findings pertaining to hospital use in New York City are important:

1. In 1957, 44 percent of the patients discharged from general-care hospitals in New York City were Blue Cross subscribers and 27 percent were public charges. However, government paid for more patient days than Blue Cross. One fifth of the patient days paid for by government were for the indigent and four fifths were for the medically indigent.

2. The same proportion of Puerto Rican patients as of non-white patients received care in the ward—90 percent. This was three times as high as the proportion of all non–Puerto Rican white patients who receive care in the ward. Among ward patients a majority of non–Puerto Rican whites (60 percent) use voluntary hospitals and a majority of Puerto Ricans and of nonwhites (60 percent of more) use municipal hospitals. A higher proportion of nonwhite ward patients than of Puerto Rican ward patients use municipal hospitals.

3. When income is held constant—in order further to isolate the ethnic factor—the three ethnic groups have approximately the same proportion of ward patients (perhaps slightly lower for the non–Puerto Rican whites). There is, however, a large difference between nonwhites, on the one hand, and Puerto Ricans and non–Puerto Rican whites, on the other hand, in the use of wards in municipal hospitals.

4. Within the municipal hospital system the proportion of nonwhite patients is much higher in the younger ages than in the older. In age class 15–44 the numbers of nonwhite and white discharges are approximately equal. In age class 65 and over white discharges exceed nonwhites by six to one.

5. The 1957 estimates confirm findings in earlier studies that in New York City nonwhites use more hospital care than other groups in the population.

6. Long-stay patients (here defined as 21 days and over) comprise 11 percent of all discharges and use 42 percent of all patient days. If the total stay of these patients is divided into two segments

(before and after 21 days), the first part of the stay accounts for 21 percent of all patient days and the second part for the remaining 21 percent.

Table 3.17 brings together the salient comparisons between patients in the wards of voluntary hospitals and in municipal hospitals. For all the characteristics of patients listed in this table, the

Table 3.17. RATE PER 100 DISCHARGES OR PER 100 IN ONE-DAY PATIENT CENSUS FOR SELECTED PATIENT CHARACTERISTICS IN WARDS OF VOLUNTARY AND MUNICIPAL GENERAL-CARE HOSPITALS, NEW YORK CITY, 1957 OR 1958

Patient Characteristic	Voluntary Hospital Wards	Municipal Hospitals
Pay status (discharges)		
Associated Hospital Service subscribers	23	9
Public charges	44	85
Public-assistance recipients	11.5	20
Ethnic status (discharges)		
Puerto Ricans	15	20
Nonwhites	19	38
Other Whites	66	42
Nonresidents (discharges)	4	1
Aged (one-day census)		
All ward patients	23.5	29
Public charges	26	29
Public-assistance recipients	30	44
Length of stay (discharges)		
Old Age Assistance recipients, 30 days or more	25	33

differences between the two ward services are large, or at least substantial.

It was not possible to make a direct comparison between the patients in the two ward services by various lengths of stay and by diagnostic category, because these items were not reported separately for the private and ward services of voluntary hospitals. However, available data on average length of patient stay and on the distribution of Old Age Assistance recipients by days of stay suggest that the municipal hospital wards are likely to have a higher proportion of long-term patients than the voluntary hospital wards.

The discussion of patients no longer in need of hospital care yields no conclusions on their current number or proportion in either hospital system. This is an important problem that calls for continuing attention.

The finding that there are certain striking differences in patient composition between the two ward services has significant implications for planning. A ward bed in one system is not interchangeable with a ward bed in the other system. Whatever the reasons may be for the existing differences—historical, traditional, cultural, geographic, administrative, or some combination of two or more—municipal hospitals have larger proportions of poor patients, old patients, patients from minority groups, and long-stay patients than the wards of voluntary hospitals. Any attempt to coordinate the services rendered by the two hospital systems must rest on the premise of an equitable, perhaps random (that is, arrived at by chance, without selection), distribution of patients between them. This means that individual hospitals may have to forego some of their autonomy in selecting—and rejecting—patients for admission. In turn, the ability of hospitals to become less selective will depend, to some degree, on the availability of appropriate related facilities to receive patients discharged from the hospital after their definitive treatment is completed. The willingness and ability of voluntary hospitals to become less selective may hinge on the adequacy of payment for the care of public charges.

Appendix 3.A

ESTIMATING THE NUMBER OF PUBLIC-ASSISTANCE RECIPIENTS IN VOLUNTARY AND MUNICIPAL GENERAL-CARE HOSPITALS AND THE PROPORTION OF AGED AMONG THEM, NEW YORK CITY, 1957

Until certain research studies became available in 1960 from the New York State Department of Social Welfare, there was no direct information on the hospitalization of public-assistance recipients in New York City. Financial information developed in this report for other purposes seemed to be the only basis for calculating patient days used by public-assistance recipients. Data on patients were unattainable for voluntary hospitals and looked uncertain for municipal hospitals.

When the new data from the State Department of Social Welfare became available, the estimates of patient days had already been completed. The two sets of data were reasonably close. It was decided to present the estimated data for two reasons: (1) they included recipients of home relief, whereas the new data did not; (2) they pertained to a single calendar year, whereas the new data reflected the total hospital stay of discharged patients, however long.

The new data were, however, a unique source of information on discharges from voluntary hospitals for the four Federal categories of public-assistance recipients.

TOTAL NUMBER OF PUBLIC-ASSISTANCE RECIPIENTS

The amount of money spent by government in voluntary and municipal hospitals for the care of the indigent (recipients of public assistance) is calculated in Chapter 16 of this report. The financial figures serve as a starting point for estimating the number of patient days, as follows:

Patient Days: Voluntary Hospitals. Payments for the indigent were related to total gross payments by government for the care of inpatients. The quotient is the proportion of indigent patient days to total public-charge patient days. This proportion was applied to one half of all ward days, because in 1957 public-charge days constituted one half of total patient days in the ward.

Patient Days: Municipal Hospitals. Here receipts for the care of the indigent were divided by 93 percent to reflect the fact that reimbursement from the State of New York fell short of computed patient-day cost by 7 percent. The denominator for calculating the ratio of indigent to total patient days was obtained by eliminating the cost of mental hygiene clinics from gross inpatient cost, as published in the Annual Cost Statement of the New York City Department of Hospitals.

Patients: Municipal Hospitals. The proportion of public assistance recipients to total patients is taken from the data compiled by the Division of Collections of the Departments of Hospitals on the potential reimbursement status of patients.

Patients: Voluntary Hospitals. Data recently became available from the New York State Department of Social Welfare for recipients of Old Age Assistance, Aid to the Blind, Aid to the Totally and Permanently Disabled, and Aid to Dependent Children.[32] An adjustment was introduced for recipients of Home Relief.

NUMBER AND PROPORTION OF AGED

Patients. All recipients of Old Age Assistance are 65 and over. All recipients of Aid to the Disabled, Home Relief (including Veterans

Relief), and Aid to Dependent Children are under 65. Among all recipients of Aid to the Blind in New York State 43 percent were 65 or over in 1957.[33] Data on the proportion of aged among patients in New York City hospitals in receipt of Aid to the Blind recently became available from the State Department of Social Welfare.

Patient Days. In each hospital system a ratio was computed of the sum of expenditures in behalf of recipients of Old Age Assistance plus 50 percent of expenditures in behalf of recipients of Aid to the Blind to total expenditures for public assistance recipients. The basic data here employed represent claims submitted to the State by the Department of Welfare of the City.

Appendix 3.B

ESTIMATING NONRESIDENTS IN GENERAL-CARE HOSPITALS BY OWNERSHIP AND BY TYPE OF ACCOMMODATION, NEW YORK CITY, 1957

The proportion of nonresidents in New York City hospitals was estimated through scatter diagrams drawn separately for each hospital system.

Over a period of more than five years the Hospital Council of Greater New York accumulated data on the proportion of nonresidents to total patients admitted to 63 voluntary, municipal, and proprietary hospitals. Beginning in 1956 the New York City Department of Health has prepared several special tabulations of births and deaths in hospitals by area of residence.

For each hospital the proportion of nonresident admissions was plotted against its proportion of nonresident deaths. A line of best fit was then drawn. The proportion of nonresident admissions for each hospital system was read off the vertical axis to correspond to the system's proportion of nonresident deaths.

Within the voluntary system the proportion of nonresident patients admitted to the private (including semiprivate) and ward services was obtained directly from the Hospital Council's admission surveys.

The results yielded by the scatter diagrams were checked through the following means:

1. Comparison with the findings of the Hospital Discharge Study. The increase in the proportion of nonresident admissions between 1933 and 1957 in each type of accommodation was much smaller than in the voluntary hospital system as a whole.

2. For a number of voluntary hospitals, the Hospital Council had admission data for intermediate years, such as 1945. In these hospitals the trend in the proportion of nonresident admissions was consistently upward in each time interval, both in the private service and in the hospital as a whole.

3. Data on births in New York City to residents of Nassau County showed large increases through the year 1955. Since then a small decline has set in.

4. In 1956 the proportion of nonresident births in hospitals in New York City was 8 percent. Analysis by the Hospital Council shows that maternity patients tend to travel shorter distances to the hospital than do other diagnostic categories of general-care patients in the same accommodation. The proportion of nonresidents may be expected to be higher for all general hospital patients than for births (or for maternity patients).

5. Recently certain data have become available that seem consistent with the estimates presented in this chapter.

(a) *Voluntary Hospitals.* In the nine general hospitals affiliated with Federation of Jewish Philanthropies nonresident patients constituted 10 percent of all patients in 1959—13 percent in the private (including semiprivate) service and 5 percent in the ward.[34]

(b) *Municipal Hospitals.* In fiscal year 1958–59 nonresidents accounted for almost 1 percent of the discharges from municipal general hospitals.[35]

Appendix 3.C

ESTIMATING THE DISTRIBUTION BY ETHNIC
STATUS OF ADMISSIONS TO GENERAL-CARE
HOSPITALS, NEW YORK CITY,
1951 AND 1957

Estimates of admissions to general-care hospitals by hospital ownership and by ethnic status are presented in the text for two years, 1951 and 1957. Certain differences between the two sets of estimates should be noted.

1. The data for 1951 pertain only to the city's residents. The data for 1957 pertain to all patients admitted to, or discharged from, voluntary, municipal, and proprietary hospitals in New York City. A large proportion of nonresident patients in New York City hospitals consists of non–Puerto Rican whites.

2. The data for 1951 are based on a household survey, whereas those for 1957 are based on hospital records. A household survey lacks information on persons who died in the hospital during the survey

period. Since deaths in hospitals occur in disproportionate numbers among older age groups, it is the non–Puerto Rican white population that is chiefly affected.

3. The data for 1951 are for admissions to all hospitals whereas the data for 1957 are only for general-care or short-term hospitals. However, long-term hospitals account for a small fraction of all hospital admissions.

4. The data for 1951 are based on a sample, with known variance. The data for 1957 pertain to all hospital admissions or discharges. The method of estimating the 1957 distribution, described below, is subject to some degree of error, whose magnitude is unknown.

5. The data for 1951 are available only by hospital ownership group. The data for 1957 are also available by type of accommodation. This significant improvement in detail was made possible by the division of admissions to voluntary hospitals into private (including semiprivate) and ward.

ESTIMATES FOR THE YEAR 1951

The data for 1951 derive from tabulations of punch cards that were furnished by the Health Insurance Plan of Greater New York. These cards are intended to reflect the hospitalization experience of a representative sample of the population of New York City in a single year.

One adjustment has been made in the original data: patients admitted to hospitals in New York City with ownership unknown were combined with patients admitted to municipal hospitals. This was justified by the obvious understatement of the relative importance of the municipal hospital system in the sample, in comparison with the known distribution of all discharges from New York City hospitals in 1951, as reported by hospitals. One result of the adjustment was to reduce the proportion of nonwhites in municipal hospitals, bringing it closer to the proportion reported for the year 1952 by the exploratory project in Hospital Morbidity Reporting; [36] even so, it was still too high.

ESTIMATES FOR THE YEAR 1957

The estimates for the year 1957 were made in two steps:

1. For the general care hospitals in each hospital ownership group a percentage distribution of patients by ethnic status was developed.

2. The percentages were applied to the corresponding number of discharges reported by each hospital system and type of accommodation in 1957.

The data employed to estimate the ethnic composition of patients in each hospital system were chiefly the following: (1) surveys of samples of patients admitted to individual hospitals in New York City, performed by the staff of the Hospital Council in recent years for 63 hospitals, of which 27 yielded information on ethnic composition; (2) a one-day patient census in 1959 in nine general hospitals affiliated with Federation of Jewish Philanthropies, which was compiled by the staff of the subcommittee on hospitals and health agencies; (3) special tabulations prepared for the Hospital Council by the Department of Health showing both ethnic status of the patient and identity of the hospital for live births occurring during three-month intervals in 1956 and 1959 and deaths occurring during three-month intervals in 1956 and 1958; and (4) discharges from municipal hospitals, reported by the Hospital Morbidity Reporting Project, operated jointly by the Department of Health and the Department of Hospitals of the City of New York. The precise technique of estimating the ethnic composition of patients for the three hospital systems varied in accordance with the availability of data.

Municipal Hospitals. The Hospital Morbidity Reporting Project furnished a breakdown between white and nonwhite discharges for 1957, 1956, and also for 1952. The problem was to estimate the number and proportion of Puerto Rican patients. A threefold breakdown of admissions by ethnic status was available for seven municipal hospitals through the Hospital Council's own admission surveys. (It is recognized that the data on Puerto Ricans are not always complete or accurate.)

For these seven hospitals the proportion of Puerto Rican to total admissions was plotted on a scatter diagram against the proportion of Puerto Rican live births to total and separately against the proportion of Puerto Rican deaths to total. In each instance a line of best fit was drawn, and the proportion of Puerto Rican admissions to municipal general-care hospitals was read off the vertical axis for the corresponding value of the proportion of Puerto Rican live births or of Puerto Rican deaths in the system.

An adjustment was then made in the proportion of nonwhite discharges reported by the Hospital Morbidity Reporting Project, on the assumption that 10 percent of all Puerto Rican patients are nonwhite.

Voluntary Hospitals. For these hospitals a threefold distribution of patients (one-day census) by ethnic status became available only for general hospitals affiliated with Federation of Jewish Philanthropies. It could not be assumed that these hospitals were representative of all voluntary hospitals.

Accordingly, it was decided to plot on a scatter diagram the proportion of Puerto Rican admissions against the proportion of Puerto Rican births and separately against the proportion of Puerto Rican deaths for those hospitals for which ethnic information on admissions or patients was available; the same was done for nonwhites. For the breakdown between private and ward services in voluntary hospitals only the information on births in 1959 was useful.

One check applied to the results obtained from the scatter diagrams was consistency between the estimated proportions of Puerto Rican and of nonwhite admissions to each type of accommodation with the proportion of Puerto Rican and of nonwhite admissions to the hospital system as a whole. Comparison with the findings of the Federation one-day census was also helpful.

Proprietary Hospitals. For lack of a sufficient number of hospitals for which the Hospital Council had ethnic information on admissions, the technique of the scatter diagram was not suitable.

The method finally employed was that of analogy. For all three hospital systems ethnic information was available for live births and for deaths. For voluntary and municipal hospitals estimates of the ethnic composition of patients had been developed. The proportion of Puerto Rican admissions and of nonwhite admissions to proprietary hospitals was the missing term in a proportion in which the other three terms were known (for example, Puerto Rican to total births in proprietary hospitals and Puerto Rican to total admissions and Puerto Rican to total births in the private service of voluntary hospitals).

Appendix 3.D

ESTIMATING THE DISTRIBUTION OF PATIENTS
BY AGE, GENERAL-CARE HOSPITALS,
NEW YORK CITY, 1958

A number of separate distributions by age were available for discharges and for a one-day patient census. All were useful in developing the estimated distribution by age of a one-day census for the year 1958 (this is equivalent to a distribution of patient days by age).

AVAILABLE DATA AND SOURCES

For convenience the available data on the age composition of patients in New York City hospitals are listed by year of occurrence. Sources are given, the quality of the data is assessed, and pertinent tables are presented.

1933. Discharges from all municipal hospitals and most voluntary hospitals. Proprietary hospitals did not participate in the Hospital Discharge Study. The result was a complete count of patients discharged from the participating hospitals, performed by a professional staff assisted by Works Progress Administration (WPA) workers. The results were published in two volumes.[37]

The distributions of hospital discharges by age in the year 1933 are of historical interest. They are therefore presented in Table 3.18 for general hospitals.

Table 3.18. DISTRIBUTION BY AGE GROUP OF DISCHARGES FROM
VOLUNTARY AND MUNICIPAL GENERAL HOSPITALS,
NEW YORK CITY, 1933

Age Group (Years)	Voluntary	Municipal
Number (all ages)	254,956	182,835
Percent		
0–14	23.3	16.2
15–44	55.5	56.3
45–64	16.5	21.0
65 and over	4.7	6.5
	100.0	100.0

SOURCE: Neva R. Deardorff and Marta Fraenkel, *Hospital Discharge Study* (2 vols.; New York, 1942), Appendix IX.

1951. Admissions to voluntary, municipal, and proprietary hospitals in New York City, based on interviews of a sample of households conducted by the Health Insurance Plan of Greater New York (HIP). The punch cards containing the hospitalization experience were furnished to the Hospital Council. The note on the ethnic status of patients describes the adjustment made in the data for municipal hospitals. Hospitalization data by age obtained from a household survey suffer from certain limitations, since the deaths missed by the survey occur disproportionately among aged persons. By comparison with the data for 1933, given above, or with the data for municipal hospitals for 1952, given below, the proportion of aged patients in the HIP data is far too low.

The data for 1951 are presented for the record, since they are not elsewhere available.

Table 3.19. DISTRIBUTION BY AGE GROUP OF RESIDENT
ADMISSIONS TO VOLUNTARY, MUNICIPAL, AND
PROPRIETARY HOSPITALS, NEW YORK CITY, 1951

Age Group (Years)	Total	Voluntary	Municipal	Proprietary
Number in sample (all ages)	861	500	203	158
Percent				
0–14	17.6	15.6	24.6	14.6
15–44	58.0	58.2	55.7	60.7
45–64	17.3	17.6	14.3	20.3
65 and over	7.1	8.6	5.4	4.4
	100.0	100.0	100.0	100.0

SOURCE: Punch cards from Household Survey conducted by Health Insurance Plan of Greater New York.

1952. All discharges from municipal hospitals for six months, May through October, 1952. This was an exploratory study in hospital morbidity reporting in which participation by voluntary hospitals was also attempted but did not succeed. This study was published.[38]

Selected data are presented below for comparative purposes (see year 1957).

1953. A one-day census of patients in voluntary, municipal, and proprietary hospitals. The data for New York City are derived from machine record tabulations furnished to the Hospital Council by the American Medical Association, which collected the information nation-wide. The limitations of the data have to do with an unevenness in response rates by different hospital groups. Editing of returns at the national level may also constitute a weakness.

The findings of this survey for general-care hospitals in New York City are presented in Table 3.8.

1955. A one-day census of one fifth of all patients in municipal hospitals. Excluded from the original study were patients in obstetrical units, premature infant units, and tuberculosis units of general hospitals. These exclusions are consistent with the purposes of the study.

Certain adjustments were made in the original data in order to develop a complete age distribution of patients. The place of obstetrical patients and of premature infants in the age distribution is obvious. For tuberculosis patients the age distribution for the three general hospitals involved was taken from the Tuberculosis Hospital Survey of 1958.[39]

Table 3.20 presents the original distribution of patients by age and the more complete distribution as adjusted.

Table 3.20. DISTRIBUTION BY AGE GROUP OF ONE-DAY PATIENT
CENSUS IN MUNICIPAL GENERAL HOSPITALS,
NEW YORK CITY, 1955

	Original Data	*Adjusted Data*
Number in sample (all ages)	1,479	1,761
Percent		
0–14	13.4	13.4
15–44	21.2	27.0
45–64	29.2	27.2
65 and over	36.2	32.4
	100.0	100.0

SOURCE: Howard M. Rusk, John E. Silson, Joseph Novey, and Michael M. Dasco, *Hospital Patient Survey* (New York, 1956), p. 26; and adjustments.

1956. Discharges from municipal hospitals only. The source is the Hospital Morbidity Reporting Project (see year 1957 for data).

1957: Municipal Hospitals. Total discharges from municipal hospitals. The source is the same as for 1956.

Table 3.21 presents the age composition of patients discharged from all municipal hospitals in 1952, 1956, and 1957.

Table 3.21. DISTRIBUTION BY AGE GROUP OF DISCHARGES FROM ALL MUNICIPAL HOSPITALS, NEW YORK CITY, 1952, 1956, AND 1957

Age Group (Years)	1952	1956	1957
Number (all ages)	121,952	235,047	242,528
Percent			
0–14	15.1	14.2	13.7
15–44	48.6	47.7	48.4
45–64	20.1	20.0	19.7
65 and over	16.2	18.1	18.2
	100.0	100.0	100.0

SOURCES: Marta Fraenkel and Carl L. Erhardt, *Morbidity in the Municipal Hospitals of New York City* (New York, 1955); and Hospital Morbidity Reporting, Joint Project of the New York City Departments of Health and Hospitals, *Bulletins*, 1–11, special reports, and tabulations, prepared by Marta Fraenkel (New York, 1957–58; mimeographed).

1957: Voluntary Hospitals. Admissions to voluntary general hospitals. This is a complete count for a sample of 28 hospitals in New York City that subscribed to the Central Tabulating Service Bureau of the United Hospital Fund. The data were especially tabulated for the Hospital Council.

The sample seems to be representative of all voluntary general hospitals in New York City, except for the underrepresentation of large hospitals (500 beds or more). Since better data became available for 1958, those for 1957 are not presented.

1958: Voluntary Hospitals. (1) Admissions. A complete count for a sample of 33 hospitals, as described for 1957 above. The large hospitals were better represented in this sample. The data are presented in Table 3.9. (2) One-Day Patient Census. A one-day patient census was conducted in 12 hospitals by Associated Hospital Service, which furnished the final tabulation for the group as a whole to the Hospital Council.

1958: Municipal Hospitals. A one-day patient census conducted by the Department of Hospitals for the Office of the City Administrator. Patients were counted as 65 and over or under 65.

1958: Proprietary Hospitals. A one-day patient census. This is a complete count prepared in the summer of 1958 by the Department of Hospitals for the Office of the City Administrator. The distribution of patients age 45 and over conforms to the class intervals employed in this chapter, but age class under 45 was not broken down.

1959. A one-day patient census. This was performed in 9 voluntary general hospitals affiliated with Federation of Jewish Philanthropies. The survey was performed by the staff of the subcommittee on hospitals and health agencies of Federation's Study Committee.

ESTIMATE OF ONE-DAY PATIENT CENSUS, 1958

Estimates were prepared separately for each of the three hospital systems and by type of accommodation. In every instance a percentage distribution by age was applied to patient days (this is equivalent to a one-day patient census, which may be defined as patient days divided by 365) in general-care hospitals, as classified by the United Hospital Fund. Under this classification psychiatric and tuberculosis units of municipal hospital centers are excluded. One adjustment to the data for proprietary hospitals was made in order to eliminate a psychiatric hospital (see Chapter 2).

The percentage distributions by age were developed as follows:

Voluntary Hospitals. The 1958 one-day patient census prepared by Associated Hospital Service and the 1959 one-day patient census prepared by Federation of Jewish Philanthropies were combined. Two hospitals were deleted to avoid duplication.

Municipal Hospitals. The count of patients 65 years old and over was taken directly from the report issued by the Department of Hospitals. The distribution of patients below age 65 was determined in relation to the available distributions of patients in 1953 and 1955 (Tables 3.8 and 3.20) and in relation to the trend in discharges between 1952 and 1957 (Table 3.21).

Proprietary Hospitals. The distribution for ages 45 and over was taken from the report of the one-day patient census furnished by the Office of the City Administrator. Age class under 45 was split into two classes on the basis of the one-day patient census in 1953, with due allowance for the decline in the number and relative importance of obstetrical patients.

4   USE OF WARD SERVICE BY
HEALTH INSURANCE SUBSCRIBERS

Health insurance increases the ability of subscribers to pay for hospital care. One of the results anticipated from the expansion of voluntary health insurance enrollment was a reduction in the use of the ward service. This result has been achieved only partially.

For New York City estimates of health insurance enrollment are available for two separate years, 1952 and 1958. During the six-year interval the proportion of the city's residents with some insurance for the cost of hospital care increased from 56 [1] to 71 percent [2] (see Chapter 1); at the same time the proportion of general-care patients in the city's hospitals receiving care in the ward declined from 45 to 41 percent. [3]

Comparison between New York City and the United States as a Whole

In New York City the proportion of patients in the ward is considerably higher than in the nation, although the two have approximately the same proportion of population enrolled under hospital-care insurance—70 percent. In the year 1953, for which data are available both for New York City and the United States, the proportion of ward patients in the former was 45 percent, compared with 33 percent in the latter. [4]

The figure for New York City is for general-care patients discharged from its voluntary, municipal, and proprietary hospitals. For New York City's residents discharged from short-term (general-care) hospitals the proportion of ward patients is somewhat higher. There are two reasons for this. One is largely statistical, namely, that most beds in psychiatric, tuberculosis, and long-term facilities in voluntary general-care hospitals are allocated to ward patients (see Chapter 2), as are all such facilities in municipal hospitals. The other is that New York City's hospitals care for a considerable number of nonresident general-care patients (more than 90,000), 90 percent of whom are in the private (including semiprivate) service (see Chapter 3). As a result, the proportion of ward patients among the city's residents in 1958 was 45 percent.

Furthermore, the rate of decline in the proportion of ward patients in the 1950s was lower than indicated by the above figures. In the past decade two new Veterans Administration hospitals were built in New York City. The three hospitals in this system report that approximately 85 percent of their patients come from the city (see Chapter 2). That the local Veterans Administration hospitals play a relatively larger role in hospitalizing veterans than the Veterans Administration hospital system as a whole is evidenced by the fact that the former care for 60 percent of all veterans hospitalized in New York City for non-service-connected medical and surgical conditions, whereas the latter care for 45 percent of the corresponding total.[5]

AHS Patients in Wards

Many patients in the wards of local hospitals have hospital-care insurance. For reasons stated elsewhere (see Chapter 17), it is not possible to obtain complete data on hospitalized patients with commercial insurance. The statistical analysis in this chapter will, therefore, focus on patients with Blue Cross (Associated Hospital Service, that is, AHS) membership.

In dealing with AHS patients in the ward it is necessary to exercise care with the data. The AHS concept of ward is somewhat broader than that employed by hospitals in this area. In hospital statistics a ward patient is one who does not have—and does not pay—a private physician but is under the care of a clinical department of the hospital (see Chapter 2). AHS adds to this category the patient who has—and pays—a private physician but occupies a bed in a room with more than six beds. Unless otherwise specified, it is the hospitals' definition of a ward patient that is followed in this book.

The hospitals report that one eighth of all AHS patients in New York City occupy the ward. The voluntary hospitals report

Table 4.1. PROPORTION OF AHS PATIENTS IN WARD, VOLUNTARY AND MUNICIPAL GENERAL-CARE HOSPITALS, NEW YORK CITY, 1958

Hospital Ownership	Total AHS Patients (in Thousands)	AHS Patients in Ward	
		Number (in Thousands)	Percent of Total AHS
All hospitals	454.9	55.2	12.1
Voluntary	326.9	37.2	11.4
Municipal	19.3	18.0	93.4
Proprietary	108.7	0	0

SOURCE: Total patients: Tables 17.8, 17.9, and 17.10. Ward patients: voluntary hospitals—United Hospital Fund of New York, Central Tabulating Service Bureau, unpublished tabulations for 33 subscribing general hospitals in New York City, 1958; municipal hospitals—Associated Hospital Service of New York.

that more than 11 percent of all AHS patients occupied ward accommodations in 1958; according to its own definition, AHS reports that almost 17 percent of all AHS patients in United Hospital Fund member general hospitals occupied the ward that year. The difference of 5 percentage points is attributable to patients with their own physician in rooms with more than six beds.

This table also shows that there are twice as many AHS patients in the wards of voluntary hospitals as in municipal hospitals. Since over-all there are fewer ward patients in voluntary general-care hospitals than in municipal hospitals, it follows that AHS subscribers cared for in the ward are more than twice as likely to be in voluntary hospitals than in municipal hospitals (see also Chapter 3).

Possible Explanatory Factors

EXTENT OF INSURANCE AGAINST DOCTOR BILLS

One reason usually advanced for the fact that an insured person receives care in the ward is lack of insurance against doctor bills. Today, however, 63 percent of the population of New York City have some kind of medical-care insurance,[6] only 8 percentage points fewer than have hospital-care insurance. Although questions may be raised regarding the completeness and adequacy of benefits provided by the several types of medical-care insurance, the difference between the numbers of persons holding hospital-care and medical-care insurance has undoubtedly narrowed in the past decade, both here and in the nation. This is particularly true of insurance against surgeons' (including obstetricians') bills. During the period 1952–58, whereas the proportion of ward patients in New York City declined by 4 percentage points, the proportion of residents with medical-care insurance rose by an estimated 25 percentage points.

Moreover, even among subscribers to the Health Insurance Plan of Greater New York (HIP), who have complete protection against doctor bills (with the possible exception of the anesthesiologist's), a certain number are to be found in hospital wards. One study found that 4 percent of HIP subscribers hospitalized in 1955 (who also had membership in AHS) were admitted to municipal hospitals.[7]

Finally, data from three large voluntary teaching hospitals in New York City indicate that perhaps one fourth of their AHS patients in the wards are also known to carry Blue Shield insurance. This figure is probably higher than in the typical community voluntary general hospital.

It would appear that, although lack of insurance against doctor bills may deter a patient from taking a semiprivate bed, the presence of such insurance does not guarantee that he will. Also at play are other influences, which may be grouped under three headings: the physician-patient relationship; financial considerations; and a miscellaneous category, comprising organizational factors on the one hand and sociocultural factors on the other. Some factors can be classified under more than one heading.

PHYSICIAN-PATIENT RELATIONSHIP

During field interviews conducted in the course of this study with physicians, hospital administrators, and social workers, a number of reasons were advanced why insured patients obtain care in the ward. Some of these bear on the relationship between the patient and his physician and between the physician and hospitals.

1. The patient may have a physician who lacks a staff appointment at a hospital with the privilege of admitting private patients. This is true of many Negro physicians. It has been suggested in a report on hospital care in another city that perhaps one factor

in the relatively high use of ward beds by Negro patients is lack of staff appointments for their physicians.[8]

2. A physician who wishes to further the teaching program of his hospital may prefer to refer a patient to its ward service rather than to another physician.

3. A person without a family physician may rely on a neighboring hospital to refer him to a physician, when needed. In 1951 a household survey found that more than one fifth of the families in New York City did not have a family physician.[9] Although every hospital will, upon request, furnish a list of physicians to whom the patient may turn, some hospitals will not take the initiative. Here, too, an important reason would be the hospital's desire to increase the number of ward patients available for teaching. This factor is likely to be of some importance as long as the ward service remains the focal point of medical education programs in hospitals (see Chapter 6).

4. Because they need patients for whom the chief resident of a clinical service can assume complete responsibility, certain large teaching hospitals admit to their ward patients without a private physician who have both Blue Cross and Blue Shield insurance. It has been suggested that medical fees collected from insurance plans are a logical source of supplementary financial support for graduate medical education. Blue Shield does not share this view and has stopped paying bills for services rendered by residents in some hospitals.

5. Traditionally, a person who receives his medical care in the outpatient department of a voluntary hospital receives his inpatient care in its ward. Such a person may jeopardize his status in the clinic by accepting a semiprivate accommodation. Since the emphasis in voluntary health insurance policies is on protection against the costs of hospitalization, it is possible for a person who is insured against the cost of illness in the hospital not to be insured against the cost of illness outside. If so, he may wish to attend the outpatient department, in order to avoid the cost of private medical care, including physicians' services and drugs. It it known that the cost of medical care on an ambulatory basis can loom large to the individual and his family.[10]

The last reason also involves finances, which received frequent mention in the interviews.

FINANCIAL CONSIDERATIONS

Under the heading of finances are grouped those factors that would entail out-of-pocket expenses by the patient at the time of illness.

1. The patient with hospital-care insurance may lack insurance against doctor bills. Although insured for surgery, he may be admitted to the hospital for a medical condition.

2. The patient may carry Blue Shield insurance. If his income exceeds the ceiling for full-service benefits, he would be subject to an additional fee, unpredictable in amount. (Depending on the type of contract held, the income ceiling of the local Blue Shield Plan is $4,000 or $6,000 per family.) In surgery there is also a bill to be paid for anesthesia when it is not administered by a hospital employee.

3. If the patient's prognosis indicates a long hospital stay, full AHS benefits will run out. During the discount period a semiprivate patient is expected to pay one half of the hospital's regular charges. The relative importance of this is suggested by the fact that in the member general hospitals of the United Hospital Fund the proportion of discount to patient days is more than twice as high for AHS ward patients as for AHS semiprivate patients.

4. Even for a short illness, expenditures may sometimes be anticipated in a semiprivate accommodation that do not occur in the ward. An example is the cost of private-duty nursing, currently more than $50 a day. For the ward patient the hospital assigns a special-duty nurse if needed and usually pays her or, under certain programs, obtains assistance from the City. Also to be considered are the cost of blood and radiotherapy, both of which are excluded from benefits under the existing AHS contract. Some voluntary hospital administrators consider it a responsibility of the hospital to protect the patient against assuming excessive financial burdens.

5. Services rendered by and through medical social workers are generally more readily available to ward patients than to semi-

private patients. It is easier to arrange for ward patients such services as housekeeping, taxis, convalescent care, or prostheses, if
needed after discharge from the hospital.

6. Maternity patients with AHS receive a cash benefit of $80,
but this does not come close to meeting the hospital bill. Those
who cannot pay the difference may seek care in the ward. However, the difficulty with this explanation is that AHS maternity
patients have behaved differently from all maternity patients.
Whereas the proportion of ward patients among AHS maternity
patients has declined almost to the same extent as among AHS
nonmaternity patients, the proportion of ward patients among
all maternity patients in the city has increased.[11] The last trend
contrasts, of course, with that for all nonmaternity general-care
patients. The comparative data are as follows:

Category of Admission	Terminal Years	Change in Proportion (Percent) of Ward to Total		
		From	To	Difference
AHS maternity	1951–59	23	15	− 8
AHS nonmaternity	1951–59	24	17	− 7
All maternity	1952–58	33	38	+ 5
All general-care patients	1952–58	45	41	− 4

An important factor in the increase in the proportion of ward
maternity patients is the rising share of births contributed by
Negroes and Puerto Ricans. With relatively low average income,
they have a higher birth rate than the rest of the population.[12]

At this point the financial factors begin to merge with the
social or cultural.

SOCIAL AND ORGANIZATIONAL FACTORS

1. There are groups, particularly among the new arrivals in
the city, who have no tradition of being cared for in the hospital
by their own physicians. One labor union, almost half of whose
members are Negro or Spanish-speaking, purchases AHS coverage
for all dependents. In 1958, 56 percent of the dependents hospitalized were accommodated in the ward—16 percent in municipal
hospitals and 40 percent in voluntary hospitals.[13] Similarly,
whereas 10 to 15 percent of all white patients with AHS in one
group of voluntary general hospitals were in the ward, the com-

parable figure for Negro patients was more than 50 percent, and for Puerto Rican patients, 70 percent [14] (see Chapter 3).

2. Some persons have a marked and conscious preference for the ward service of a particular hospital, voluntary or municipal. They know the hospital and trust it and do not like to be referred elsewhere. This is one of the problems encountered by the pilot project at one of the municipal hospitals (Metropolitan) that aims to find and refer insured patients to neighboring voluntary hospitals.

3. Some persons do not know they are insured. Others know but do not know what benefits are provided by their policies. It is conceivable that increasing reliance on employer payment of health insurance premiums, when not accompanied by adequate education of employees, may serve to extend the area of ignorance.

4. A patient with insurance or other means to pay for his hospital care may find himself in a municipal hospital in an emergency. An emergency patient who can pay is less likely to occupy a ward bed in a voluntary hospital, because he can be transferred to the more appropriate accommodation during his hospital stay. Just what proportion of total admissions to municipal hospitals consists of emergency patients is a moot question. The figures cited range all the way from 10 to 90 percent of all admissions; the correct figure cannot be ascertained without study. It is reasonable to speculate that the true figure is closer to the middle of the range than to either extreme. The true figure may be higher today than formerly, because municipal hospitals are providing an increasing share of the city's emergency services, as measured in ambulance calls and in emergency department visits (see Chapter 2).

5. A patient with insurance or other means to pay for hospital care may find himself in a municipal hospital for still another legitimate set of reasons. The municipal hospital system may have a unique facility, as exemplified by a unit for patients with cerebral palsy.

6. Finally, particularly in winter, there may be a shortage of semiprivate beds in the community, so that insured persons in need of hospitalization must accept ward accommodations. Although this reason is frequently cited, its effect is believed to be

limited, particularly when the patient is admitted to a voluntary hospital. If patients who are potentially semiprivate go to the ward when semiprivate accommodations are overcrowded but do not do so during periods of normal or low semiprivate occupancy, it would be reasonable to expect a high semiprivate census in the summer months and a low ward census. In fact, the semiprivate patient census is high when the ward patient census is high and both are low at the same time. The drop in census from peak to trough is greater for semiprivate accommodations than for ward accommodations.

This is not to say that there is no shortage of semiprivate beds in the community. But if there is, it will not express itself through a high ward census, because patients with their own physicians who occupy a ward bed, whether temporarily or permanently, are classified and reported by hospitals as semiprivate patients (see Chapter 2).

Discussion and Implications of Analysis

As the Hospital Council stated in its annual report of 1958–59: "Corrective measures designed to bring about a shift of patients from ward to semiprivate accommodations more nearly comparable to the growth in hospital insurance must be as varied as are the factors that have brought about the existing situation." [15] Among the preliminary suggestions made at the time were that efforts should be made to educate policy holders about the provisions of their policies; expand insurance for physicians' services and broaden hospital care insurance benefits; influence a larger proportion of patients to seek semiprivate accommodations; and educate the public to rely on a family physician in preference to an outpatient clinic, as this might also lead to an increased use of semiprivate accommodations.

On the basis of the discussion in this chapter additional steps are indicated. One is provision of hospital staff appointments with private patient privileges for more practicing physicians (see Chapter 5). Another is expansion of medical teaching in private (including semiprivate) accommodations, with the cooperation of patients and their physicians (see Chapter 6).

The Hospital Council believes that the proportion of ward

patients in New York City hospitals should be reduced.[16] One model that deserves further investigation is the pattern of hospital use in one of the five boroughs of New York City, namely, Richmond (Staten Island). In 1955, when the Hospital Council studied the hospitalization needs of Staten Island, the proportion of ward admissions in the voluntary and proprietary general hospitals of this borough was 20 percent—less than one half of the city-wide figure of 42 percent that year.[17] By 1958 the proportion for Staten Island was 17 percent and for the city 41 percent. Since Staten Island is largely self-sufficient in providing hospital care to its residents,[18] the 17 percent figure applies to the residents, as well as to the hospitals, of the borough. A small understatement of the true proportion of ward patients results from the presence on the Island of the United States Public Health Service Hospital, which renders some services to local residents.

Absence of a municipal general hospital on Staten Island may contribute to the relatively low proportion of ward patients. Other influences in the same direction are the low proportion of Puerto Rican and nonwhite population, who for reasons of income, health insurance status, and other factors tend to be heavy users of ward service. Concentration on Staten Island of employees of the City with membership in HIP further reduces the demand for ward accommodations.

Certain characteristics of the local hospitals and medical profession probably contribute to the prevailing emphasis on semi-private care. None of the three voluntary hospitals on the Island is a major teaching center with a demand for large numbers of ward patients for teaching. None is supported by substantial philanthropic contributions or earnings on investments. As to the physicians, a relatively larger proportion than elsewhere in the city are in general practice, earning correspondingly lower fees. A large majority of the total (with few specific exceptions) have one or more hospital staff appointments with private patient privileges, through which they earn part of their income.

Summary

1. Between 1952 and 1958 the proportion of New York City's population with hospital-care insurance rose from 56 to 71 per-

cent, whereas the proportion of ward general care patients in local hospitals declined from 45 to 41 percent.

2. The proportion of New York City residents receiving care in the ward is 45 percent, substantially higher than in the nation as a whole.

3. Twelve percent of all AHS patients are in wards, as reported by hospitals. The proportion reported by AHS is higher, because it encompasses not only patients without a private physician but also patients with a private physician in a room with more than six beds.

4. One reason that persons with AHS insurance receive care in the ward is lack of medical-care insurance. This factor is, however, of declining importance. It is reported that 63 percent of the residents of New York City have some type of insurance against the cost of doctor bills.

5. Factors favoring the use of ward accommodations by persons with hospital-care insurance, as advanced in field interviews, are enumerated and discussed. Broadly, these fall in three groups: physician-patient relationship; financial; and other, including social and organizational. Available information is introduced to appraise the relative weight of the several factors.

6. The implications of the analysis are that corrective measures must be as varied as the factors that have brought about the existing situation.

7. It is suggested that the experience of Richmond (Staten Island) might be examined as a possible model for reducing the proportion of ward patients in New York City.

Part II. PERSONNEL, PLANT, AND
ORGANIZATION

5   ATTENDING STAFF

Hospital care is rendered by people: it takes physicians, nurses, and others, making use of various facilities and equipment, to give care to patients. It is reasonable to think that well-trained, experienced personnel, working with superior facilities and equipment, are capable of providing better care than personnel with lower qualifications, working with inferior facilities and equipment. It is also reasonable to think that more effective organization can both increase the volume of services produced by a given combination of people and plant and improve the quality of care rendered. This capability may not invariably be translated into performance (see Chapter 10).

This and subsequent chapters in Part II deal, in order, with physicians as attending staffs of hospitals, physicians as interns and residents, nurses, physical plant, and hospital organization and management. These are followed by chapters on quality of care and on hospital coordination.

Significance of Staff Appointments

THE ATTENDING STAFF OF A HOSPITAL

In New York City the term attending staff has traditionally referred to physicians in practice who contribute their services in hospital wards and outpatient departments. In return, they receive an opportunity to keep abreast of new clinical knowledge and enjoy the privilege of admitting patients to private and semi-private accommodations. Patients in the general ward are considered the responsibility of the particular clinical department rather than of an individual physician, and attending physicians caring for them neither submit a bill nor receive payment from the hospital (see Chapter 4). There is no doctor fee to patients in the outpatient department either, but there is an increasing tendency for some hospitals, especially the municipal, to pay physicians for serving there. Since the end of World War II a number of nonuniversity voluntary hospitals in New York City have instituted a system of full-time directors of clinical service, under which incumbents spend all their time in the hospital and earn their income in a variety of ways (see Chapter 9). University hospitals have had full-time physicians on their staffs for a generation or two.

The attending staffs of hospitals are largely drawn from physicians in practice in the community. Physicians in training (interns and residents) and retired physicians are excluded. Physicians in related fields (industry, insurance, and administration) may or may not seek hospital staff appointments. Whether it is appropriate to exclude certain categories of practicing physicians from access to hospital staffs is a moot question in actuality, if not in theory.

RESPONSIBILITY OF HOSPITAL TO THE COMMUNITY

The Hospital Council of Greater New York addressed itself to this problem at length in its report *Hospital Staff Appointments of Physicians in New York City*.[1] Its position can be stated briefly.

The central question is whether hospitals should aim to appoint to their attending staffs a cross section of the medical practitioners in the community or limit their staffs to full specialists or diplomates certified by specialty boards. (A full specialist is one who reports that he limits his practice to a single field of medicine. A diplomate is one who has passed certain examinations posed by a board of specialists in his field, having qualified for admission to the examination by training and experience). The issue is not whether a member of a hospital's attending staff should perform only the diagnostic and treatment procedures for which he is qualified; this goes without saying. The issue is whether to appoint to the staff only the best qualified physicians in the community or to afford every practicing physician an opportunity to learn and grow, meanwhile carefully supervising what he does and limiting his activity in the hospital to what he is equipped to do.

In a country like England a sharp line is drawn between physicians who practice in the hospital and physicians who practice in the community. In New York City no such line exists, although some hospitals take pride in having only full specialists on their staffs.

The Hospital Council believes that hospitals are the best place for transmitting to the practicing physician information on medical advances. If the physician is to have a systematic opportunity to keep abreast of developments in medical knowledge and to improve his performance, he must have access to the organized staff of a hospital.

Most physician services are rendered outside the hospital. A physician who cannot qualify to work in the hospital, where supervision is available, is not qualified to practice outside the hospital, where supervision does not exist. It is the obligation of hospitals to the nonhospitalized public to reach out to the community and to afford to every physician who practices there an opportunity to join a hospital's staff and participate in its work within the limits set by his experience and competence. Hospitals do not discharge this obligation by appointing only the best qualified physicians to their staffs.

Physicians and Staff Appointments in New York City

TREND IN NUMBER OF PHYSICIANS, 1950–58

The American Medical Association reports that between 1950 and 1958 the total number of physicians in New York City declined from 19,700 to 18,700, or by 1,000. The decline in the number of physicians in private practice was even greater, 1,300.

The reduction of 336 in the group in temporary service with the federal government is a result of a change in classification in the Medical Directory. Today the same physicians would be charged to the federal service, not to the areas of their permanent residence. Another difference between the 1950 and 1958 counts is that the former excludes one recent class of graduates from

Table 5.1. NUMBER OF PHYSICIANS BY TYPE OF PRACTICE,
NEW YORK CITY, 1950 AND 1958

Type of Practice	1950	1958	Change
Total physicians	19,695	18,696	− 999
In private practice	15,412	14,115	− 1,297
In hospital (in training or institutional service)	3,222	3,597	+ 375
In practice in related fields	341	567	+ 226
Retired or not in practice	384	417	+ 33
Temporarily with federal government	336	0	− 336

SOURCE: American Medical Association, Directory Department, *Survey of Number of Physicians in the United States by County, Dependencies and Canada, March 1, 1950* (Chicago, 1950), pp. 77–78; and its *Physician-Population Counts in the United States by County, 1958* (Chicago, 1958), pp. 64–65.

United States and Canadian medical schools, whereas the latter excludes two.

To make the counts of physicians in the two years comparable, the following adjustments are necessary:

1. 1950, total reported	19,695	
Less: temporarily with federal government	336	
Adjusted, 1950		19,359
2. 1958, total reported	18,696	
Plus: 1957 graduates from United States and Canadian medical schools in voluntary and municipal hospitals, New York City (see Chapter 6)	550	
Adjusted, 1958		19,246
3. Change 1950 to 1958, adjusted basis		− 113

Between 1950 and 1958 the total number of physicians in New York City is shown to have declined by approximately 100, rather than by 1,000. The several adjustments do not affect the size of the decline in the number of physicians in private practice, which remains at 1,300 (see Appendix 5.A).

The decline in the number of physicians in private practice, who are by far the predominant source of physicians seeking and holding hospital staff appointments, is consistent with the cessation of growth in the city's population during this period and with the increase in population in neighboring suburban counties. In part, it may also reflect the fact that physicians' incomes in New York City are relatively low. In 1949 the average net income of practicing physicians in New York City was reported by the United States Department of Commerce to be lowest among the 32 largest cities in the country. It was then 25 percent below the national average, compared with 11 percent in 1941.[2] It is interesting that New York City ranks second or third from the top among 20 large cities in the level of certain selected specialists' fees, as measured by the United States Bureau of Labor Statistics.[3] Helping to reconcile a tendency toward low average physicians' income and high fees are the high ratio of physicians to population and the large proportion of ward to total hospital patients, for whose care physicians receive no payment.

TREND IN PHYSICIANS' APPOINTMENTS IN TWO
HOSPITAL SYSTEMS, 1948–58

For this study an analysis was made of the staff appointments of a 10 percent sample of physicians listed in the *Medical Directory of New York State,* as of 1958. In so far as possible the classification of physicians by type of practice was made comparable with that developed for the year 1948 for all physicians in New York City. As the *Directory* does not list courtesy staff appointments in voluntary hospitals or any appointments in proprietary hospitals, these were eliminated from the 1948 data. The figures for both years pertain to physicians with regular staff appointments in voluntary and municipal hospitals.

Table 5.2. PHYSICIANS WITH REGULAR STAFF APPOINTMENTS IN VOLUNTARY OR MUNICIPAL HOSPITALS, OR BOTH, NEW YORK CITY, 1948 AND 1958

Hospital Ownership	1948	1958	Change
Total physicians with regular staff appointments	10,600	10,890	+ 290
a. In voluntary hospitals only	5,990	5,610	– 380
b. In municipal hospitals only	1,890	1,520	– 370
c. In voluntary and municipal hospitals	2,720	3,760	+ 1,040
Total in voluntary hospitals (a + c)	8,710	9,370	+ 660
Total in municipal hospitals (b + c)	4,610	5,280	+ 670

SOURCE: Hospital Council of Greater New York, *Hospital Staff Appointments of Physicians in New York City* (New York, 1951), pp. 30–31; and study of staff appointments, 1958.

Table 5.2 shows that (1) although the numbers of physicians with staff appointments in voluntary hospitals only and in municipal hospitals only declined, the number of physicians with appointments in both systems increased; (2) as a result, each hospital system had an increase in its attending staff. The numerical increase was the same in both hospital groups, but the relative increase was twice as great in municipal hospitals as in voluntary hospitals—15 percent compared with 7.5 percent.

Attending Staffs of Municipal Hospitals

How do these statistical findings accord with what is known of the difficulties encountered by hospitals in New York City in attracting physicians to their attending staffs? In many interviews it was reported that in certain specialties, such as pediatrics, most hospitals in Manhattan, Brooklyn, and the Bronx, voluntary or municipal, have difficulty in recruiting new staff members. At all municipal hospitals it is increasingly necessary to pay physicians for attendance in the outpatient department. At municipal hospitals without university affiliation, the common report was of difficulty in recruiting in every specialty. Their attending staffs are declining by attrition, for lack of replacements at the bottom step of the promotion ladder. If nothing is done to improve recruitment, the rate of decline is likely to accelerate.

The remainder of this chapter concentrates on the staffing situation in municipal hospitals, with particular emphasis on hospitals without university affiliation. It will be found that the available data bear out the common report. Presentation of data is followed by a discussion of the factors that might account for prevailing trends, concluding with an attempt to assess their implications for the future.

TRENDS AND COMPARISONS

Appointments in Municipal Hospitals. To ascertain in which municipal hospitals the increase in the total number of attending physicians took place, a comparison was made between the number of staff appointments in the system in 1948 and in 1958. Such a comparison differs from a comparison of physicians holding appointments (shown in Table 5.2) in two ways: (1) physicians with offices outside the city who are on the staffs of the hospitals are included, and (2) physicians who hold appointments in two or more municipal hospitals are counted more than once.

Exclusive of consultants' positions, the number of appointments increased from 5,270 in 1948 to 6,450 in 1958. Most of this increase is accounted for by university hospitals and by the opening of new hospitals. Of the municipal general hospitals without university affiliation, 9 out of 11 suffered reductions in size of staff. The two hospitals with increases in staff occupy new buildings.

Duplicate Appointments. A physician who holds appointments in two or more hospitals may favor one over the other. If so, the burden of possible neglect associated with duplicate staff appointments is likely to fall more heavily on a municipal hospital than on a voluntary. One reason is that, whereas 71 percent of the physicians in municipal hospitals are also on the staffs of voluntary hospitals and must be responsive to their demands, only 40 percent of the physicians in voluntary hospitals also serve in municipal hospitals and must respond to their demands. Another reason is that the voluntary hospital is in a better position to induce attendance through its control over beds for physicians' private (including semiprivate) patients.

There has been an increase in the number of physicians with duplicate appointments within the municipal hospital system. It is estimated that in 1948 the number of attending appointments in the municipal hospital system exceeded the number of physicians holding them by 500; in 1958 the correspoding figure was 1,000. The rules of the Department of Hospitals that formerly tended to reduce the number of duplicate appointments between municipal general hospitals at ranks higher than clinical assistant have been relaxed. The Commissioner of Hospitals has the authority to approve duplicate staff appointments between any two hospitals and at any rank for a medical specialist in a field in which recruitment is difficult.

Data on staff appointments do not convey anything about trends in frequency of attendance by physicians at the hospital nor about the length of their visits. Meaningful data pertaining to these items are not available.

Caliber of Physicians. The very extent to which the attending staffs of the two hospital systems overlap, as shown in Table 5.2, raises the question whether there can be much of a difference in their caliber. At first impression the answer seems to be negative.

The following data for 1958 compare the proportion of attending staff in each hospital system who are diplomates, full specialists, or graduates from American (United States and Canadian) medical schools.

	Proportion (Percent) to Total Attending Staff	
Status of Physician	Voluntary Hospitals	Municipal Hospitals
Diplomate of specialty board	48.2	46.5
Full specialist	69.9	68.6
Graduate of American medical school	72.5	68.5

Differences between the two groups of hospitals in the proportion of physicians with given status are very small.

Larger differences appear, however, when the same comparison is made among three categories of physician: those with appointments in one system or in the other and those with appointments in both.

	Proportion (Percent) to Total Attending Staff		
Status of Physician	Both Voluntary and Municipal Hospitals	Voluntary Hospitals Only	Municipal Hospitals Only
Diplomate	56.9	42.0	20.4
Full specialist	77.9	64.2	45.1
Graduate of American medical school	75.3	70.4	51.4

Physicians with municipal hospital appointments only have the lowest proportion of diplomates, full specialists, and graduates of American medical schools. The reason is that almost three fourths of them are at non-medical-school hospitals. By contrast, of the physicians with appointments in both systems, only one half are associated with non-medical-school municipal hospitals.

Hospitals in First and Third Teaching Classes. The data on staff appointments permit certain comparisons between the two hospital systems for corresponding teaching classes of hospital. Class I teaching hospitals are defined for this purpose as comprising those with a medical school affiliation for undergraduate teaching and approved residency training programs in more than 10 specialties; Class II teaching hospitals are defined as having the same type of medical school affiliation and approved residencies in 6 or more specialties but fewer than 10; and Class III teaching hospitals are all hospitals not classified as Class I or Class II. It turned out that the number of Class II teaching hospitals in the municipal system was too small to permit valid comparisons with Class II teaching hospitals in the voluntary system. The comparisons that follow are therefore limited to Class I and Class III teaching hospitals.

1. *Diplomate Status.* What proportion of staff appointments is held by certified diplomates?

Hospital Teaching Class	Proportion (Percent) of Diplomates to Total Attending Staff		
	Voluntary Hospitals	Municipal Hospitals	Difference
Class I	65.5	64.2	+ 1.3
Class III	43.4	37.0	+ 6.4

The proportion of staff appointments held by diplomates is considerably lower in Class III hospitals than in Class I. The difference between the two systems in Class I teaching hospitals is small. In Class III it is considerably greater.

2. *Full Specialists.* A similar comparison was made of the proportion of staff appointments held by full specialists.

Hospital Teaching Class	Proportion (Percent) of Full Specialists to Total Attending Staff		
	Voluntary Hospitals	Municipal Hospitals	Difference
Class I	80.0	82.9	− 2.9
Class III	64.7	59.4	+ 5.3

The proportion of appointments held by full specialists is again much lower in Class III hospitals than in Class I. Within Class I the proportion of full specialists is higher in municipal hospitals. Within Class III voluntary hospitals have the higher proportion.

3. *Age. The Medical Directory of New York State* does not report the age of physicians. It does report the year of graduation from medical school, and this can serve as an index of age. The following data show, in each teaching class of hospitals, the proportion of appointments held by physicians who have been gradu-

ated from medical school since 1941, the year this country entered World war II.

Hospital Teaching Class	Proportion (Percent) of Graduates since 1941 to Total Attending Staff		
	Voluntary Hospitals	Municipal Hospitals	Difference
Class I	34.1	33.6	+ 0.5
Class III	26.3	21.0	+ 5.3

The findings here are similar to those for diplomate status. They indicate that (1) Class I hospitals are better able to attract young physicians to the atttending staff than are Class III hospitals; and (2) within Class III, municipal hospitals are at a considerable disadvantage.

In summary, Class I teaching hospitals consistently display a more favorable position than Class III in attracting physicians to the attending staff. In Class I teaching hospitals the difference between the two systems is small and may favor either one. In Class III teaching hospitals the difference is considerable, and it is consistently unfavorable to the municipal system.

Relative Attractiveness. An attempt was made to examine the relative attractiveness of staff appointments in voluntary and municipal hospitals. This was done by correlating for each physician with appointments in both systems the teaching class of the voluntary hospital and of the municipal hospital with which he is affiliated. Excluded from the analysis were consultants' appointments and attending appointments in closely associated voluntary and municipal hospitals.

The number of physicians associated with Class II municipal hospitals is again too small to permit analysis. For the others,

Table 5.3. CROSS-CLASSIFICATION BY TEACHING CLASS OF HOSPITAL OF STAFF APPOINTMENTS HELD BY PHYSICIANS AFFILIATED WITH BOTH HOSPITAL SYSTEMS, NEW YORK CITY, 1958

Municipal Hospital Teaching Class	Voluntary Hospital Teaching Class			
	Total	Class I	Class II	Class III
Total appointments	4,280	830	770	2,680
Class I	1,860	450	380	1,030
Class II	260	60	70	130
Class III	2,160	320	320	1,520

SOURCE: Hospital Council of Greater New York, study of staff appointments, 1958.

despite variation, there is a tendency for a physician to accept appointment in a voluntary hospital of lower teaching class than that of his municipal appointment.

This is conveyed by the fact that while 55 percent (1,030 of 1,860) of all appointments in Class I municipal hospitals are associated with Class III voluntary hospitals, 39 percent (320 of 830) of all appointments in Class I voluntary hospitals are associated with appointments in Class III municipal hospitals.

The ranks held by physicians in the two systems were also compared. A higher rank in a given teaching class of hospital in one system than in the other may be taken as an indication of a lower degree of attractiveness, and conversely for a lower rank.

Table 5.4. COMPARISON BETWEEN RANKS HELD IN VOLUNTARY AND MUNICIPAL HOSPITALS OF SPECIFIED TEACHING CLASS BY PHYSICIANS WITH APPOINTMENTS IN BOTH SYSTEMS, NEW YORK CITY, 1958

Teaching Class of Hospital of Appointment	*Total Physicians*	*Physician's Rank in Municipal Hospital*		
		Higher	*Equal*	*Lower*
Municipal, Class I and:				
Voluntary, Class I	450	160	190	100
Voluntary, Class III	1,030	190	400	440
Municipal, Class III and:				
Voluntary, Class I	320	270	30	20
Voluntary, Class III	1,520	460	600	460

SOURCE: Hospital Council of Greater New York, study of staff appointments, 1958.

Physicians with appointments in Class III teaching hospitals in both systems have approximately the same rank in each, with just as many having the higher rank in one as in the other. Physicians with appointments in Class I municipal hospitals and Class III voluntary hospitals are more likely to have the same or lower rank in the former than the same or higher rank (the odds are 10 to 7). Similarly, as may be expected, physicians with appointments in Class I voluntary hospitals and Class III municipal hospitals are more likely to have the same or lower rank in the former than the same or higher rank (6 to 1). Physicians with appointments in Class I teaching hospitals in both systems are more likely to have the same or higher rank in the municipal hospital than in the voluntary (6 to 5).

Although none of these comparisons yields a large difference between the two hospital systems, each points in the same direction, namely, toward a relatively lower attractiveness on the part of Class III municipal hospitals. The nature of the differences—small and always in the same direction—is consistent with the reports encountered in interviews that this is a period of mounting difficulty for these hospitals.

TREND IN PAYMENT OF PHYSICIANS FOR ATTENDANCE
IN OUTPATIENT DEPARTMENT

The foregoing conclusion receives support from another set of facts, namely, the rapid increase in the number of paid outpatient department sessions in municipal hospitals. Between 1955 and 1958 the number of paid sessions (including those for anesthesiologists, psychiatrists, and physicians in public-home infirmaries) doubled, with the result that today more than one half of all outpatient department sessions in municipal hospitals are paid for, mostly at $15 per session. In voluntary hospitals such payment is rare.

Payment to physicians for service in the outpatient departments of municipal hospitals began in the mid 1930s. It was then limited to certain clinics, such as tuberculosis, venereal disease, and refraction. As the range of clinics in which payment could be made was expanded, limitations on the rank of the physician who might be paid were slowly removed. Today a physician of any rank may receive payment for working in the outpatient department, and many physicians of senior rank request payment as a means of qualifying for old age benefits under the Social Security Act.

Substantial differences exist among municipal hospitals in the proportion of all outpatient department sessions paid for, ranging from approximately 20 percent to 90 percent or higher. In general, there is a tendency for nonuniversity hospitals to pay for a higher proportion of sessions than university hospitals.

Although the number of physicians with appointments in municipal hospitals has increased, they are apparently not so available as formerly to render free care in the outpatient department. Aggravating the situation is the expansion in the volume of visits, which has increased the demand for physicians' services.

There was a time, not more than a generation ago, when staff appointments to the wards of municipal hospitals in New York City were highly sought after by young physicians. Here one could develop proficiency in medicine and maintain it over the years, keeping abreast of advances in medical knowledge. Today, municipal hospitals without medical school affiliation seem to have lost their attraction for young physicians. How has the change come about?

In interviews with physicians and hospital administrators a number of reasons were advanced. These are presented in order of increasing importance.

Departmental Rule. The rule of the Department of Hospitals that a staff member above the rank of clinical assistant can hold only one general hospital appointment, unless authorized to the contrary by the Commissioner, tends to militate against municipal hospitals without medical school affiliation. When a physician must choose between an appointment in a university affiliated general hospital and an unaffiliated one, he is likely to take the former.

Decline in Attraction of Teaching. With the advent and expansion of house staff who were graduated from foreign medical schools, the morale of the attending staff who supervise graduate education has been impaired. For some attending physicians, it was reported, a municipal hospital without medical school affiliation no longer offers a stimulating environment for teaching.

Decline of House Staff as Source of Attending Staff. With the rising proportion of foreign exchange students on the house staff, most of the alumni return to their countries of origin and do not become potential recruits to the attending staff. This point is independent of the question whether these men would be considered qualified to receive such appointments. Moreover, a present member of the attending staff would consider that he has lost the prospect of receiving referrals from the men he has trained when they enter practice.

Relative Scarity of Certain Specialists in the City. Throughout the city hospitals report difficulty in recruiting pediatricians and obstetricians to their attending staffs. It was also frequently mentioned that it was difficult to attract specialists in ophthalmology and otolaryngology. Oftentimes similar difficulties were reported by neighboring voluntary and municipal hospitals and by both nonuniversity and university hospitals. There is, however, a difference in degree.

Decline in Number of Physicians in Practice. As previously shown, there has been a significant decline in the number of physicians in private practice in New York City. In two of the boroughs, the Bronx and Brooklyn, the rate of decline is above the city-wide average.

Economic Pressures and Incentives. At the time they complete their training, the majority of physicians today have families and must earn a living (see Chapter 6). They cannot afford to give their time to a municipal hospital without compensation in money or private patient privileges. Their families also put a heavy demand on their leisure time, so that they cannot spend as much time at hospitals as their predecessors did.

Moreover, there exist opportunities for earning money, such as service at Veterans Administration hospitals and outpatient clinics, in union health centers and industrial concerns, and in insurance companies. Office practice is more lucrative than it was a generation ago, with the average number of physicians' services per person per year estimated to have doubled since 1929.[4]

Finally, for contributing his services in the ward or outpatient department of a voluntary hospital, the physician gains an opportunity to earn a good part of his livelihood. He receives no such return when he makes a similar contribution in a municipal hospital.

The net result is that even when the physician is on the attending staff of a hospital, he visits less often. It was further reported that, whereas in the past a physician would come to the hospital and spend two or three hours at a time on the ward, today "he comes and runs."

Transformation of Training from Apprenticeship to Residency. Thirty or so years ago attendance in hospital wards was the only way a physician could acquire proficiency in a field on the basis of which he would qualify as a specialist. This was particularly true in surgery. In local hospitals promotion from the staff of the outpatient department to that of the inpatient service was a significant step in a man's career. Promotion was not readily forthcoming and had to be earned.

Today a physician qualifies as a specialist through residency training. The young physician in practice has less to gain than his predecessor from an appointment in the ward of a municipal hospital, because he is already fairly proficient by the time he enters practice. Moreover, the opportunity to gain in proficiency is not so great as in the past, because the specialty boards expect the senior residents to assume full responsibility for the care of patients.

Another consequence of the transformation of medical training is that as graduate training has become longer and more formal, it calls for larger resources in men and materials. These the City of New York has failed to provide to its hospitals. In an affiliated municipal hospital this lack is not so apparent, because the medical school affords considerable supplementation in personnel, salaries, and equipment. As a result, the nonaffiliated hospitals are without important support and leadership in the effort to raise standards of care and education.

A BALANCED VIEW

Nevertheless, the fact is that senior men on the attending staff do remain at municipal hospitals without medical school affiliation to perform the necessary work, and that some younger men, apparently in insufficient numbers, do join them. When the question is asked why they do so, in view of all the adverse factors enumerated above, the answer frequently given is that physicians enjoy the association with the hospital and the prestige. There may be, in addition, a small financial return from service in the outpatient department. These favorable factors do not seem to be of great weight, in comparison with the adverse factors.

What is a balanced view of the current status of the attending staff in municipal hospitals without medical school affiliation? In the course of interviews several physicians suggested that municipal hospitals without medical school affiliation may be better off today than they were twenty or thirty years ago. Today the specialist members of the attending staff are well trained and are not, as formerly, acquiring proficiency by practicing on ward patients. The important question is whether enough well-trained men are being recruited into the system to replace the men leaving it through resignation and retirement.

Almost every hospital in New York City has difficulty in attracting certain medical specialists, such as pediatricians and obstetricians, who follow the young middle-class population to the suburbs. It is true, nevertheless, that municipal hospitals without medical school affiliation seem to have difficulty across the board in replacing senior men with new appointees at the bottom of the promotion ladder. Many members of the senior attending staff find it necessary to work longer and harder than their predecessors did. Some are, moreover, working beyond their strength. Possibilities are nearly exhausted for reducing the size of attending staff by consolidating two medical or surgical services in a hospital into one or for increasing available manpower by lengthening the annual period of service of attending staff members.

One physician-administrator summarized the possibilities for attracting physicians to the attending staffs of municipal hospitals as follows: it is easier for hospitals with a medical school affiliation than for hospitals without such affiliation; it is easier for hospitals with new buildings, facilities, and equipment than for hospitals with obsolete buildings, facilities, and equipment; it is easier for hospitals with good nursing service than for hospitals with poor nursing service or similar frustrations—at least to retain the attending staff that they have; it is easier for hospitals with adequate parking areas and accessible to expressways than for hospitals without these conveniences. Above all, in his opinion, the determining factor is the interest, loyalty, zeal, and leadership of the chief of service.

The evidence suggests that the gradual, probably accelerating, attrition of attending staff at some of the non-medical-school municipal hospitals is the greatest single threat to their ability to continue to provide care of adequate quality. Drastic steps may be required to arrest and reverse recent trends.

It will not be simple to find a solution to this problem, if the factors involved are as varied and as deep-seated as stated above. Any effort at solution must, of course, take into account other aspects of the problem, including the pattern of financing hospital care in New York City. Alternative approaches are discussed elsewhere (see Chapters 9, 11, and 21).

Summary

1. Every physician in practice should have the opportunity to join the attending staff of a hospital and to participate in its work within the limits set by his experience and competence. Hospitals do not fulfill this obligation to the community by appointing to their staffs only the best qualified physicians.

2. Between 1950 and 1958 the number of physicians in private practice in New York City declined by 1,300, or 8 percent. This decline is consistent with the cessation of population growth in the city and the relatively low average income earned by its practitioners.

3. Between 1948 and 1958 the number of physicians with staff appointments increased in each hospital system. This increase has come about through an increase in the number of physicians who have appointments in both hospital systems, more than offsetting the decline in the number of physicians with appointments in one system only.

4. The entire increase in staff appointments in the municipal system has occurred in hospitals with medical school affiliation or with new physical plant. Among municipal general hospitals without medical school affiliation 9 of 11 have had decreases in size of staff; the two with increases occupy new buildings.

5. A comparison was made of the caliber of physicians in the two hospital systems, as expressed in the proportion of diplomates, full specialists, and graduates from American medical schools. Appreciable differences were found among physicians with voluntary hospital appointments only, municipal hospital appointments only, and appointments in both systems. This is important, because the physicians with appointments in municipal hospitals only tend to be concentrated in non-medical-school hospitals.

6. Similar comparisons were made between the staffs of Class I and Class III teaching hospitals in the two systems. The teaching class of a hospital, defined in the text, is determined by the scope

of its teaching program. The data show that attending staffs in Class I hospitals had higher qualifications than staffs in Class III hospitals; and that within Class III hospitals the staffs of voluntary hospitals had the higher qualifications. The latter have also been more successful in recruiting young physicians to their attending staffs.

7. Although most of these differences are small, all point in the same direction. They are consistent with the view that this is a time of mounting difficulty for municipal hospitals without medical school affiliation.

8. Today more than one half of all outpatient department sessions in municipal hospitals are paid for. Non-medical-school hospitals tend to pay for a larger proportion of their sessions than medical school hospitals. In both the trend is upward.

9. In the course of interviews a number of explanations were advanced for the fact that municipal hospitals without medical school affiliation have lost their attractiveness for young physicians. Among the important factors are: the decline in the number of physicians in practice in the city, which is accentuated in certain specialties; economic pressures and incentives that draw physicians elsewhere; and the transformation of graduate medical training from apprenticeship to residency, which has reduced the young practitioner's dependence on municipal hospitals.

10. Municipal hospitals without medical school affiliation are not recruiting enough young men to replace the older men leaving through resignation and retirement. The attrition of the attending staffs at some of these hospitals poses the greatest single threat to their ability to continue to provide care of adequate quality.

Appendix 5.A

TREND IN NUMBER OF LICENSED PHYSICIANS AND
OF THOSE IN PRIVATE PRACTICE
IN NEW YORK CITY

Despite, and perhaps because of, the plethora of data on physicians in New York City, it proved difficult to determine whether the number of private practitioners had remained constant or declined during the 1950s. It was not until data were obtained from the Directory Department of the American Medical Association that a firm conclusion could be reached. (It should be noted that these differ from the data in the published *Directory of the American Medical Association*, because of a difference in timing.)

TOTAL NUMBER

The Medical Directory of New York State [5] presents a table in its preface on the number of licensed physicians listed in each borough in New York City. Between 1948 and 1958 the total for the city fluctuated as follows:

Date	Number
June 1, 1948	17,554
November 15, 1950	17,761
March 1, 1953	17,591
December 1, 1954	17,864
October 1, 1956	17,712
September 15, 1958	17,756

Available data from other sources show the following numbers of physicians in New York City in 1950:

Directory Department, AMA [6]	19,695
Special study by AMA [7] (computed)	17,920
U.S. Public Health Service and Census [8]	19,188

One factor that helps to explain the differences among all these figures is the extent to which resident physicians are included. This depends, at least in part, on the provisions of the State licensure law applicable to residents, which change from time to time (see Chapter 6).

It is also noteworthy that the lowest of all the figures, that of the *Medical Directory of New York State*, contains a large number of duplicate listings for physicians with offices in two or more boroughs. On the basis of a 10 percent sample the extent of duplication is estimated at 870 for private practitioners and at a larger number for all physicians.

IN PRIVATE PRACTICE

The Hospital Council had performed a study of hospital staff appointments for physicians in 1948 [9] and wished to perform a similar one for 1958. The former was a total count of physicians; the latter, it was decided, would be a 10 percent sample of the physicians listed in the *Medical Directory of New York State*. The *American Medical Directory* would provide supplementary information on the physicians, as needed.[10]

The point of departure of a study of hospital staff appointments is the number of physicians in practice (mostly private practice). On the basis of the published data for 1948 [11] and the sample survey for 1958, the change in the distribution of physicians appeared to be as follows:

	1948	1958	Change 1948–58
Total	17,703	17,690	− 13
Not in practice	2,853	2,320	− 533
In practice	14,850	15,370	+ 520

These figures were not consistent with what is known from other sources about trends in the number of physicians not in practice. There was reason to suspect the completeness of the count for this group. Nevertheless, there was no basis for determining the true direction of trend in the number of physicians in practice until the unpublished data from the Directory Department of the American Medical Association became available. They count a person only once, at the address of his choice.

The complexity of the task of estimating the true trend is illustrated by the finding that between 1950 and 1958 the number of private practitioners declined by 1,300, although the total number of licensed physicians may have declined by only 110 (see page 146).

6   INTERNS AND RESIDENTS

Interns and residents have become important members of the staff of the modern hospital. In New York City 64 voluntary hospitals, 18 municipal hospitals, and 1 proprietary hospital have approved training programs for interns (newly graduated physicians in their first year of full-time hospital experience) or residents (physicians in the second and subsequent years of training in a specialized field of medicine) or both. The presence of interns and residents helps a hospital provide medical services around the clock and maintain an educational environment, both of which increase patients' prospects of receiving care of high quality (see Chapter 10).

The twin objectives of rendering service to patients through young physicians and of educating the latter are closely linked. One program may attach too much weight to the hospital's present service requirements to the neglect of the young physicians' education; whereas another may attach too much weight to medical education and research to the detriment of patient care. An authority recently stated: "Too much service may mean too little education. But too much emphasis on research and education may also result in a type of patient care which is impersonal and lacking in understanding of the real needs of the patient." [1]

The two extremes should be avoided. Although the primary objective of intern and residency training is to educate the young physician,[2] rendering service to patients is an "inevitable, proper and necessary" element of such education.[3] Working under the supervision of experienced physicians, the young physician is expected to assume progressively increasing responsibility in patient care.

Every hospital should aim for an educational atmosphere. A hospital that cannot be approved for intern or residency training or, if approved, is unable to recruit trainees with appropriate educational background, can still foster a good teaching program for its attending staff.[4] It is important for the practicing physician to keep abreast of advances in medical knowledge, and the best way —perhaps the only practical way—for him to do this is by participating in the work of an active hospital staff.

Statement of Problem

The Hospital Council's *Master Plan for Hospitals and Related Facilities for New York City* states that there are three major factors to be considered in planning hospital facilities and services: care of patients, medical education, and medical research.[5] The first two are emphasized. The number of hospital beds in a community should be determined by the needs of the population for care; the distribution of beds among individual hospitals is determined by (1) the geographic distribution of the population and (2) the need to concentrate in one place sufficient numbers of patients for training residents in the various medical specialties. A major consideration in setting the minimum size of new general hospitals in New York City at 200 beds was the desire to have every general hospital offer residency training in at least the four basic medical fields—internal medicine, general surgery, obstetrics, and pediatrics. Large hospitals, drawing on larger population groups, would in addition offer training in other specialties.[6]

Looking ahead, the *Master Plan* anticipated that private patients, as well as ward patients, would come to be employed for teaching. In residency training, particularly in the surgical specialties at the senior level, teaching with private patients poses certain problems that require continuing attention. In any event, as long as ward patients exist in sizable numbers, they should serve as the core of medical education programs.

The *Master Plan*, published in 1947, was developed at a time of apparently inexhaustible demand by young physicians for house staff positions in hospitals. It was believed that for every hospital in New York City to offer residency training would improve the quality of care given to patients and maintain the preeminent position of local hospitals in graduate medical education in this country. The reform of undergraduate medical education in the United States had borne fruit, so that few applicants for internships and residencies were graduates of unapproved medical schools. Experience before World War II in training graduates of foreign medical schools had been limited largely to graduates of schools in Western Europe, many of them American citizens who had gone abroad for their medical education. Immediately after the war residency training in this country expanded rapidly, and there was reason to expect the trend to continue, in line with the acceleration of specialization in medical practice. Hitherto, there had been few vacant house staff positions. There were no grounds for anticipating that additional house staff positions in New York City hospitals would go unfilled.

Accordingly, the *Master Plan's* recommendations on graduate training in hospitals were received in a favorable climate. A recent review by the Hospital Council shows that in the decade 1947–57 the number of hospitals in New York City with approved residency training programs in all four basic medical specialties doubled, increasing from 17 to 35. This occurred during a period when the total number of general hospitals with 200 beds or more increased by 10 percent, from 57 to 63.

Among voluntary hospitals alone the record was even more favorable: the number with residency training programs in all four basic fields tripled between 1947 and 1957, increasing from 8 to 24, while the number with 200 beds or more increased only by 2, from 43 to 45. The number of voluntary hospitals with residency training in three basic fields also increased during this period, while the number of hospitals with two or fewer programs declined, the last most dramatically.

A closer view of postwar developments in residency training in New York City shows, however, that not every hospital with expanded training programs has been able to recruit graduates of American (United States and Canadian) medical schools for its residency positions. Of the 16 voluntary hospitals that attained approval for residency training in all four basic fields during the period 1947-57, only 2 reported recently that graduates of American medical schools constituted 70 percent or more of all their residents. Two more hospitals reported that such graduates constituted between 50 and 70 percent of their residents. On the other hand, 2 hospitals reported that all of their residents were graduates of foreign medical schools, and in 5 hospitals foreign graduates constituted more than 80 percent of all residents.

In many hospitals in New York City—and throughout the country—recruitment of house staff for approved training programs has become a struggle, recurring annually and often with disappointing outcome. Early in the 1950s there was a high rate of vacancies in intern and residency positions. Recently relatively few positions in local hospitals have gone unfilled. However, many hospitals have large numbers of house staff who attended medical school abroad; these physicians frequently lack the qualifications of graduates of American medical schools, with resultant problems in the provision of medical care of adequate quality. (Their additional impact on the attending staff was discussed in Chapter 5.) Imminent is a period of decline in the number of eligible candidates for house staff positions; this will accentuate the difficulties in recruitment facing some hospitals.

How the present situation in New York City came about can best be understood against the background of developments in graduate medical education in the country, examined both for the similarities and differences that obtain between this city and the United States as a whole. Detailed findings for New York City then follow, with major emphasis on a comparison between the voluntary and municipal hospital systems. Finally, alternative proposals for action are discussed.

Developments in the Nation

The first hospitals in this country were established to care for the sick poor. From the beginning it was recognized that they needed the services of physicians around the clock and that their wards provided an unexcelled opportunity for training young physicians. Throughout the first century of house staff history in this country the number of physicians involved was small. Most physicians went directly into practice, whereas only a few attained the coveted position of hospital attending through prolonged training on the house staff.[7]

PRE-WORLD WAR II PHASE

The expansion of house staff training has occurred since 1900.[8] In its modern form and extent, however, it is of fairly recent origin. One medical educator gives 1935 as the beginning of the present pattern of graduate medical education in this country.[9]

In 1914, for the first time, a state (Pennsylvania) required the hospital internship as a prerequisite for licensure.[10] It was also in 1914 that the first complete listing of internships in this country was issued. Thereafter, increasing numbers of physicians took an internship as a means of acquiring assurance and skill in clinical medicine, though some did not. (By 1935 fewer than 1 percent of the physicians who had been graduated from New York City's medical schools between 1919 and 1931 lacked an internship.)[11] In 1920 there were enough internship positions to provide one for every graduate of United States medical schools, had every internship been of one year's duration. The balance between the total number of internship positions and the annual number of graduates of United States medical schools remained close and precarious until 1926, when a sizable excess of the former (750) occurred for the first time.[12] By World War II the excess had risen to 2,900, but 2,000 of the positions were held by second-year interns.[13]

Expansion of residency training came later. Formerly, a physician became a specialist by cultivating a special interest or skill in his practice and then limiting himself to it; by apprenticeship to such a specialist; or, less often, by training in Europe. Then came the postgraduate schools of medicine and the hospitals' residency training programs.[14] In 1926 the first complete listing of approved residency training programs showed 1,780 residency positions, a number equal to 36 percent of the internship positions offered that year (4,950).[15] The formation of certifying and examining boards in the specialties, which contributed greatly to the establishment of residency training as the chosen route to specialization, reached a peak in the 1930s. In that decade 12 of the 19 speciality boards now in existence were established, 9 in the three-year period 1934-37.[16] By 1940 there were 4,880 residency positions, or 60 percent of the number of internship positions (8,180).[17]

THE POSTWAR PHASE

World War II and its aftermath brought a rapid transformation in graduate medical education in this country. There were two simultaneous developments in intern training: (1) the total number of positions continued to increase, rising by 52 percent between 1940 and 1958 (from 8,180 to 12,469)[18] and (2) the number with a two-year term declined from 25 percent of the total in 1940 to 10 percent in 1949[19] and to less than 1 percent in 1958. The Korean War brought the virtual abandonment of the two-year internship.[20] Although the number of graduates of American medical schools continued to increase, it was far from sufficient to fill all positions. Vacancies continued to increase, until they were stabilized by the influx of foreign-educated physicians.

The armed forces gave considerable stimulus to residency training when they took account of a physician's diplomate status in classifying and assigning him. After World War II many discharged physicians sought residencies for refresher training or in preparation for a specialist's career. In 1945, for the first time, the number of residency positions offered exceeded the number of internships, 8,930 to 8,430. By 1949 the number of residency positions had doubled to 18,670; and by 1955 tripled to 26,520. In 1958 their number reached 31,800.[21] The number of residency positions was now 250 percent of the number of intern positions, compared with 60 percent in 1940 and 106 percent in 1945.

The number of interns and residents holding positions in approved programs in this country can be presented beginning in 1930. Between 1930 and 1958 the number of interns in this country nearly doubled, whereas the number of residents increased eighteen fold. In 1930 there were one fourth as many residents as interns; in 1940, one half; and in 1958, the ratio was better than two and one half to one. In the single decade of the 1940s the ratio of residents to interns was reversed from one half to two. (Indeed, the shift in ratios was even sharper in the five-year period 1945-50; but 1945 was an abnormal year and should

Table 6.1. INTERNS AND RESIDENTS IN APPROVED TRAINING
PROGRAMS, UNITED STATES, 1930–58

Year	Total	Interns	Residents	Residents per 100 Interns
1930	7,000	5,500	1,500	27
1940	11,453	7,553	3,900	52
1945	8,364	6,300	2,064	33
1950	21,416	6,821	14,595	214
1957	35,174	10,198	24,976	245
1958	37,110	10,352	26,758	258

SOURCE: 1930, 1940, 1950, and 1957—Frank Bane (for the Surgeon General's Consultant Group on Medical Education), *Physicians for a Growing America* (Washington, D.C., 1959), p. 9; 1945—U.S. Public Health Service, Division of Public Health Methods, *Health Manpower Source Book, Section 9* (Washington, D.C., 1959), p. 25, and letter from Frank G. Dickinson, then with American Medical Association, to Herbert E. Klarman, March 27, 1951; and 1958—American Medical Association, Council on Medical Education and Hospitals, *Directory of Approved Internships and Residencies, 1960*, reprinted from *Journal of American Medical Association*, CLXXIV, No. 6 (October 8, 1960), p. 583.

not serve as a base.) Although the number of interns in approved training programs has continued to increase, the number of residents is increasing at a faster rate and the ratio of residents to interns continues to rise. This indicates prolongation of medical training.

FACTORS IN EXPANSION OF HOUSE STAFF

The number of hospitals in this country with approved training programs and the average number of physicians per hospital house staff have both increased. Among the factors contributing to the higher demand by hospitals for house staff are the following:

1. Reduction in the average length of patients' stay in hospitals. As a result, a higher proportion of house staff time than formerly is devoted to patients' initial examinations upon admission. This calls for a larger house staff at a given time to maintain a given degree of thoroughness of examination.

2. Increased activity in caring for ambulatory patients, especially in the emergency departments of hospitals in large cities.

3. Continuing proliferation of medical specialties and subspecialties, accompanied by the desire of hospitals to cover as many services as possible with residents.

4. The requirement by most specialty boards that a year's

training in internal medicine and general surgery, the mother specialties, precede and augment training in the medical and surgical subspecialities.[22]

5. Increasing reliance by attending staff on interns and residents to render medical services to hospitalized patients, which releases the former to provide more services outside the hospital.[23]

6. The tendency for more hospitals to assign house staff to the private service. Twenty-five years ago this serivce was regarded as providing but a "meager" educational experience to the young physician.[24] In the middle 1940s it was reported that residencies in private pavilions had improved.[25] Today, assignment to the private service is an important supplement to assignment on the ward, if not a substitute for it.

7. An increase in the proportion of interns and residents who are married and have children, so that many are not so readily available as formerly for round-the-clock duty seven days a week. (A survey of the graduates of United States medical schools in 1959 shows that 63 percent of the male graduates were married; and of the married students, 24 percent had two or more children.[26] In 1959–60, 71 percent of all residents were married.) [27]

8. An increase in the number of fellows, many of whom do substantially the same kind of work as residents but follow a nine-to-five o'clock schedule.

The postwar expansion in graduate training in medicine has been made possible by (1) an increase in the number of physicians graduated from American medical schools; (2) prolongation of the average duration of graduate medical education; and (3) an influx of physicians from abroad seeking hospital training in this country.

The number of graduates from American medical schools increased from 5,100 in 1940 to 6,135 in 1951 and 6,860 in 1958.[28] For the period 1940–58 the increase was approximately 35 percent.

With an increasing number and proportion of physicians in this country engaged in specialty practice, the average duration of graduate medical education for graduates of American medical schools has lengthened from an estimated two years in 1940 to 3.25 years in 1956 (see Appendix 6.A). A recent study estimates the average duration of graduate medical education in 1958 at 3.5 years.[29] For the period 1940–58 the average duration of graduate medical education was lengthened by 75 percent.

The increase in the number of foreign-educated physicians serving as house staff in this country has taken on spectacular dimensions, particularly in the 1950s. In Appendix 6.A it is estimated that there were 2,500 of these physicians in 1951, 8,900 in fiscal year 1956, and at least 12,500 in fiscal year 1959. In less than a decade the number of foreign-educated physicians serving as house staff increased by 10,000. The principal factor is the exchange visitors program, which was authorized by the United States Information and Educational Exchange Act of 1948 and became effective in July, 1949.

THE PROBLEM OF THE FOREIGN-EDUCATED PHYSICIAN

During the period 1945–50 the rate at which new intern and residency positions were created in approved hospital training programs in this country exceeded the rate of increase in the number of candidates. The result was a rise in the number of vacant positions. The subsequent influx of large numbers of physicians educated abroad (attending medical schools outside the United States and Canada) has succeeded in curtailing the number of vacant positions but not in eliminating them. Vacancies in this country reached a peak in the year 1952—2,900 in intern positions and 5,425 in residency positions. In 1958 vacant positions were still numerous—2,120 and 5,060, respectively—despite substantial increases in the number of interns and residents. Relative to the total number of house staff positions, vacancies fluctuated from 11 percent in 1949 (the first year for which complete data are available) to 25 percent in 1952 and to 16 percent in 1958 [30] (see following section for comparison with New York City).

It is possible for numerous vacancies to exist, because no attempt is made to balance the number of intern or residency positions offered with the number of candidates. In passing on an individual program, the Council on Medical Education and Hospitals of the American Medical Association is concerned only with its educational potential (see final section of this chapter). Interns and residents, however, also render medical services to patients.

Although some graduates of foreign medical schools are well trained and capable, others have deficiencies in English or in the basic medical sciences or in clinical contact with patients.

One American student of medical education abroad has summarized the problem as follows. A vast number of students admitted to foreign medical schools lack knowledge of the basic sciences—a necessary foundation for medical education. In addition, the tradition in most foreign countries, with a few notable exceptions, of admitting to medical school all persons capable of passing from secondary school results in large classes. These preclude teaching in small groups, intimate interchange between student and teacher, and practical laboratory instruction. Finally, the organization of hospital services in other countries may serve to minimize or even eliminate contact between medical students and patients, much less assumption by the former of clinical responsibility.[31]

Medical and hospital authorities in this country have been concerned about the medical service problems resulting from the increase in the number of foreign-educated physicians on house staffs. After experimenting with a list of approved foreign medical schools, which could not be kept current, a decision was reached in 1956 to establish the Educational Council for Foreign Medical Graduates (ECFMG) which would evaluate every graduate of a foreign medical school (except Canadian and the University of Puerto Rico) who applied for an internship or residency in the United States. The evaluation consists principally of an examination in medicine, modeled after the National Board examinations, and a screening for comprehension of English. The organization was established in 1957, and the tests were inaugurated in the spring of 1958 and given twice a year thereafter. By December, 1960, 41 percent of the candidates had passed with a standard certificate (grade of 75 or higher) and 25 percent had obtained a temporary certificate (grade of 70–74) that entitled them to receive training in this country for two years.[32] Beginning January 1, 1961, hospitals in this country have been requested not to appoint or retain as interns or residents physicians without a state license who lack a certificate from ECFMG. In the immediate future the number of exchange visitors serving as house staff in approved training programs in this country is likely to decline; the probable size of the decline is discussed in the final section of the chapter.

Comparison between New York City and the United States

The long term trend in training physicians in hospitals in New York City resembles that in the United States but is not identical with it. Similarities lie chiefly in the expansion in residency training and in the influx of large numbers of physicians educated abroad.

A major difference between the two geographic areas is that twenty-five years ago graduate medical education in New York City was considerably advanced over most other parts of the country. The intervening years have witnessed some catching up by the latter and a lag in the rate of expansion of house staff training in New York City compared with that in the nation. The lag in the internship is particularly noteworthy.

Table 6.2 shows the increase in interns and residents in approved programs in all hospitals in New York City and the United States between 1935 and fiscal year 1959. (The data for the United States in 1935 show the number of internship and residency positions, rather than the number of persons filling them, because the latter could not be ascertained. The error resulting from this substitution is believed to be small, since relatively few positions were then vacant.) The 1959 data for New York City are based on a special house staff questionnaire by the Hospital Council to which every hospital with an approved program responded.

New York City had the same number of hospitals approved for internship training in 1935 and in 1959 and approximately the same number of interns—60 hospitals and 1,230–1,240 interns. (The hospitals involved were not identical. Three programs were discontinued before or during the war and at least six after the war,[33] so that a minimum of nine new ones were established.) In the United States the number of hospitals with approved internships increased from 697 [34] to 853,[35] and the number of interns increased by one half. New York City's proportion of all interns in this country declined from 18 percent in 1935 to 12 percent in fiscal year 1959.

Table 6.2. INTERNS AND RESIDENTS IN APPROVED TRAINING
PROGRAMS IN NEW YORK CITY AND UNITED
STATES, 1935 AND FISCAL 1959

			Change	
Place	*1935*	*1959*	*Number*	*Percent*
Interns and Residents				
New York City	1,759	4,990	+ 3,231	+185
United States	9,599	37,110	+27,511	+287
Interns				
New York City	1,239	1,226	– 13	– 1
United States	6,759	10,352	+ 3,593	+ 53
Residents				
New York City	520	3,764	+ 3,244	+625
United States	2,840	26,758	+23,918	+845

SOURCE: 1935—American Medical Association, *Medical Education in the United States
and Canada, 1934–35*, reprinted from *Journal of American Medical Association*, CV,
No. 9 (August 31, 1935), pp. 699, 709, and Appendix 6.B; and 1959—American
Medical Association, Council on Medical Education and Hospitals, *Directory of Ap-
proved Internships and Residencies, 1960*, reprinted from *Journal of American
Medical Association*, CLXXIV, No. 6 (October 8, 1960), p. 583, and Hospital Council
of Greater New York, questionnaire survey of house staff in hospitals in New York
City, April 20, 1959.

The number of hospitals in New York City with approved residencies increased from 53 in 1935 to 88 in 1959, and the number
of residents increased more than sevenfold. In the country as a
whole the number of hospitals with approved programs increased
from 392 [36] to 1,265,[37] and the number of residents increased nine
and one half times. New York City's proportion of the nation's
residents in approved programs declined from 18 percent in 1935
to 14 percent in fiscal year 1959.

While the number of physicians serving as house staff in New
York City almost tripled between 1935 and 1959, it increased almost fourfold in the United States. New York City's share of
house staff training in this country is, therefore, smaller today
than it was a generation ago, 13 percent compared with 18 percent.

A second difference between New York City and the nation,
which has undoubtedly influenced local thinking about solutions
to current problems, is the much larger role that the two-year internship formerly played here. In the classic study of internships
in New York City in the middle 1930s it was found that in 40 of
50 hospitals with rotating internships (then accounting for 72 percent of all internships) the length of training was two years or
longer. It was one and one half years in 3 hospitals, and in only 7

hospitals was it one year.[38] At that time the two-year internship was the direct route to medical practice for many local physicians, who subsequently acquired further and specialized skill in clinical medicine as volunteer members of the attending staffs of hospitals [39] (see Chapter 5).

By 1941, at the beginning of World War II, approximately two thirds of all internships in New York City were for two years; [40] this compares with one fourth, as previously noted, for the United States. Since the two-year internship is equally rare today in New York City and in the nation, its decline has been much faster here.

A third difference between New York City and the nation is the former's much larger proportion of house staff graduated from foreign medical schools. In New York City almost one half of all physicians serving as house staff in approved programs in 1959 were graduates of foreign medical schools; the corresponding proportion for the United States is estimated at one third. Also pointing to a sizable difference between New York City and the United States in this respect is the fact that the former has 6 of the 10 hospitals in the country with 50 or more foreign exchange visitors on the house staff.[41]

It was possible to develop detailed estimates for fiscal year 1956 of the composition of house staff in the United States by location of medical school of graduation and by citizenship status (see Appendix 6.A). Table 6.3, for fiscal year 1959, shows numerical data for New York City and an approximate percentage distribution, as derived in Appendix 6.A, for the United States. It should be noted that citizenship status is shown only for graduates of foreign schools. The number of noncitizens among graduates of American schools is believed to be small.

There are wide differences between New York City and the nation in the relative importance of temporary visitors with exchange visas and of United States citizens who attended medical school abroad.

The proportion of house staff in New York City hospitals educated abroad has increased from 7.5 percent in 1935 [42] to 48 percent in 1959. The corresponding figure for the United States in 1935 is not known; on the plausible assumption that it was certainly no higher than in New York City, the difference between the two areas has widened in the past twenty-five years.

Table 6.3. DISTRIBUTION OF HOUSE STAFF IN APPROVED TRAIN-
ING PROGRAMS BY LOCATION OF MEDICAL SCHOOL
OF GRADUATION AND BY CITIZENSHIP STATUS,
NEW YORK CITY AND UNITED STATES,
FISCAL YEAR 1959

Location of School and Citizenship Status	New York City		United States
	Number	Percent	Percent
Total	4,990	100.0	100
Graduates of American schools	2,602	52.1	66
Graduates of foreign schools	2,388	47.9	34
United States citizens	526	10.6	3
Permanent immigrants	376	7.5	10
Temporary visitors	1,486	29.8	21

SOURCE: Hospital Council of Greater New York, questionnaire survey of house staff in hospitals in New York City, April 20, 1959, and Appendix 6.A.

The fifth difference, which may be associated with the proportion of house staff educated abroad, is the lower rate of vacant
positions in New York City. The rate of vacancy in internship or
residency programs in a hospital or group of hospitals cannot be
computed precisely, because of complications introduced by
several factors. Among them are (1) interchangeability between
internship and junior residency positions, depending on the availability of suitable candidates; (2) variation in counting, or excluding, fellows, whose duties may closely resemble those of residents
or differ substantially from them; (3) differences between the
number of positions listed for a program and the number budgeted, with certain positions continued to be carried for future contingencies; and (4) discrepancies between the number of positions
vacant and the number of house staff reported as still needed.[43]
In addition, the number of vacancies may increase during the academic year as physicians leave and are not replaced. It is clear,
nevertheless, that in 1959 the rate of vacancy in approved training
programs in New York City was of the order of 5 + percent, or
one third of the nation-wide rate of 16 percent.

Rates (percent) of vacancy in internships and in residencies
were as follows:

	New York City [44]	United States [45]
Internship	7	17
Residency	5	16

In the voluntary hospital system in New York City the majority of vacancies occur in hospitals affiliated with medical schools. Apparently some hospitals have vacancies because they do not choose to fill them with the candidates who are available.

A sixth difference between New York City and the United States is in the proportion of house staff concentrated in affiliated hospitals. In New York City the relative importance of hospitals associated with medical schools has declined in the past generation. Nevertheless, these hospitals still provide a larger share of house staff training in New York City than they do in the country as a whole (see Tables 6.4 and 6.5, below).

An affiliated hospital may be classified as a major or minor teaching hospital. A major teaching hospital, as defined by the American Medical Association, is one that is a major unit of a medical school's teaching program and is so designated. A minor teaching hospital is one that is used to a limited extent in a medical school's teaching program. A striking difference between New York City and the United States in the training of interns is the much greater importance in the former of minor teaching hospitals.

Table 6.4. DISTRIBUTION OF INTERNS IN APPROVED TRAINING PROGRAMS BY MEDICAL SCHOOL AFFILIATION STATUS OF HOSPITALS, NEW YORK CITY, 1936 AND FISCAL 1959, AND UNITED STATES, FISCAL 1958

Affiliation Status	*New York City*		*United States*
of Hospital	*1936*	*Fiscal 1959*	*Fiscal 1958*
Number	1,369	1,226	10,198
Percent	*100.0*	*100.0*	*100.0*
Major teaching	35.7	36.7	37.3
Minor teaching	26.5	20.0	6.8
Unaffiliated	37.8	43.3	55.9

SOURCE: Jean Alonzo Curran (for the Committee on the Study of Hospital Internships and Residencies), *Internships and Residencies in New York City, 1934–1937; Their Place in Medical Education* (New York, 1938), pp. 18, 24; Hospital Council of Greater New York, questionnaire survey of house staff in hospitals in New York City, April 20, 1959; and American Medical Association, Council on Medical Education and Hospitals, *Directory of Approved Internships and Residencies, 1958,* reprinted from *Journal of American Medical Association*, CLXVIII, No. 5 (October 4, 1958), p. 523.

Nation-wide data on the distribution of residents by the affiliation status of hospitals recently became available for the first time. These do not distinguish between major and minor teaching hospitals.

Table 6.5. DISTRIBUTION OF RESIDENTS IN APPROVED TRAINING
PROGRAMS BY MEDICAL SCHOOL AFFILIATION STATUS
OF HOSPITALS, NEW YORK CITY, 1936 AND FISCAL 1959,
AND UNITED STATES, FISCAL 1960

Affiliation Status	New York City		United States
of Hospital	1936	Fiscal 1959	Fiscal 1960
Number	545	3,764	27,531
Percent	100.0	100.0	100.0
Major teaching	48.4	43.6	} 60.3
Minor teaching	34.2	29.1	
Unaffiliated	17.4	27.3	39.7

SOURCE: Jean Alonzo Curran (for the Committee on the Study of Hospital Internships and Residencies, *Internships and Residencies in New York City, 1934–1937,
Their Place in Medical Education* (New York, 1938), pp. 18, 24; Hospital Council of
Greater New York, questionnaire survey of house staff in hospitals in New York
City, April 20, 1959; and American Medical Association, Council on Medical Education and Hospitals, *Directory of Approved Internships and Residencies, 1960*, reprinted from *Journal of American Medical Association*, CLXXIV, No. 6 (October 8,
1960), p. 548.

Residency training is concentrated in medical school affiliated hospitals to a greater extent than intern training. Otherwise, both the trend in New York City and the contrast with the country as a whole are similar to those shown for interns.

Usually affiliated hospitals attract higher proportions of graduates of American medical schools than do unaffiliated hospitals.[46] A situation in which New York City has both a higher proportion of foreign-educated physicians than the United States and a higher proportion of house staff in affiliated hospitals offers something of a paradox, which cannot be explained with existing knowledge. It may be that medical school affiliation has a different significance here from elsewhere; or that the proportion of foreign-educated physicians in unaffiliated hospitals is much higher in New York City than in other parts of the country; or that the proportion of foreign-educated physicians is higher here in each class of hospitals.

Comparison between Voluntary and Municipal Hospitals

Between 1935 and 1959 the number of interns and residents in approved training programs in New York City increased almost threefold (Table 6.2). The rate of increase in voluntary and municipal hospitals was somewhat lower, two and one half times, as the number of interns and residents in federal and state hospitals in New York City increased almost ninefold (from 60 to 525). Proprietary hospitals in New York City play a negligible role in graduate medical education; currently two such hospitals are approved for a single residency each, one in pathology and one in psychiatry.

Through the cooperation of New York City Headquarters of the Selective Service System the Hospital Council was able to compile data on the size of house staff in voluntary and municipal hospitals in 1951 and 1955. These supplement the data for 1935 and 1959.

TRENDS, 1935–59

Table 6.6 shows the number of physicians in approved training programs in the two major hospital systems for selected years.

Table 6.6. HOUSE STAFF IN APPROVED TRAINING PROGRAMS IN VOLUNTARY AND MUNICIPAL HOSPITALS, NEW YORK CITY, 1935, 1951, 1955, AND 1959

Year	All Hospitals	Voluntary Hospitals	Municipal Hospitals
Number			
1935	1,700	920	780
1951	2,929	1,776	1,153
1955	3,873	2,180	1,693
1959	4,465	2,510	1,955
Percent increase			
1935–59	163	173	151
1935–51	72	93	48
1951–59	52	41	69
1951–55	32	23	47
1955–59	15	15	15

SOURCE: 1935—Appendix 6.B; 1951 and 1955—Hospital Council of Greater New York, tabulations from reports on house staff filed with New York City headquarters of Selective Service System; and 1959—Hospital Council of Greater New York, questionnaire survey of house staff in hospitals in New York City, April 20, 1959.

The distribution of house staff by hospital system in 1935 was estimated from several sources, as shown in Appendix 6.B.

The size of house staff increased in each of the intervals shown. During the sixteen-year span 1935–51 the increase amounted to almost three fourths of the 1935 total, and in the eight-year span

1951–59 it amounted to one half of the 1951 total. In the 1950s the rate of increase in the first half of the decade was twice that in the second half.

For the period 1935–59 the two hospital systems had the same rates of increase, but they differ in the timing of the increases. Between 1935 and 1951 the size of house staff almost doubled in voluntary hospitals, while it increased only one half in municipal hospitals. Between 1951 and 1959 the size of house staff increased by seven tenths in municipal hospitals and by four tenths in voluntary hospitals. In the 1950s the entire difference in rate of increase was confined to the first half of the decade.

Interns. Figures for total house staff reflect changes in the number of interns and of residents. Changes in the two categories did not follow the same pattern.

Table 6.7 shows the number of interns in the two major hospital systems in selected years. During the period 1935–59 the

Table 6.7. INTERNS IN APPROVED TRAINING PROGRAMS IN VOLUNTARY AND MUNICIPAL HOSPITALS, NEW YORK CITY, 1935, 1951, 1955, AND 1959

Year	All Hospitals	Voluntary Hospitals	Municipal Hospitals
Number			
1935	1,205	615	590
1951	870	463	407
1955	998	547	451
1959	1,182	683	499
Percent change			
1935–59	– 2	+ 11	– 15
1935–51	– 28	– 25	– 31
1951–59	+ 36	+ 48	+ 22
1951–55	+ 15	+ 18	+ 11
1955–59	+ 18	+ 25	+ 11

SOURCE: 1935—Appendix 6.B; 1951 and 1955—Hospital Council of Greater New York, tabulations from reports on house staff filed with New York City headquarters of Selective Service System; and 1959—Hospital Council of Greater New York, questionnaire survey of house staff in hospitals in New York City, April 20, 1959.

number of interns in the two major hospital systems actually declined. A substantial reduction occurred between 1935 and 1951, which was not offset by the increase between 1951 and 1959.

The general pattern, first decline then recovery, held true in both hospital systems. However, voluntary hospitals had the smaller decline and the greater recovery.

Residents. Large increases in the number of residents occurred in each hospital system. Between 1935 and 1959 the number of

Table 6.8. RESIDENTS IN APPROVED TRAINING PROGRAMS
IN VOLUNTARY AND MUNICIPAL HOSPITALS,
NEW YORK CITY, 1935, 1951, 1955, AND 1959

Year	All Hospitals	Voluntary Hospitals	Municipal Hospitals
Number			
1935	495	305	190
1951	2,059	1,313	746
1955	2,875	1,633	1,242
1959	3,283	1,827	1,456
Percent increase			
1935–59	563	500	665
1935–51	316	331	293
1951–59	60	39	95
1951–55	40	24	67
1955–59	14	12	17

SOURCE: See Table 6.7.

residents in voluntary and municipal hospitals increased more than six and one half times. The rate of increase was much greater from 1935 to 1951 than from 1951 to 1959; and it was greater in the first half of the 1950s than in the second half.

Each hospital system followed the general pattern. Voluntary hospitals had, however, the higher rate of increase in the earlier period and the lower rate in the later period and in each of its segments. This contrast between the two hospital systems in the 1950s is surprising, since the number of approved residency training programs in municipal hospitals has declined since 1948, whereas the number in voluntary hospitals has increased almost 80 percent (from 188 to 336). The difference in the latter system between an increase of approximately 40 percent in residents and an increase of 80 percent in residency programs is one measure of the growth of specialty and subspecialty training programs in New York City hospitals.

The principal source of the increase in residents in New York City in the 1940s must have been the expansion of American medical schools, accompanied by extension of the length of graduate medical training. In the 1950s the principal, though not exclusive, source of additional residents (as well as of interns) was graduates of foreign medical schools seeking house staff appointments in this country.

TREND IN ROLE OF FOREIGN-EDUCATED PHYSICIANS, 1951–59

United States Public Health Service hospitals accept only graduates of United States and Canadian medical schools. Veterans Administration hospitals follow the same pattern, except that they also accept graduates of foreign medical schools who are United States citizens.[47] In the three Veterans Administration hospitals in New York City one fourth of the house staff, all of them residents, are United States citizens who attended medical school abroad and three fourths are graduates of American medical schools. In 1959 the proportion of house staff in voluntary and municipal hospitals graduated from foreign medical schools was 51 percent (Table 6.15), compared with 48 percent in all hospitals, including federal (Table 6.3).

For years other than 1959 house staff cannot be divided into graduates of American and foreign schools. Since the data for the years 1951 and 1955 originate in reports filed with the Selective Service System, physicians are classified as American citizens or aliens. The former group includes United States citizens educated abroad, whereas the latter includes graduates of Canadian medical schools. The number of graduates of Canadian medical schools in approved training programs in voluntary and municipal hospitals in New York City is small—less than 2 percent of total house staff —and can be disregarded in an analysis of trends. The increase in the number of aliens represents, therefore, a minimum estimate of the increase in foreign-educated physicians, so long as the number of United States citizens educated abroad does not decline.

Numerical Changes in Total House Staff. Table 6.9 shows data on house staff classified by citizenship status within each hospital system for the years 1951 and 1959.

Between 1951 and 1959 the number of United States citizens rose one seventh (14 percent), while the number of aliens rose

Table 6.9. HOUSE STAFF IN APPROVED TRAINING PROGRAMS BY CITIZENSHIP STATUS IN VOLUNTARY AND MUNICIPAL HOSPITALS, NEW YORK CITY, 1951, 1955, AND 1959

Citizenship Status	1951	1955	1959
All hospitals	2,929	3,873	4,465
United States citizens	2,233	2,408	2,539
Aliens	696	1,465	1,926
Voluntary hospitals	1,776	2,180	2,510
United States citizens	1,343	1,383	1,570
Aliens	433	797	940
Municipal hospitals	1,153	1,693	1,955
United States citizens	890	1,025	969
Aliens	263	668	986

SOURCE: 1951 and 1955—Hospital Council of Greater New York, tabulations from reports on house staff filed with New York City headquarters of Selective Service System; and 1959—Hospital Council of Greater New York, questionnaire survey of house staff in hospitals in New York City, April 20, 1959.

two and three quarter times. Table 6.10 shows the numerical changes in each hospital system during the period 1951–59 and during each four-year segment. The number of aliens added to house staff in the 1950s amounted to four times the number of United States citizens added—1,230 compared with 306. For both citizens and aliens approximately three fifths of the increase took place in the first half of the decade and two fifths in the second half.

The increase in United States citizens was divided as follows: three fourths accrued to voluntary hospitals and one fourth to mu-

Table 6.10. CHANGES IN HOUSE STAFF IN APPROVED TRAINING PROGRAMS BY CITIZENSHIP STATUS IN VOLUNTARY AND MUNICIPAL HOSPITALS, NEW YORK CITY, 1951–59, 1951–55, AND 1955–59

Citizenship Status	1951–59	1951–55	1955–59
All hospitals	+ 1,536	+ 944	+ 592
United States citizens	+ 306	+ 175	+ 131
Aliens	+ 1,230	+ 769	+ 461
Voluntary hospitals	+ 734	+ 404	+ 330
United States citizens	+ 227	+ 40	+ 187
Aliens	+ 507	+ 364	+ 143
Municipal hospitals	+ 802	+ 540	+ 262
United States citizens	+ 79	+ 135	− 56
Aliens	+ 723	+ 405	+ 318

SOURCE: Table 6.9.

nicipal. In the first half of the decade both hospital systems reported increases; in the second half voluntary hospitals gained more than in the first half, while municipal hospitals lost.

The increase in aliens was distributed differently, with two fifths accruing to voluntary hospitals and three fifths to municipal. In the first half of the decade municipal hospitals received 53 percent of the total increase and in the second half 68 percent.

Changes in Proportion of Alien Physicians. Although municipal hospitals gained a majority of the additional aliens, voluntary hospitals also gained more aliens than United States citizens in the 1950s. The proportion of alien physicians increased, therefore, in each hospital system. In 1951 the municipal system had a slightly

Table 6.11. PERCENTAGE OF ALIEN PHYSICIANS IN APPROVED
TRAINING PROGRAMS IN VOLUNTARY AND
MUNICIPAL HOSPITALS, NEW YORK CITY,
1951, 1955, AND 1959

Year	All Hospitals	Voluntary Hospitals	Municipal Hospitals
1951	23.8	24.4	22.8
1955	37.9	36.5	39.2
1959	43.1	37.5	50.3

SOURCE: Table 6.9.

lower proportion of alien physicians than the voluntary; in each system the proportion was one fourth or less. In 1955 the difference between the two systems was still small—less than three percentage points—but the municipal system had the higher proportion of aliens. By 1959 the difference between the two systems had widened to 13 percentage points, as the proportion of aliens in municipal hospitals rose markedly while that in voluntary hospitals scarcely changed.

Separate Data on Interns and Residents. In the 1950s the number of interns increased by 220 in voluntary hospitals and by 90 in municipal hospitals. The number of residents also increased in each system, but by a smaller number in voluntary hospitals than in municipal—510 compared with 710. The latter reflects the establishment of the Bronx Municipal Hospital Center, which had 182 residents (and 34 interns) in 1959.

The data on house staff in approved programs in New York

City hospitals in the years 1951, 1955, and 1959, by citizenship status, are shown for interns in Table 6.22 and for residents in Table 6.23.

In two respects the trends in interns and in residents are similar: (1) the number of alien physicians in each physician category increased in each hospital system between 1951 and 1959; and (2) between 1955 and 1959 the number of United States citizens in each category increased in voluntary hospitals and declined in municipal hospitals. The difference in trend between interns and residents was this: between 1951 and 1955 the number of U.S. citizens serving as residents increased in each hospital system, whereas the number serving as interns remained constant (voluntary system) or declined (municipal system).

The changes in numbers are reflected in shifts in the proportion of alien physicians. In 1951 voluntary hospitals had the higher

Table 6.12. PERCENTAGE OF ALIEN PHYSICIANS AMONG INTERNS AND RESIDENTS IN APPROVED TRAINING PROGRAMS IN VOLUNTARY AND MUNICIPAL HOSPITALS, NEW YORK CITY, 1951, 1955, AND 1959

Year	All Hospitals	Voluntary Hospitals	Municipal Hospitals
Interns			
1951	24.1	29.8	17.7
1955	35.5	40.4	29.5
1959	40.8	37.5	45.6
Residents			
1951	23.6	22.5	25.6
1955	38.7	35.3	43.0
1959	44.0	37.4	52.2

SOURCE: Tables 6.22 and 6.23.

proportion of alien physicians among interns and municipal hospitals had the higher proportion among residents. In 1955 the proportion of alien physicians was higher than in 1951 for interns and for residents in each hospital system; but the relationships described for 1951 still prevailed. By 1959 municipal hospitals had the higher proportion of alien physicians in each category.

COMPOSITION OF HOUSE STAFF, 1959

For the year 1959 alien physicians can be divided into graduates of Canadian medical schools, temporary visitors on exchange visas, and permanent immigrants; and United States citizens can be further divided into graduates of United States and foreign medical schools. The data on house staff in the two hospital systems can then be regrouped in the manner of Table 6.3.

Table 6.13 shows the numerical and percentage distributions of interns and of residents in voluntary and municipal hospitals in 1959 by location of medical school of graduation and, for graduates of foreign medical schools, by citizenship status. Tables 6.20 and 6.21 below show the distribution of each physician category (graduates of American medical schools, United States citizens educated abroad, and so forth) among hospitals, classified by ownership and by degree of affiliation with a medical school.

In 1959 foreign-educated physicians constituted 51 percent

Table 6.13. DISTRIBUTION OF INTERNS AND RESIDENTS IN APPROVED TRAINING PROGRAMS BY LOCATION OF MEDICAL SCHOOL OF GRADUATION AND BY CITIZENSHIP STATUS FOR GRADUATES OF FOREIGN SCHOOLS IN VOLUNTARY AND MUNICIPAL HOSPITALS, NEW YORK CITY, 1959

Location of School and Citizenship Status	All Hospitals		Voluntary Hospitals		Municipal Hospitals	
	Number	Per cent	Number	Per cent	Number	Per cent
Interns and Residents	4,465	100.0	2,510	100.0	1,955	100.0
American medical schools	2,187	49.0	1,422	56.7	765	39.1
Foreign medical schools	2,278	51.0	1,088	43.3	1,190	60.9
American citizens	437	9.8	196	7.8	241	12.4
Permanent immigrants	369	8.3	130	5.2	239	12.2
Temporary visitors	1,472	32.9	762	30.3	710	36.3
Interns	1,182	100.0	683	100.0	499	100.0
American medical schools	571	48.3	357	52.3	214	42.9
Foreign medical schools	611	51.7	326	47.7	285	57.1
American citizens	136	11.5	72	10.5	64	12.8
Permanent immigrants	95	8.0	55	8.1	40	8.0
Temporary visitors	380	32.2	199	29.1	181	36.3
Residents	3,283	100.0	1,827	100.0	1,456	100.0
American medical schools	1,616	49.2	1,065	58.3	551	37.8
Foreign medical schools	1,667	50.8	762	41.7	905	62.2
American citizens	301	9.2	124	6.8	177	12.2
Permanent immigrants	274	8.3	75	4.1	199	13.7
Temporary visitors	1,092	33.3	563	30.8	529	36.3

SOURCE: Hospital Council of Greater New York, questionnaire survey of house staff in hospitals in New York City, April 20, 1959.

of the house staff in the two major hospital systems, whereas alien physicians constituted 43 percent (Table 6.11). The difference of 8 percentage points is accounted for by United States citizens educated abroad offset in part by graduates of Canadian medical schools. United States citizens educated abroad constituted 12 percent of house staff in municipal hospitals and 8 percent in voluntary hospitals.

Temporary visitors on exchange visas constituted the largest group of physicians educated abroad—one third of total house staff and almost two thirds of house staff educated abroad. The relative importance of temporary visitors in the two hospital systems can be expressed in two ways:

	Proportion (Percent) of Temporary Visitors to	
	Total Home Staff	Foreign-Educated House Staff
Voluntary hospitals	30	70
Municipal hospitals	36	60

The greatest difference between the two hospital systems is in the proportion of permanent immigrants—5 percent in voluntary hospitals and 12 percent in municipal. The entire difference is attributable to residents, owing to certain provisions of the New York State licensure law (discussed later in this chapter).

Affiliation Status and Success in Recruiting Interns. Analysis of the composition of house staff in terms of hospital ownership alone obscures the influence of other facts on recruitment of graduates of American medical schools. Table 6.14 shows the degree of success in attracting interns attained by voluntary and municipal hospitals in each medical school affiliation class. A hospital is either very successful or unsuccessful in attracting interns from American medical schools. While 7 hospitals reported that all of their interns were graduates of American medical schools, 32 had no such interns.

Two sets of facts may explain the concentration of hospitals at the extreme ends of the distribution. (1) Most hospitals have a single intern training program, the rotating internship, in which the intern in typically assigned to the four major clinical services during the year. This program either does or does not attract

Table 6.14. DISTRIBUTION OF VOLUNTARY AND MUNICIPAL HOSPITALS WITH APPROVED INTERNSHIPS BY PERCENTAGE OF TOTAL BUDGETED POSITIONS FILLED BY GRADUATES OF AMERICAN MEDICAL SCHOOLS AND BY MEDICAL SCHOOL AFFILIATION, NEW YORK CITY, 1959

Percent Graduates of American Medical Schools to Total Internships	All Hospitals			Medical School Affiliation					
				Major Teaching		Minor Teaching		Unaffiliated	
	Total	Voluntary	Municipal	Voluntary	Municipal	Voluntary	Municipal	Voluntary	Municipal
90 and over	11	10	1	2	1	8	0	0	0
70–89.9	4	4	0	2	0	2	0	0	0
50–69.9	4	2	2	2	2	0	0	0	0
30–49.9	2	2	0	0	0	0	0	2	0
10–29.9	2	1	1	0	0	1	0	0	1
Under 10	35	26	9	0	0	0	2	26	7
Total	58	45	13	6	3	11	2	28	8

SOURCE: Hospital Council of Greater New York, questionnaire survey of house staff in hospitals in New York City, April 20, 1959.

senior medical students in American medical schools. (2) In a hospital with several types of internship (rotating, all internal medicine, and all general surgery) the tendency seems to be for all programs to succeed or fail together. In New York City in 1959 there were only four instances in which a hospital succeeded in recruiting graduates of American medical schools in one program and failed in another.[48] In other areas the straight internship is reported to be much more successful than the rotating internship in attracting graduates of American medical schools.[49]

Table 6.14 above, as well as Table 6.15 following, shows how the hospitals in New York City fared in a single year, 1959. Over a longer time span less concentration at the extreme ends of the distribution is to be expected, since individual hospitals experience some degree of fluctuation in their ability to attract American graduates. In the borough of Brooklyn in recent years voluntary hospitals have tended to attract varying shares of a fairly constant total. Since the National Intern Matching Program was inaugurated in 1952, 10 of the unaffiliated hospitals in New York City—5 voluntary and 5 municipal—have dropped markedly in their recruitment of graduates of American medical schools.

The concentration of hospitals at the upper or lower end of the distribution is associated with, though not fully determined by, the presence or absence of a medical school affiliation. Among unaffiliated hospitals all but two fall in the bottom group of six. Conversely, among affiliated hospitals one half are in the top group and another one third are in the next two groups.

In each affiliation class voluntary hospitals have an advantage over municipal hospitals. The advantage is negligible among unaffiliated hospitals, moderate among major teaching hospitals, and marked among minor teaching hospitals. It is noteworthy that a higher percentage of voluntary minor teaching hospitals than of voluntary major teaching hospitals got 70 percent or more of their interns from American medical schools.

Certain observations may help explain the above findings. Not every affiliation between a hospital and a medical school, whether designated as major or minor, is equally close. Some affiliations are tenuous or even nominal, whereas others entail close contact and much interaction. Some affiliations involve all or most departments of an institution, whereas others involve only one department or a few. These differences contribute to the variation among hospitals with similar medical schools affiliation status in recruiting house staff (see Chapter 11). A minor teaching hospital may possess considerable strength of its own, which in some instances exceeds that of a major teaching hospital. It may be this very advantage that brought the hospital to a medical school's attention in the first place and led to affiliation. Finally, in a major teaching hospital three groups of students are present—undergraduates, interns, and residents—with the interns sometimes caught in an "apparent squeeze." [50] In a minor teaching hospital undergraduates are likely to be present in smaller numbers and less regularly, taking elective courses only. Under certain conditions an internship in a minor teaching hospital may be considered to offer the superior training opportunity.

Differences between affiliated and unaffiliated hospitals in recruiting interns were known from the published results of the National Intern Matching Program (NIMP). (A close relationship exists between a hospital's proportion of American-educated interns and its proportion of interns obtained through NIMP. Although graduates of foreign medical schools are allowed to participate in NIMP, the number participating has been relatively small. In 1958, 376 graduates of foreign medical schools, other than Canadian, participated in the program, of whom 224 were matched. In 1959, when prior screening by the Educational Council for Foreign Medical Graduates was required, only 4 participated, all of whom were matched.) [51]

A recent study of interns in one group of voluntary hospitals in New York City indicates that hospitals with 100 percent success in the matching program, or close to it, are most likely to recruit as interns graduates from leading American medical schools and from the top third of the senior class. Within a group of hospitals that achieve the same degree of success, there may be differences in the ranking of medical schools and in the percentile of graduating classes from which interns are drawn. [52] Such differences have apparently little to do with the nature and degree of the affiliation between the hospital and a medical school but reflect a hospital's own reputation as a teaching center.

Affiliation Status and Success in Recruiting Residents. There was no way, however, of anticipating from published data the extent to which affiliation with a medical school, or lack of it, affects a hospital's ability to recruit residents. A priori the affiliated hospital may be expected to offer several advantages over the unaffiliated one, including quality of teaching program, presence of research, greater choice among fields of specialization, and perhaps additional technical and clerical assistance.

Table 6.15, dealing with residents, shows some similarities to Table 6.14 but also certain differences.

There are two similarities between Tables 6.14 and 6.15. (1) In each table a higher proportion of major or minor teaching hospitals than of unaffiliated hospitals is at the upper end of the distribution—signifying relative success in attracting graduates of American medical schools. Conversely, most unaffiliated hospitals are at the lower end of the distribution—signifying relative failure. (2) In each type of affiliation class voluntary hospitals have an advantage over municipal. Even so, because of their large number, 21 of the 30 hospitals in the bottom group in Table 6.15, as well as 26 of 33 in the bottom group in Table 6.14, are under voluntary control.

There are several differences between the two tables. (1) Voluntary major teaching hospitals are more successful than voluntary minor teaching hospitals in attracting graduates of American medical schools as residents, whereas the converse is true for interns. (2) Among voluntary unaffiliated hospitals a few are highly successful and another few are moderately successful in attracting graduates of American medical schools as residents. By contrast, no unaffiliated hospital recruited many American graduates as interns. (3) In every type of affiliation the distribution of hospitals by the percentage of total residents graduated from American medical schools is more dispersed than the corresponding distribution of hospitals for interns. This means that affiliated hospitals have less success in attracting graduates of American medical schools as residents than as interns, whereas unaffiliated hospitals have more success in attracting such graduates as residents than as interns.

Several factors help to explain the last difference. In the first

Table 6.15. DISTRIBUTION OF VOLUNTARY AND MUNICIPAL HOSPITALS WITH APPROVED RESIDENCIES BY PERCENTAGE OF TOTAL BUDGETED POSITIONS FILLED BY GRADUATES OF AMERICAN MEDICAL SCHOOLS AND BY MEDICAL SCHOOL AFFILIATION, NEW YORK CITY, 1959

Percent Graduates of American Medical Schools to Total Residencies	All Hospitals			Medical School Affiliation					
				Major Teaching		Minor Teaching		Unaffiliated	
	Total	Voluntary	Municipal	Voluntary	Municipal	Voluntary	Municipal	Voluntary	Municipal
90 and over	4	4	0	2	0	1	0	1	0
70–89.9	6	6	0	2	0	3	0	1	0
50–69.9	14	11	3	2	3	7	0	2	0
30–49.9	7	5	2	3	1	0	1	2	0
10–29.9	18	14	4	0	0	4	1	10	3
Under 10	30	21	9	0	0	1	4	20	5
Total	79	61	18	9	4	16	6	36	8

source: Hospital Council of Greater New York, questionnaire survey of house staff in hospitals in New York City, April 20, 1959.

place, specialty hospitals, whether or not affiliated with a medical school, may be successful in recruiting graduates of American medical schools. In 1959 of the 4 voluntary unaffiliated hospitals reporting that their resident staffs had 50 percent or more graduates of American medical schools, 3 were specialty hospitals. Moreover, in a general hospital it is possible to have a few weak residency programs in a generally favorable teaching environment or one or more strong residency programs in a generally unfavorable environment; the chief of service can make the difference. Finally, several fields of residency training fail today to attract graduates of American medical schools; these programs must, therefore, rely on graduates of foreign medical schools.

For example, exchange visitors fill one half or more of all positions offered in anesthesia and thoracic surgery in voluntary and municipal hospitals in this city; between two fifths and one half in plastic surgery, dermatology, urology, otolaryngology, pediatrics, and pathology; and between one third and two fifths in radiology. Only in psychiatry do exchange visitors fill a small proportion of total positions, one tenth.[53]

Even in major teaching hospitals foreign exchange visitors fill one quarter or more of the positions in anesthesia, radiology, urology, general surgery, and pathology in the voluntary system, and in dermatology, thoracic surgery, neurology, otolaryngology, radiology, and pathology in the municipal system. In voluntary minor teaching hospitals foreign exchange visitors fill one quarter or more of the positions in anesthesia, pediatrics, otolaryngology, neurology, urology, pathology, and radiology.

Summary Ratios. The data on interns and residents for 1959 can be summarized in terms of the proportion of graduates of American medical schools in hospitals classified by degree of affiliation with a medical school. In each hospital system unaffiliated hospitals have a higher proportion of graduates of American medical schools among residents than among interns. In affiliated hospitals the reverse is true, except in municipal minor teaching hospitals, which follow the pattern for municipal unaffiliated hospitals. In voluntary minor teaching hospitals the composition of house staff resembles that of voluntary major teaching hospitals. Only major teaching hospitals in both systems and voluntary minor teaching hospitals have three fourths or more of all interns

Table 6.16. PERCENTAGE OF TOTAL INTERNS AND RESIDENTS IN
APPROVED PROGRAMS WHO GRADUATED FROM
AMERICAN MEDICAL SCHOOLS, BY HOSPITAL
OWNERSHIP AND BY MEDICAL SCHOOL
AFFILIATION, NEW YORK CITY, 1959

		Medical School Affiliation		
	All	Major	Minor	
Hospital Ownership	Hospitals	Teaching	Teaching	Unaffiliated
Voluntary and Municipal				
Interns	48.3	77.5	84.2	3.1
Residents	49.2	65.3	50.3	16.4
Voluntary				
Interns	52.3	82.1	95.1	2.7
Residents	58.3	77.1	63.8	20.1
Municipal				
Interns	42.9	74.7	0.0	3.6
Residents	37.8	56.0	11.5	11.6

SOURCE: Hospital Council of Greater New York, questionnaire survey of house staff
in hospitals in New York City, April 20, 1959.

graduated from American medical schools. Among residents this
proportion of graduates of American medical schools is attained
only by voluntary major teaching hospitals; in voluntary minor
teaching hospitals the proportion of American graduates is 64
percent and in municipal major teaching hospitals, 56 percent.

*Correlation between Success in Recruiting Residents and
Interns.* Since the data on residents by location of medical school
of graduation are available for individual hospitals only for the
year 1959, whereas those on interns have been available from
NIMP for almost a decade, it seems worth while to juxtapose the
two sets of data to examine the relationship between the composition of a hospital's residency staff and that of its intern staff.

The diagonal line, which slopes downward to the right, con-
nects hospitals that have the same proportion of American educated residents as of interns. The data indicate that (1) in general,
the proportion of a hospital's graduates of American medical
schools among residents varies directly with its proportion of such
graduates among interns; (2) at the low end of the distribution (upper left of table) the proportion of graduates of American medical
schools among residents is likely to exceed that among interns;
and (3) near the high end of the distribution (lower right of table)
the proportion of such graduates among residents is likely to fall
below that among interns. Findings (2) and (3) are consistent with

Table 6.17. JOINT DISTRIBUTION OF VOLUNTARY AND MUNICI-
PAL HOSPITALS WITH APPROVED TRAINING PRO-
GRAMS BY PERCENTAGE OF AMERICAN GRADUATED
INTERNS AND AMERICAN GRADUATED RESIDENTS,
NEW YORK CITY, 1959

Percent American Educated Interns to Total	Percent American Educated Residents to Total										
	All Hospitals	0–10	11–20	21–30	31–40	41–50	51–60	61–70	71–80	81–90	91–100
All hospitals	57	25	6	6	3	2	3	7	2	2	1
0– 10	31	20	6	4	1	—	—	—	—	—	—
11– 20	5	5	—	—	—	—	—	—	—	—	—
21– 30	—	—	—	—	—	—	—	—	—	—	—
31– 40	2	—	—	1	—	1	—	—	—	—	—
41– 50	—	—	—	—	—	—	—	—	—	—	—
51– 60	2	—	—	—	1	—	1	—	—	—	—
61– 70	2	—	—	—	1	—	—	1	—	—	—
71– 80	1	—	—	—	—	—	1	—	—	—	—
81– 90	4	—	—	1	—	1	1	1	—	—	—
91–100	10	—	—	—	—	—	—	5	2	2	1

SOURCE: Hospital Council of Greater New York, questionnaire survey of house staff in hospitals in New York City, April 20, 1959.

the findings previously derived from Tables 6.14 and 6.15. Finding (1) suggests that the earlier findings are applicable not only to a group of hospitals but also to an individual hospital, provided that an ample allowance is made for variation. The direction of the allowance—as much as 30 percentage points—depends on how successful the hospital in question is in attracting interns.

Success in recruiting graduates of American medical schools as interns should imply success in recruiting them as residents, if a hospital's interns were the exclusive or predominant source of its resident staff. A recent study of a group of voluntary hospitals in New York City shows that only 30 percent of the residents had their internship in the same hospital.[54] If this finding is typical, it suggests that recruiting interns and residents are usually distinct processes, with the outcome depending on the reputation of each of the hospital's training programs.

PROPORTION OF ALIEN PHYSICIANS IN AFFILIATED AND
UNAFFILIATED HOSPITALS, 1951 AND 1959

There is a marked difference today between affiliated and unaffiliated hospitals in New York City in the proportion of house staff positions filled by graduates of American medical schools. Perhaps some difference also existed in the past; the question is whether the size of the difference has changed and, if so, in which direction and by how much.

Unfortunately, available data do not permit a comparison between 1959 and 1935. It is known, however, that several municipal unaffiliated hospitals which today have no American-educated interns and few, if any, applicants from American medical schools had as many as 20 or more such applicants per intern position before World War II.

Comparisons in composition of house staff can begin with the year 1951, with citizenship status used as an approximation for location of medical school of graduation. The numbers of interns

Table 6.18. CHANGES BETWEEN 1951 AND 1959 IN NUMBER OF INTERNS AND OF RESIDENTS IN APPROVED TRAINING PROGRAMS, BY MEDICAL SCHOOL AFFILIATION OF HOSPITAL AND BY CITIZENSHIP STATUS OF PHYSICIAN, IN VOLUNTARY AND MUNICIPAL HOSPITALS, NEW YORK CITY

Hospital Ownership and Citizenship Status	Medical School Affiliation			
	All Hospitals	Major Teaching	Minor Teaching	Unaffiliated
Interns and Residents				
Voluntary	+734	+118	+311	+305
United States citizens	+227	+81	+172	−26
Aliens	+507	+37	+139	+331
Municipal	+802	+509	+49	+244
United States citizens	+79	+242	−74	−89
Aliens	+723	+267	+123	+333
Interns				
Voluntary	+220	+32	+63	+125
United States citizens	+102	+39	+67	−4
Aliens	+118	−7	−4	+129
Municipal	+92	+3	−1	+90
United States citizens	−63	−7	−7	−49
Aliens	+155	+10	+6	+139
Residents				
Voluntary	+514	+86	+248	+180
United States citizens	+125	+42	+105	−22
Aliens	+389	+44	+143	+202
Municipal	+710	+506	+50	+154
United States citizens	+142	+249	−67	−40
Aliens	+568	+257	+117	+194

SOURCE: Tables 6.24, 6.25, and 6.26.

and residents in each hospital system, distributed by citizenship status of house staff and by affiliation status of hospital, are presented in Tables 6.24, 6.25, and 6.26 at the end of the chapter. Table 6.18 shows changes in these categories between 1951 and 1959.

Interns increased in number in each affiliation class in the voluntary system and in the unaffiliated hospitals of the municipal system. United States citizens serving as interns increased only in voluntary major and minor teaching hospitals; they decreased slightly in municipal major and minor teaching hospitals and in voluntary unaffiliated hospitals and substantially in municipal unaffiliated hospitals. Alien interns increased substantially in the unaffiliated hospitals of both systems and slightly in municipal major and minor teaching hospitals and declined slightly in voluntary teaching hospitals.

Alien, as well as total, residents increased across the board. United States citizens increased substantially in municipal major teaching hospitals and moderately in voluntary major and minor teaching hospitals and declined in municipal minor teaching hospitals and in both groups of unaffiliated hospitals.

In the voluntary system minor teaching hospitals gained two thirds of the gross increase in United States citizens serving as house staff, and major teaching hospitals gained one third, whereas unaffiliated hospitals incurred a loss. The increase in alien house staff in the voluntary system was distributed as follows: two thirds in unaffiliated hospitals, more than one fourth in minor teaching hospitals, and a small fraction in major teaching hospitals.

In the municipal system major teaching hospitals gained 240 United States citizens. They were drawn in almost equal numbers from a net increase of 79 in the system and from losses by minor teaching hospitals and by unaffiliated hospitals. Each class of hospitals registered substantial gains in alien house staff.

The numerical changes are reflected in shifts in the proportion of alien physicians to total. The proportion of alien physicians among residents increased in each type of hospital affiliation and ownership class. Among interns it increased in each type of municipal hospital and in voluntary unaffiliated hospitals, but decreased in voluntary major and minor teaching hospitals.

Table 6.19. PERCENTAGE OF ALIEN PHYSICIANS AMONG INTERNS AND RESIDENTS IN APPROVED TRAINING PROGRAMS, BY HOSPITAL OWNERSHIP AND BY MEDICAL SCHOOL AFFILIATION, NEW YORK CITY, 1951 AND 1959

| Hospital Ownership and Year | All Hospitals | Medical School Affiliation | | |
		Major Teaching	Minor Teaching	Unaffiliated
Interns and Residents				
Voluntary, 1951	24.4	15.7	15.9	52.0
1959	37.5	17.9	25.4	75.8
Difference, 1951–59	+ 13.1	+ 2.2	+ 9.5	+ 23.8
Municipal, 1951	22.8	15.0	47.6	20.1
1959	50.3	31.7	83.2	73.0
Difference, 1951–59	+ 27.5	+ 16.7	+ 35.6	+ 52.9
Interns				
Voluntary, 1951	29.8	9.9	5.2	69.0
1959	37.5	4.0	1.8	83.6
Difference, 1951–59	+ 7.7	− 5.9	− 3.4	+ 14.6
Municipal, 1951	17.7	12.8	66.7	16.5
1959	45.4	16.2	89.7	80.8
Difference, 1951–59	+ 27.7	+ 3.4	+ 23.0	+ 64.3
Residents				
Voluntary, 1951	22.5	17.1	19.4	40.7
1959	37.4	21.5	32.5	70.4
Difference, 1951–59	+ 14.9	+ 4.4	+ 13.1	+ 29.7
Municipal, 1951	25.6	16.6	44.8	22.1
1959	52.1	36.7	82.5	68.6
Difference, 1951–59	+ 26.5	+ 20.1	+ 37.7	+ 46.5

SOURCE: Tables 6.24, 6.25, and 6.26.

LIMITATIONS OF DATA ON APPROVED PROGRAMS

Changes in the approval status of training programs can usefully supplement data on changes in the composition of house staff in approved programs. Changes in approval status may or may not be reflected in the lists published by the Council on Medical Education and Hospitals. When an intern or residency program loses approval, it is deleted from the list; this occurs even when the loss is temporary. When a program is shifted from full to probationary approval, or conversely, the published list remains unchanged, and no comment is offered.

From published sources it is known that at least 9 approved internships were discontinued in New York City between 1935 and 1958: 5 in voluntary hospitals, 3 in municipal hospitals, and 1 in proprietary hospitals. Between 1948 and 1958 approximately 15 approved residency training programs in half a dozen specialties were discontinued in the municipal system, whereas an increase of 150 took place in voluntary hospitals. Although the initiative for seeking approval of a program always originates with the hospital, the initiative for discontinuance may come from the Council on Medical Education and Hospitals or from the hospital.

The Consolidated List of Approved Internships provides ready information on past lapses in approval. It these are short in duration—a year or less—they may be taken as indicative of difficulty in meeting standards. During the period 1914–55, 14 hospitals in New York City experienced brief lapses in approval, 11 voluntary and 3 municipal. Two of the latter occurred after World War II, compared with 3 of the former. In the voluntary system 5 of the lapses occurred in wartime.[65]

A shift from full to probationary approval can only be learned about from the hospital involved. In this respect there is a significant difference between a voluntary and municipal hospital, to the latter's disadvantage. More is likely to be known about developments in the municipal system, because budgetary hearings may be entailed, a tradition of public discussion exists, and a central headquarters compiles information on its member hospitals.

It is public knowledge, for example, that one municipal hospital has in recent years lost approval for all its graduate training programs. It is also known that five municipal hospitals have recently experienced difficulty in retaining approval for residency training in internal medicine. Drastic efforts had to be exerted to retain or regain approval, full or probationary.

If similar developments take place in voluntary hospitals, they are not so likely to be known. Through informal conversations during this study it was learned that approximately the same number of voluntary as municipal hospitals in New York City have recently experienced difficulty in retaining full approval for one or another residency training program. The information on voluntary hospitals is necessarily less complete than that on municipal hospitals.

Discussion of Future Policy

So far the data have been presented in terms of composition of house staff by medical school of graduation and by citizenship. Comparisons have been made between a recent year and one in the past, between New York City and the United States, between voluntary and municipal hospitals in the city, and between hospitals with and without medical school affiliation. To lay a basis for discussing the probable impact of alternative policies, the data will now be presented in terms of the distribution of American and foreign medical school graduates among hospitals. In which hospitals in New York City do graduates of American medical schools serving in approved training programs tend to concentrate? Do the patterns of distribution differ for United States citizens who attended medical school abroad, for permanent immigrants, and for temporary visitors on exchange visas?

DISTRIBUTION OF INTERNS AND RESIDENTS AMONG HOSPITALS
BY MEDICAL SCHOOL AFFILIATION

Tables 6.20 and 6.21 for interns and residents, respectively, show separately for each group of medical school graduates the ownership and medical school affiliation status of the hospitals in which they trained in 1959.

Few graduates of American medical schools serve in unaffiliated hospitals in New York City, and none serve in municipal minor teaching hospitals. Of the United States citizens educated abroad, however, one half intern in unaffiliated hospitals and the other half in teaching hospitals. More than four fifths of alien physicians, whether permanent immigrants or temporary visitors, intern in unaffiliated hospitals.

The distribution of residents is similar to that of interns for graduates of American medical schools, but not for the three groups of physicians educated abroad. Each category of residents educated abroad is more widely distributed than the corresponding group of interns. Stated another way, unaffiliated hospitals have a lower proportion of the foreign-educated residents than of interns; and, conversely, affiliated hospitals have a higher proportion of foreign-educated residents than of interns. These tendencies are

Table 6.20. DISTRIBUTION OF INTERNS IN APPROVED TRAINING
PROGRAMS (AMERICAN MEDICAL SCHOOL GRADU-
ATES AND OTHERS BY CITIZENSHIP STATUS)
AMONG HOSPITALS, BY OWNERSHIP AND
BY MEDICAL SCHOOL AFFILIATION,
NEW YORK CITY, 1959

Hospital Ownership and Medical School Affiliation	Graduates of American Medical Schools		U.S. Citizens Educated Abroad		Permanent Immigrants		Temporary Visitors	
	Num- ber	Per- cent	Num- ber	Per- cent	Num- ber	Per- cent	Num- ber	Per- cent
All hospitals	571	100.0	136	100.0	95	100.0	380	100.0
Voluntary	357	62.5	72	52.9	55	57.9	199	52.4
Municipal	214	37.5	64	47.1	40	42.1	181	47.6
Major teaching	*349*	*61.1*	*55*	*40.4*	*13*	*13.7*	*33*	*8.7*
Voluntary	142	24.8	24	17.6	3	3.2	4	1.1
Municipal	207	36.3	31	22.8	10	10.5	29	7.6
Minor teaching	*207*	*36.3*	*11*	*8.1*	*4*	*4.2*	*24*	*6.3*
Voluntary	207	36.3	8	5.9	2	2.1	0	0
Municipal	0	0	3	2.2	2	2.1	24	6.3
Unaffiliated	*15*	*2.6*	*70*	*51.5*	*78*	*82.1*	*323*	*85.0*
Voluntary	8	1.4	40	29.4	50	52.6	195	51.3
Municipal	7	1.2	30	22.1	28	29.5	128	33.7

SOURCE: Hospital Council of Greater New York, questionnaire survey of house staff in hospitals in New York City, April 20, 1959.

especially true of permanent immigrants and of temporary visitors.

Another marked difference between the resident and intern distributions pertains to United States citizens educated abroad and to permanent immigrants and is that municipal hospitals have a much higher proportion of residents in these categories than of interns. This difference reflects the operation of the New York State Licensure Law, which does not apply to interns. Every resident is required by law to have a license or to be certified as eligible for admission to the licensing examination, unless he works in a governmental hospital. Temporary visitors on exchange visas are exempt from the requirement.

In the foreseeable future the most likely changes in the availability of young physicians to serve as house staff in local hospitals are (1) an increase in the number of graduates of American med-

Table 6.21. DISTRIBUTION OF RESIDENTS IN APPROVED TRAIN-
ING PROGRAMS (AMERICAN MEDICAL SCHOOL GRAD-
UATES AND OTHERS BY CITIZENSHIP STATUS)
AMONG HOSPITALS, BY OWNERSHIP AND
BY MEDICAL SCHOOL AFFILIATION,
NEW YORK CITY, 1959

Hospital Ownership and Medical School Affiliation	*Graduates of American Medical Schools*		*U.S. Citizens Educated Abroad*		*Permanent Immigrants*		*Temporary Visitors*	
	Num- ber	*Per- cent*	*Num- ber*	*Per- cent*	*Num- ber*	*Per- cent*	*Num- ber*	*Per- cent*
All hospitals	1,616	100.0	301	100.0	274	100.0	1,092	100.0
Voluntary	1,065	65.9	124	41.2	75	27.3	563	51.5
Municipal	551	34.1	177	58.8	199	72.7	529	48.5
Major teaching	*999*	*61.8*	*121*	*40.1*	*125*	*45.7*	*287*	*26.3*
Voluntary	517	32.0	33	10.9	18	6.6	103	9.4
Municipal	482	29.8	88	29.2	107	39.1	184	16.9
Minor teaching	*490*	*30.3*	*62*	*20.7*	*50*	*18.2*	*372*	*34.1*
Voluntary	461	28.5	45	15.0	16	5.8	201	18.4
Municipal	29	1.8	17	5.7	34	12.4	171	15.7
Unaffiliated	*127*	*7.9*	*118*	*39.2*	*99*	*36.1*	*433*	*39.6*
Voluntary	87	5.4	46	15.3	41	14.9	259	23.7
Municipal	40	2.5	72	23.9	58	21.2	174	15.9

SOURCE: Hospital Council of Greater New York, questionnaire survey of house staff in hospitals in New York City, April 20, 1959.

ical schools and (2) a decrease in the number of temporary visitors. Changes in the number of United States citizens educated abroad and in permanent immigrants are not so readily subject to control and cannot be anticipated over a short period.

Any increase in the number of graduates of American medical schools will probably occur gradually. In this area the Downstate Medical Center in Brooklyn is shortly slated to expand its capacity from 150 to 200 new students annually. Recently a proposal was advanced for the State University of New York to add two or three medical schools,[56] at least one of which would presumably be located in this area. If prevailing patterns in the distribution of house staff persist, the major teaching and voluntary minor teaching hospitals may be expected to gain.

To the extent that foreign physicians are unable to pass the test given by ECFMG, there is likely to be a decline in the number of temporary visitors. A reduction in interns from this source would primarily affect the unaffiliated hospitals, hitting the voluntary and municipal systems with equal force. A reduction in residents would hurt the unaffiliated hospitals in both systems and the municipal minor teaching hospitals. A weak house staff is likely to have a greater impact on the care provided at a municipal hospital than at a voluntary hospital, because the former has traditionally been more dependent on its house staff for medical services.

The size of the probable decline in temporary visitors has been variously estimated at 15,[57] 33,[58] and 50 percent.[59] The 33-percent figure approximates the rate of failure so far experienced in the ECFMG examinations administered in this country. The 50 percent figure is somewhat above the rate of failure in the examinations when taken abroad. It has been suggested that the decline in the number of foreign graduates available for internships and residencies may be temporary and that it will be reversed if medical education abroad improves and more qualified physicians take the examinations.

Whatever the reduction in the number of foreign exchange visitors proves to be, its adverse impact on unaffiliated hospitals is likely to be greater than the prevailing distribution of such physicians implies. The reasons are twofold. (1) Frequently, though not always, a higher proportion of candidates from unaffiliated hospitals than from affiliated hospitals fail the ECFMG examination; and (2) by passing the examination or obtaining a temporary certificate a physician has improved his qualifications. Upon termination of his existing contract, he may have enlarged opportunities in this or other hospitals, including affiliated ones.

POSSIBLE SOLUTIONS

Hospitals without approved training programs must resort to other means to provide physicians' services around the clock. The Council on Medical Education and Hospitals has offered certain suggestions for providing medical service on a twenty-four-hour basis to the hospitals unable to qualify for internship approval: (1) employ young physicians who have just completed hospital training and pay them an adequate salary; (2) rotate night and weekend duty among junior members of the attending staff or the entire staff; (3) hire junior members of the attending staff on a part-time basis; and (4) train nurses and technicians to perform certain procedures.[60]

It has previously been pointed out that a hospital without approved training programs need not be a hospital without a teaching program. Any medical staff that strives for better patient care must constantly be teaching itself. Recently a proposal was advanced that hospitals without intern and residency programs be rated for the quality of care rendered, with special consideration given to the teaching program carried on by and for the attending staff.[61]

One analysis of the medical staff situation in municipal hospitals in New York City proposed that (1) university hospitals replace interns with clinical clerks, leaving the training of interns to other hospitals (unaffiliated and minor teaching); (2) the duration of internship training be prolonged to two years; (3) hospitals with approved programs be limited in the number of physicians they may recruit for house staff; and (4) unaffiliated hospitals discontinue the internship and concentrate on improving residency training. The last is to be done by offering "realistic" salaries, employing full-time directors of clinical service or educational coordinators to supervise the program, and making attendance at hospitals more attractive to practitioners by paying them for visiting and furnishing them with beds for private and semiprivate patients. Ancillary personnel could be employed to advantage to perform the intern's nonmedical work.[62]

A more recent analysis of the problems facing municipal hospitals emphasized proposals to raise salaries for house staff and to establish intensive orientation programs for foreign-educated physicians when appointed to the house staff.[63] Still other proposals have emphasized affiliation with medical schools and co-ordination of services among hospitals, so that hospitals with superior medical resources, including house staff, would assume responsibility for an increased proportion of the patient load in New York City.[64]

Several of these proposals are dealt with elsewhere in this report. Employment of full-time directors of clinical service, along with improvement of ancillary services, is discussed in Chapter 9;

provision in municipal hospitals of facilities for private and semi-private patients in Chapter 11; and affiliation with medical schools and coordination of hospital services also in Chapter 11. The remainder of this chapter discusses the other proposals in this order:

1. Discontinue the internship in university hospitals
2. Limit the number of positions per approved program
3. Prolong internship training to two years
4. Raise salaries of house staff
5. Provide an intensive program of orientation for graduates of foreign medical schools.

Discontinue Internship Training in University Hospitals. The proposal is to eliminate the internship in university hospitals and to divide its duties between clinical clerks (undergraduate medical students) and residents. It is expected that this would make more interns available for minor teaching and unaffiliated hospitals.

In New York City the several hospitals affiliated with one medical school (New York Medical College) discontinued the internship beginning in 1953. Not many hospitals here or elsewhere have taken this step.

An intensive study of the role of the internship in medical education was completed in 1953 by the Advisory Committee on Internships to the Council on Medical Education and Hospitals. This Committee found that developments in other phases of medical education had created problems for internship training. It decided, however, not to recommend major changes, such as elimination of the internship in hospitals with undergraduate clinical clerks. The Committee concluded: "Clerks and residents, with duties appropriately assigned, add rather than detract from the internship's value." [65]

Any proposal to modify the internship, whether pertaining to its location or duration, must obviously be assessed in terms of the training needs of the young physician. It is not tenable to view interns merely as a source of supply of medical services to be allocated in accordance with the needs of hospitals.

The Council on Medical Education and Hospitals does not undertake to balance the total number of positions offered by approved training programs in this country with the number of potential applicants for them. The existence of an over-all surplus of positions gives the young physician a choice and tends to make programs competitive. Competition is desirable, if it stimulates hospitals to improve the educational value of their programs.

Limit the Number of Positions per Approved Program. The proposal is that hospitals be limited to recruiting only the number of interns or residents that is warranted by the number of patients participating in the educational program. It is expected that this would divert young physicians from hospitals with a surplus and promote a wider distribution of the graduates of American medical schools.

In support of this proposal it has been observed that some hospitals that are successful in attracting graduates of American medical schools tend to recruit them in increasing, perhaps excessive, numbers. Although the Council on Medical Education and Hospitals has the opportunity of looking at the number of positions in a program when it grants initial approval and at the regular three-year review, it leaves to the hospital the decision on the number of physicians to seek from year to year.[66] In certain programs there are guidelines for determining the number of physicians needed per training program. For example, in the internship the stated range is 15–25 beds per intern.[67] Quantitative requirements per resident are given for training in obstetrics and gynecology and in pathology, but not in the other medical specialties.[68]

The difficulty with this proposal is that it is not a simple matter to determine the appropriate number of interns or residents in a given program. The number of physicians a hospital is capable of training well does not depend solely on the number of ward patients or on the total number of inpatients. Other factors are also important. A hospital may or may not assign house staff to services for ambulatory patients, may or may not provide a substantial amount of training in the basic sciences, may or may not enlist a large number of attending physicians for teaching, and may or may not offer opportunities in medical research. With so much variation in the content of training programs, it is not possible to determine whether a surplus (or shortage) of house staff exists by applying a numerical formula. Whether the size of house staff is in excess of a hospital's training capabilities can only be determined by the judgment of experienced persons, once they agree on the content of a desirable program.

No hospital should have a larger house staff than it can properly train. This calls for self-restraint on the part of hospitals with advantages in recruitment. Outside agencies can only provide an element of review in extreme cases.

Prolong the Duration of the Internship. Formerly two thirds of the internships in New York City were of two years' duration, a much higher proportion than in the nation. For hospitals to return to this length of training would be equivalent to increasing the number of physicians available for internships. It would then be possible to replace some foreign-educated interns with graduates of American medical schools.

There is no consensus that one year is the best length of internship training, particularly for the purpose of preparing the young physician for general practice. This year the American Medical Association is launching an experiment in a two-year program for family practice.[69]

Since the residency has become the designated route to specialization, prolongation of the internship would have to be meshed with the length of the residency. Most specialty boards would be reluctant to surrender one year in their fields in exchange for an additional year of internship. At the same time it must be recognized that young physicians who intend to limit their practice to a specialty are eager to proceed with the residency. A recent survey in the municipal hospital system reports that 95 percent of the interns intend to specialize.[70]

Any hospital or group of hospitals that lengthened the internship while others did not would be at a disadvantage in recruitment. An unintended result of adopting this proposal might be a loss of house staff by the very hospitals it is supposed to help.

Higher Salaries for House Staff. After many years of free service by house staff, the City of New York began to pay interns in municipal hospitals $15 a month in July, 1936. Today remuneration for interns and residents is an accepted practice. Competition among hospitals in terms of stipend alone is, however, frowned upon. "Excessive salaries" raise a question of the adequacy of the educational program.[71]

Two opposing points of view are expressed on the effect of the amount of stipend on a hospital's success in recruitment. One view is that stipend does not significantly influence the outcome,[72] whereas another holds specifically that a lag in the amount of stipend has impaired the recruitment potential of municipal hospitals in New York City.[73] Both points of view receive some support from an analysis of the relationship between amount of stipend and degree of success in the National Intern Matching Program (NIMP).

The conclusion that stipend does not affect recruitment is based on the finding that hospitals with small stipends match a higher proportion of interns than hospitals with large stipends.[74] Most hospitals with low stipends are, however, affiliated with medical schools, whereas most hospitals with high stipends are unaffiliated. The variable "stipend" may be masking the influence of the variable "affiliation status" to an unknown extent. It would be helpful to have an analysis of the degree of association between success in the NIMP and amount of stipend for each type of medical school affiliation class and perhaps also by hospital ownership. Stipend should be defined to reflect room and board and other fringe benefits.

That small stipends have impaired the ability of municipal hospitals in New York City to recruit house staff is supported by 1958 data for a group of unaffiliated hospitals under city or county ownership throughout the nation, all of which provide full maintenance. The data were compiled by the Committee of Interns and Residents of the New York City Municipal Hospitals and show that municipal hospitals outside the city, paying an average monthly stipend of $169, filled 50 percent of their positions under the NIMP, whereas New York City's municipal unaffiliated hospitals, paying $105 monthly, matched 1 percent.[75] (Today municipal hospitals in New York City pay interns $175 a month.) An analysis by this Committee of recruitment in five large cities shows that unaffiliated and minor teaching hospitals tend to be most successful where stipends are highest, despite uniformly effective competition from major teaching hospitals.[76] In both of these analyses no effort was made to explore variables other than amount of stipend that make for success, or lack of it, in recruiting interns.

Hospitals with the same amount of stipend may have different degrees of success in recruiting graduates of American medical schools. On the basis of experience and interviews conducted during this study, it is concluded that the quality and reputation of a teaching program are a more important factor than stipend. Other factors being equal, however, the amount of stipend is important in many instances and decisive in some. The last is particularly true when the young physician's financial resources fall short of his family obligations.

A voluntary hospital can adjust the amount of stipend it offers from year to year, in line with its experience in recruitment and with the views of its board of trustees. Although affiliated hospitals tend to pay lower stipends than unaffiliated hospitals, this is not true of every member of each group. In New York City several voluntary hospitals with major medical school affiliation are among those paying the highest stipends.

In the municipal system every hospital pays the same stipend. This places the unaffiliated hospitals at a disadvantage. In the future, in addition to keeping the amount of stipend in line with general trends, the Department of Hospitals may wish to consider establishing a differential that varies inversely with a hospital's degree of affiliation with a medical school.

Intensive Training for Foreign Physicians. This proposal pertains to interns and residents in municipal hospitals who were not able to pass the ECFMG examination, and it consists of two parts: (1) intensive instruction in English for three months and (2) a clinical clerkship for another three months. Clinical instructors would be nominated by the local medical schools and paid an adequate salary by the City.[77]

There are almost as many physicians who failed the recent ECFMG examination in voluntary hospitals in New York City as in municipal. An orientation program should not be limited to one hospital system but should aim to meet the needs of all hospitals serving the community.

Moreover, the ECFMG examination was devised to set a floor on an individual's eligibility to participate in an approved training program. In view of the differences, noted early in this chapter, between foreign and American medical schools in teaching the basic sciences and in exposing students to patients, a more intensive program of initial orientation and review for all or most graduates of foreign medical schools may be advisable.

Recently the proposal has been advanced that hospitals, acting alone or in a group, undertake to provide supervised training to foreign-educated physicians through clerkships, prior to assigning them to the house staff. The clerkship would combine a review of the basic sciences and orientation to American practices in the examination and diagnosis of patients.[78]

Providing Physicians' Services in the Absence of a House Staff. There is no way to mesh from year to year the need of hospitals for physicians' services with the need of young physicians for training. Once a surplus of positions exists, some hospitals will have to do without house staff or with fewer house staff than they seek. This may entail a difficult adjustment for hospitals that have come to rely on the services rendered by house staff. One study in a large university hospital, cited in a recent report, found that more than one half of the existing resident staff would be required just to maintain the present level of care, exclusive of any teaching or research. The same study shows that residents on the average spend only one quarter of their working time away from patient services.[79]

In the absence of house staff the attending physicians would have to do more. In some instances it may be possible to obtain physicians' services from volunteers by rotating the entire attending staff or its junior members through evening and weekend duty, as suggested in the *Essentials of an Approved Internship.* In other instances it may be necessary to pay for these services, whether per session or on part-time salary. Full-time salaried physicians may be required to perform other services, including staffing of the emergency department. It has also been suggested that hospitals provide administrative, clerical, and other personnel in support of the attending staff, so that the latter may have more time for direct services to patients.[80]

A comment is in order on the prospects that hospitals will obtain the requisite services from young practitioners working part time for pay. Traditionally, young physicians just entering practice have preferred to work in hospitals without fee. As the demand for physicians' services increases both inside and outside the hospital, the old pattern may no longer provide adequate physician coverage in the hospital. To change the traditional preference will require leadership from the medical societies and in the long run a new orientation for students in medical school.

Summary

1. The existing pattern of house staff training in this country is of fairly recent origin. A marked expansion took place after World War II, particularly in residencies. Owing to many factors outlined in this chapter, the number of positions offered by approved training programs has increased rapidly. The initial result was an increase in vacancies, despite an increase in the number of applicants. Subsequently, as the number of foreign-educated physicians rose and kept rising, there was a small decline in vacancies and, finally, stabilization at a high level.

2. Estimates are presented of the composition of house staff in hospitals in New York City and in the United States by the location of medical school of graduation (American or foreign) and by citizenship status for the foreign-educated. Differences between the city and the nation are considerable. Even larger is the difference between voluntary and municipal hospitals in New York City. The most prominent characteristic distinguishing hospitals with a high and low proportion of graduates of American medical schools is not ownership but degree of affiliation with a medical school.

3. During the 1950s, especially in the second half, the ability of hospitals in New York City without medical school affiliation to recruit graduates of American medical schools has steadily declined. Conversely, most voluntary hospitals with a minor medical school affiliation have been notably successful.

4. Implementation by January, 1961, of the program adopted in 1956, under which a physician graduating from a foreign medical school must pass the examination given by the Educational

Council for Foreign Medical Graduates before serving as an intern or resident, aggravated to the point of crisis the problem facing many hospitals that depend largely on foreign-educated house staff. The probable impact of the decline in applicants for house staff is discussed, and a number of proposals are discussed that have been offered to alleviate the situation.

5. It is concluded that certain proposals, such as reverting to the two-year internship or imposing a numerical limitation on the number of house staff per approved training program, are either undesirable or impracticable; that a difference in amount of stipend between affiliated and unaffiliated hospitals may be advisable and should be given consideration by the New York City Department of Hospitals for municipal hospitals; that an intensive orientation program for newly appointed foreign-educated house staff is indicated; and that hospitals may have to rely increasingly on attending staff and paid physicians to render medical services around the clock, as hospitals without approved training programs do.

Appendix 6.A

ESTIMATING THE COMPOSITION OF HOUSE STAFF AND LENGTH OF GRADUATE MEDICAL TRAINING, UNITED STATES

The composition of house staff by the location of medical school of graduation has an inherent interest. It is also essential for calculating the average length of graduate medical training.

In recent years the size of one component of house staff in this country has been generally known, namely, the number of physicians on exchange visitor visas, as compiled by the Institute of International Education. It is a mistake to assume, as is frequently done,[81] that the difference between total house staff and the number of exchange visitors equals the number of house staff physicians graduated from American medical schools. This difference does in fact include graduates of American medical schools; but it also includes United States citizens who attended medical school abroad and physicians who came to this country as permanent immigrants. The number of permanent immigrants serving as house staff has on occasion been estimated at 1,000,[82] but no estimate is forthcoming of the number of United States citizens educated abroad.

An accurate distribution of house staff by location of medical school of graduation and by citizenship status for graduates of foreign schools can only be derived from survey data similar to those obtained by the Hospital Council for New York City. Pending the compilation of such data, reliance must be placed on the best estimates that can be developed from the materials at hand. Fortunately, a reliable estimate can be developed for one recent year, which can serve as a point of departure for estimates for other years.

MEDICAL SCHOOL OF GRADUATION AND CITIZENSHIP STATUS

The method employed to derive the composition of house staff in approved training programs in hospitals in the United States is as follows:

1. The total number of physicians serving as house staff in approved programs is known. It is reported annually in the *Directory of Approved Internships and Residencies*, prepared by the Council on Medical Education and Hospitals of the American Medical Association.

2. The number of exchange visitors is compiled annually by the Institute of International Education, reported in its publication *Open Door*, and frequently reprinted.

3. The number of permanent immigrants can be estimated for one recent year, 1955–56, by subtracting the number of exchange visitors from the total number of aliens, as reported to the Selective Service System and adjusted (see below). This is the most recent year for which information is available both on the number of exchange visitors and the total number of aliens.

4. The number of United States citizens educated abroad is estimated separately (see below).

5. The number of graduates of United States medical schools is the difference between Item 1 and the sum of Items 2, 3, and 4.

6. The number of graduates of American medical schools (United States plus Canadian) is taken as the sum of Item 5 plus the number of Canadians holding exchange visitor visas. The latter can be found in the *Health Manpower Source Book, Section 9*, of the United States Public Health Service, Division of Public Health Methods.

Estimate for Fiscal Year 1956. The *Health Manpower Source Book*, Section 9, and "Hospital House Staff, 1950–1955," reprinted from *Hospitals*,[83] give all the necessary data, except for the adjustment factor for women. The latter corrects the tendency of reports to Selective Service to omit female graduates of foreign medical schools. The adjustment factor is derived from an article in the *Journal of the American Medical Association* on foreign physicians.[84] The computations follow:

Aliens

1.	Number reported by Selective Service System	7,873
2.	Add: Adjustment for women, 11 percent	865
3.	Total aliens, adjusted (1 plus 2)	8,738
4.	Less: Temporary visitors, reported by Institute of International Education	6,033
5.	Permanent immigrants (3 minus 4)	2,705

United States Citizens

6.	Number reported by Selective Service System	22,120
7.	Less: Above adjustment for women	865
8.	Subtotal (6 minus 7)	21,255
9.	Add: House staff in military and Public Health Service hospitals	987
10.	Total, adjusted (8 plus 9)	22,242
11.	Number educated abroad (see below)	750
12.	Graduates United States medical schools (10 minus 11)	21,492

Other data

13.	Total number of positions filled, reported by American Medical Association	31,028
14.	Number of Canadians on exchange visitor visas	584

Explanation of Line 11: $750 = 250 \times 3$ years (number of United States citizens educated abroad annually).[85]

Arranged more conveniently, the composition of house staff in fiscal year 1956 was as follows:

Total (Line 13)	*31,028*
Graduates of United States and Canadian medical schools (Line 12 plus 14 plus discrepancy, as below)	22,124
Graduates of foreign medical schools	*8,904*
United States citizens	750
Permanent immigrants (Line 5)	2,705
Exchange visitors (Line 4 minus Line 14)	5,449

Derivation of discrepancy: Line 13 does not quite equal the sum of Lines 1, 6, and 9, but exceeds it by a small number, 48, as follows:

Line 14		31,028
Less: Line 1	7,873	
Line 6	22,120	
Line 9	987	30,980
Discrepancy		48

Approximation for Fiscal Year 1959. Between 1956 and 1959 the following changes in house staff took place:

1. The total number increased by 6,080, to 37,110.

2. The number of temporary visitors increased to 8,360, or by 2,330. There was no significant change in the Canadian component.

3. The number of permanent immigrants in house staff must have increased, as the total number of permanent immigrant physicians reaching this country rose from 1,050 in calendar year 1955 [86] to 1,940 in 1958.[87] For present purposes the size of the increase in this component of house staff is set at 1,000.

4. United States citizens educated abroad also increased, conservatively by 250, to 1,000. (The figures on the number of United States citizens attending foreign medical schools are not exact.[88])

5. It follows from the above that the number of graduates of American medical schools increased by 2,500, to 24,625.

The estimated composition of house staff in fiscal year 1959 follows:

	Number	*Percent*
Total	*37,110*	*100.0*
Graduates of American medical schools	24,625	66.3
Graduates of foreign medical schools	*12,485*	*33.7*
United States citizens	1,000	2.7
Permanent immigrants	3,705	10.0
Exchange visitors	7,780	21.0

Estimate of Foreign Educated Physicians, 1951. The number of aliens serving as house staff, as reported by Selective Service, amounted to 2,100.[89] To this figure should be added (1) an allowance for women physicians—230 (a markup of 11 percent) and (2) an allowance for United States citizens educated abroad, perhaps 500 or more. To be subtracted is the number of graduates of Canadian medical schools, around 400. The resulting estimate is 2,400 to 2,500.

LENGTH OF GRADUATE TRAINING, 1955–56

The average length of graduate training is the ratio of the number of house staff to the number of physicians graduated annually. For graduates of United States medical schools the number of house staff is taken from Line 12 in the derivation for fiscal year 1956; the average annual number of graduates is derived, below.

House staff who are graduates of United States medical schools	21,492
Average annual number of graduates of United States medical schools	6,647
Ratio of house staff to annual graduates (in years)	3.24

The average annual number of graduates of United States medical schools is the arithmetic mean for four years, as follows: [90]

1952	6,080
1953	6,668
1954	6,861
1955	6,977
Total	26,586
Arithmetic mean	6,647

For the year 1940 the estimate of the average length of graduate medical education at two years is a rough approximation. Total house staff consisted of 11,450.[91] If it is assumed that the number of foreign-educated physicians approximated 1,000, graduates of United States medical schools amounted to 10,450. The latter is then divided by the number of graduates of United States medical schools, which amounted to 5,200 in 1938 and 5,100 in 1939.

Appendix 6.B

ESTIMATING THE NUMBERS OF INTERNS AND
RESIDENTS IN VOLUNTARY AND
MUNICIPAL HOSPITALS IN
NEW YORK CITY, 1935

The problem is this: one source of data appears to offer an accurate total count but fails to give a distribution by hospital ownership; another source gives a distribution by hospital ownership but seems to be too high in its total count. By comparison with other contemporary sources of information, such as the annual reports of the Department of Hospitals and of the United Hospital Fund, it would seem that the second source must have included house staff in unapproved programs.

The procedure for estimating the number of house staff in approved training programs in each major hospital system was as follows:

1. Assume that the data derived from the study of *Internships and Residencies in New York City* [92] represent correct totals.

2. Assume that the data presented in *The Hospital Survey for New York* [93] are correct for governmental hospitals—municipal, federal, and state—in that they pertain exclusively to approved programs.

3. It follows that interns and residents in approved programs in voluntary hospitals must be the difference between Items 1 and 2.

The step by step derivation follows:

1. The report by the New York Committee on the study of *Hospital Internships and Residencies* gives the following totals: [94]

Residents and fellows	520
Private assistants	20
Special interns	104
Interns	1,135
Total	1,779

The following adjustments were made:

Interns. Combine special interns (6–12 months training in a specialty) and interns. Total interns are, therefore, 1,239.

Residents. Delete private assistants.[95] Total residents are 520.

2. The distribution of interns and residents by hospital ownership, as given in *The Hospital Survey for New York,* is as follows: [98]

Hospital Ownership	Residents	Interns
Municipal	191	592
Federal and State	25	33
Subtotal, government	216	625
Voluntary	352	896
Total	568	1,521

3. The numbers of house staff in approved programs in voluntary hospitals follow:

	Residents	Interns
Total (see Item 1, above)	520	1,239
Less: Government hospitals (see Item 2, above)	216	625
Difference: Voluntary hospitals	304	614

4. The estimates follow, rounded:

Hospital Ownership	Residents	Interns	Total
Voluntary (see Item 3, above)	305	615	920
Municipal (see Item 2, above)	190	590	780
Total	495	1,205	1,700

Table 6.22. INTERNS IN APPROVED TRAINING PROGRAMS BY CITIZENSHIP STATUS IN VOLUNTARY AND MUNICIPAL HOSPITALS, NEW YORK CITY, 1951, 1955, AND 1959

Citizenship Status	1951	1955	1959
All hospitals	870	998	1,182
United States citizens	660	644	699
Aliens	210	354	483
Voluntary hospitals	463	547	683
United States citizens	325	326	427
Aliens	138	221	256
Municipal hospitals	407	451	499
United States citizens	335	318	272
Aliens	72	133	227

SOURCE: 1951 and 1955—Hospital Council of Greater New York, tabulations from reports on house staff filed with New York City headquarters of Selective Service System; and 1959—Hospital Council of Greater New York, questionnaire survey of house staff in hospitals in New York City, April 20, 1959.

Table 6.23. RESIDENTS IN APPROVED TRAINING PROGRAMS
BY CITIZENSHIP STATUS IN VOLUNTARY AND
MUNICIPAL HOSPITALS, NEW YORK CITY,
1951, 1955, AND 1959

Citizenship Status	1951	1955	1959
All hospitals	2,059	2,875	3,283
United States citizens	1,573	1,764	1,840
Aliens	486	1,111	1,443
Voluntary hospitals	1,313	1,633	1,827
United States citizens	1,018	1,057	1,143
Aliens	295	576	684
Municipal hospitals	746	1,242	1,456
United States citizens	555	707	697
Aliens	191	535	759

SOURCE: See Table 6.22.

Table 6.24. HOUSE STAFF IN APPROVED TRAINING PROGRAMS BY
CITIZENSHIP STATUS AND BY MEDICAL SCHOOL
AFFILIATION IN VOLUNTARY AND MUNICIPAL
HOSPITALS, NEW YORK CITY, 1951 AND 1959

Citizenship Status	All Hospitals	Medical School Affiliation		
		Major Teaching	Minor Teaching	Unaffiliated
1951				
Voluntary and municipal	2,929	1,355	860	714
United States citizens	2,233	1,147	650	436
Aliens	696	208	210	278
Voluntary	1,776	726	629	421
United States citizens	1,343	612	529	202
Aliens	433	114	100	219
Municipal	1,153	629	231	293
United States citizens	890	535	121	234
Aliens	263	94	110	59
1959				
Voluntary and municipal	4,465	1,982	1,220	1,263
United States citizens	2,539	1,470	748	321
Aliens	1,926	512	472	942
Voluntary	2,510	844	940	726
United States citizens	1,570	693	701	176
Aliens	940	151	239	550
Municipal	1,955	1,138	280	537
United States citizens	969	777	47	145
Aliens	986	361	233	392

SOURCE: Tables 6.25 and 6.26.

Table 6.25. INTERNS IN APPROVED TRAINING PROGRAMS BY
CITIZENSHIP STATUS AND BY MEDICAL SCHOOL
AFFILIATION IN VOLUNTARY AND MUNICIPAL
HOSPITALS, NEW YORK CITY, 1951 AND 1959

| | | *Medical School Affiliation* | | |
Citizenship Status	All Hospitals	Major Teaching	Minor Teaching	Unaffiliated
1951				
Voluntary and municipal	*870*	*415*	*184*	*271*
United States citizens	660	366	156	138
Aliens	210	49	28	133
Voluntary	*463*	*141*	*154*	*168*
United States citizens	325	127	146	52
Aliens	138	14	8	116
Municipal	*407*	*274*	*30*	*103*
United States citizens	335	239	10	86
Aliens	72	35	20	17
1959				
Voluntary and municipal	*1,182*	*450*	*246*	*486*
United States citizens	699	398	216	85
Aliens	483	52	30	401
Voluntary	*683*	*173*	*217*	*293*
United States citizens	427	166	213	48
Aliens	256	7	4	245
Municipal	*499*	*277*	*29*	*193*
United States citizens	272	232	3	37
Aliens	227	45	26	156

SOURCE: 1951—Hospital Council of Greater New York, tabulations from reports on
house staff filed with New York City headquarters of Selective Service System; and
1959—Hospital Council of Greater New York, questionnaire survey of house staff in
hospitals in New York City, April 20, 1959.

Table 6.26. RESIDENTS IN APPROVED TRAINING PROGRAMS BY
CITIZENSHIP STATUS AND BY MEDICAL SCHOOL
AFFILIATION IN VOLUNTARY AND MUNICIPAL
HOSPITALS, NEW YORK CITY, 1951 AND 1959

| | | *Medical School Affiliation* | | |
Citizenship Status	*All Hospitals*	*Major Teaching*	*Minor Teaching*	*Unaffiliated*
1951				
Voluntary and municipal	*2,059*	*940*	*676*	*443*
United States citizens	1,573	781	494	298
Aliens	486	159	182	145
Voluntary	*1,313*	*585*	*475*	*253*
United States citizens	1,018	485	383	150
Aliens	295	100	92	103
Municipal	*746*	*355*	*201*	*190*
United States citizens	555	296	111	148
Aliens	191	59	90	42
1959				
Voluntary and municipal	*3,283*	*1,532*	*974*	*777*
United States citizens	1,840	1,072	532	236
Aliens	1,443	460	442	541
Voluntary	*1,827*	*671*	*723*	*433*
United States citizens	1,143	527	488	128
Aliens	684	144	235	305
Municipal	*1,456*	*861*	*251*	*344*
United States citizens	697	545	44	108
Aliens	759	316	207	236

SOURCE: 1951—Hospital Council of Greater New York, tabulations from reports on house staff filed with New York City headquarters of Selective Service System; and 1959—Hospital Council of Greater New York, questionnaire survey of house staff in hospitals in New York City, April 20, 1959.

7 NURSING PERSONNEL

It was not feasible to study the complete staffing patterns of hospitals in New York City. It was early decided to concentrate on the staffing of the nursing service, not because of its representative character, but because the nursing service is important in itself and its adequate staffing is a difficult assignment. All the categories of nursing personnel constitute between 40 and 45 percent of the total personnel of hospitals. Recruiting nurses and organizing them to render service under prevailing conditions of "shortage" pose as challenging a set of operating problems as confront hospitals today.

This chapter deals with the staffing of nursing services in voluntary and municipal hospitals in New York City against the background of developments in the nation. Hospital schools of nursing and private duty or special nursing in hospitals in New York City receive separate consideration.

Postwar Developments in Hospital Nursing

During the depression of the 1930s there was a "surplus" of registered (professional) nurses in this country. At prevailing salaries the number of nurses available for employment exceeded the number that hospitals were prepared to hire. Since World War II, when the number of registered nurses in civilian hospitals first declined, there has been a "shortage" of registered nurses in this country, that is, at prevailing salaries the demand by hospitals exceeds the number of nurses available for employment. In recent years the shortage of full-time registered nurses, as reflected in the ratio of vacant to budgeted positions, has been somewhat relieved. Between 1953 and 1958 the nation-wide rate of vacancy declined from 15 to 11 percent.[1]

Unlike the wartime experience, the postwar shortage is not the result of a reduction in the number of registered nurses available to hospitals. During much of the postwar era recruitment of students for schools of nursing kept pace with population growth.[2] As techniques for counting nurses improved, it came to be recognized that the rate of increase in active registered nurses was exceeding the rate of increase in population in the United States. The ratio of active nurses to population has increased—from 216 per 100,000 population in 1940 to 249 in 1950 and to 268 in 1958.[3] In hospitals there has been an even larger increase in the ratio of registered nurses to average daily patient census—from 15 per 100 patients in general care hospitals in 1932 to 47 per 100 in 1958.[4]

The shortage is clearly the result of an expansion in demand in excess of the expansion in supply, owing to the reduction in the work week of graduate nurses and students, more intensive activity in hospitals, associated with faster turnover of patients (see Chapter 2), and an increase in the variety and complexity of services rendered by nurses.[5]

Reduction in the length of the work week understates the increase in demand for personnel occasioned by the improvement in working conditions in hospitals. The same period witnessed the elimination of the split shift, which as late as 1940 applied to 70 percent of the nurses in voluntary hospitals in New York City.[6] Under the split shift the working day of the nurse consisted of two tours of duty, with intervening time off that was not paid for. Without the split shift it takes three or more nurses working a seven- or eight-hour day to do the work that formerly required two persons, each paid for nine or ten hours a day.

The feeling that an acute shortage exists is aggravated by the high rate of turnover of registered nurses, especially general-duty or staff nurses. Many young graduates leave employment to marry and raise a family, not to return to nursing for some years. The very condition of shortage is conducive to a high degree of mobility from one job to another. An annual rate of turnover of the order of 67 percent [7] is costly and also wasteful of the time of those who remain on the job.

There are many inactive registered nurses today. These are not likely to return to the profession in significant numbers in the absence of a very large increase in salary.[8] Minor inducements, such as invitations to attend refresher courses, have not proved to be significant sources of additional supply.[9]

Difficulties in staffing the nursing service are accentuated by increasing reliance on part-time personnel. These pose problems in scheduling and organization of the nursing service and are not readily oriented to the goals of the institution.[10] Part-time employees constitute a rising proportion of nursing personnel and are especially important among general-duty nurses. In the latter group part-time employees constituted 30 percent of the total in 1958,[11] compared with only 12 percent in 1944.[12]

Another—partial—adjustment to the shortage is to hire auxiliary personnel, including practical nurses, nurses' aides, ward clerks, and messengers. By 1958 auxiliary personnel accounted for 54 percent of total nursing staff in short-term hospitals in this country—practical nurses 14 percent and nurses' aides and others 40 percent.[13] Registered nurses filled 46 percent of all positions— 40 percent full-time and 6 percent part-time. (Part-time nurses have been converted to full-time equivalents at a ratio of two to one.) [14] Ten years earlier registered nurses had filled 50 percent of all nursing positions, and auxiliary personnel filled the other 50 percent; and part-time registered nurses accounted for only 2 percent of the total.[15]

Many hospitals have gradually expanded the range of duties assigned to practical nurses. For example, practical nurses are increasingly being trained for service in the operating room. In some hospitals they give much of the medication; in others, none at all. There is no consistent policy on this. One practical nurse has observed a diurnal phenomenon: "Within many hospitals the practical nurse is not allowed to chart or give medicines from 7 A.M. to 3 P.M. but, by some feat of alchemy, becomes steadily more competent with the passing hours, so that by 11 P.M. she is carrying the entire nursing service on a ward." This has been called "sunshine and moonshine" nursing.[16] One advantage of employing practical nurses is their relatively low rate of turnover.[17]

In recent years a tendency has developed to promote nurses'

aides and assign them to specialized tasks. Some hospitals reward reliability and proficiency by offering aides additional training in specific procedures, so that they become technicians or assistants on the nursing floor or in the operating room.

Another adjustment made by hospitals is to try to reduce the size of the total task assigned to the nursing service. It is generally agreed that responsibilities for housekeeping, dietary, and clerical activities should be taken from the nurse and given to others.[18] There are, however, limits to the number of adjustments that can be made. Other departments of the hospital may be in no better position than the nursing service to assume the duties proposed for transfer to them.

It is not always feasible freely to substitute auxiliary personnel for registered nurses. The question has been raised whether, in terms of efficient and flexible use of personnel, the number of auxiliary nursing staff today is not excessive.[19]

With the increasing complexity of nursing procedures, it is desirable to have some specialized professional nurses doing bedside care.[20] Notwithstanding, administration and nursing education are still the most direct routes to promotion and higher pay.

Increased use of auxiliary personnel and specialization of function place a heavy burden on supervision. The major role of the professional nurse today is that of manager of nursing personnel.[21] In interviews this point of view was frequently expressed: the professional nurse must be prepared for the job of manager. The question is no longer whether this should be done, but how. This is an area in which facts are lacking and wide differences of opinion prevail among nurses and hospital administrators.[22] It seems that no area of research in hospital administration or planning promises a greater return on expenditures than that of devising ways to improve the management of the nursing service.

Nursing Personnel in Local Hospitals

Available data do not permit the tracing of a trend in the composition of hospital nursing staffs in New York City. Data for registered nurses are, however, available for selected years for all voluntary hospitals or for an important subgroup, the United Hospital Fund member hospitals, and for the municipal hospital system. For practical nurses engaged in caring for inpatients, there are data available for the year 1954. (See Appendix 7.A for the sources of data in this section.)

In voluntary hospitals there was a marked decline in the number of registered nurses during World War II. (United Hospital Fund general hospitals reported a decline from 4,600 in 1938 to 3,400 in 1945.) After the war, recovery was rapid, and the number of registered nurses rapidly climbed to a new peak. (All United Hospital Fund hospitals reported 3,900 in 1945, 5,750 in 1947, and 6,250 in 1948.) In the middle 1950s the increase was moderate. (United Hospital Fund general hospitals reported an increase from approximately 6,000 in 1953 to 6,950 in 1958.) Much of this increase took place in one year, between 1957 and 1958. (All voluntary general-care hospitals reported an increase of 700.)

In the middle 1950s the increase in general duty or staff nurses was small. (All general-care hospitals reported 3,750 in 1954 and 3,900 in 1958.) Most of the increase in registered nurses in this period was in nurses in administrative or supervisory positions, including head nurses.

The number of practical nurses in voluntary hospitals also increased in the 1950s. (General-care hospitals reported an increase from 2,250 in 1954 to 2,850 in 1958; the former figure was for inpatient care only.) As a result, there was an increase in the ratio of practical nurses to registered nurses in general-duty positions (from 60 per 100 in 1954 to 75 per 100 in 1958).

In municipal hospitals the peak number of registered nurses was reported in 1937—4,700. A marked decline took place during the war—to 3,000 in 1946—and a rapid but moderate recovery came afterward—to 3,850 in 1948. During the period 1949–56 the number of registered nurses was fairly stable, fluctuating between 3,550 and 3,750.

A decline set in in 1958 or earlier, but the timing of the decline is uncertain because of a discrepancy between the data given in the annual reports of the Department of Hospitals and those reported by the individual hospitals to the American Hospital Association. From the Department's own figures a peak of 3,900 was attained in 1957, but this number is too high in light of the revision made in 1958, both in reporting methods and in the base figure. The best estimate is that a decline of 100 registered nurses took place between 1957 and 1958 and a further decline of 50 between 1958 and 1959. The salary increase initiated in 1960 arrested the downward trend.

Between 1954 and 1958 there was a decline in the number of registered nurses on general duty in municipal hospitals. (General-care hospitals reported 1,650 in 1954 and 1,500 in 1958.) The number of nurses in administrative positions remained approximately constant. During this period several municipal hospitals became more active institutions and required additional nurses.

In the middle 1950s the number of practical nurses increased. (General-care hospitals reported 1,350 in 1954 and 2,000 in 1958; as previously, the former figure was for inpatient care only.) The ratio of practical nurses to general-duty nurses, which was already higher in municipal than in voluntary hospitals, increased still further (from 83 per 100 in 1954 to 133 per 100 in 1958). Recently the number of practical nurses in municipal hospitals has shown a small decline; this may be related to increased competition from other hospitals, particularly federal hospitals, which in 1958 for the first time reported practical nurses on their staffs.

In 1958 there were 15,300 registered nurses working in all hospitals in New York City; private-duty nurses are excluded. This number compares with 10,700 registered nurses employed in hospitals, resident in New York City, and registered in New York State during the biennium 1955–57.[23] The difference of 4,600 can be accounted for by (1) incompleteness in the early registration count, of the order of 10 percent, or 1,100; (2) the presence of 700 professional nurses in federal hospitals, who need not be registered in New York State; (3) time lag between the two sources of data; for example, between September, 1957, and September, 1958, the number of registered nurses in hospitals in New York City increased by 500; (4) time lag in registering new graduates, who are reported by hospitals as registered nurses upon graduation from school; there are 1,100 graduates from schools of nursing in New York City in a year; (5) a small number of exchange visitors, of the order of 50 to 60; (6) commuters from the suburbs, number unknown; and (7) foreign-trained nurses working in hospitals who are preparing to qualify for registration. Of the last group, few are in municipal hospitals and a significant number are in voluntary hospitals.

Of the 15,300 registered nurses working in hospitals in New York City in 1958, 1,700, or 11 percent, worked part time and 13,600 full time.

COMPOSITION OF STAFFS OF NURSING SERVICES IN 1958

In the voluntary, municipal, and proprietary general-care hospitals in New York City there were in 1958 approximately 35,000 personnel employed in the nursing service, distributed as follows:

Category of Nurse	Number	Percent
Registered nurses	13,200	37.9
Practical nurses	5,900	17.0
Nurses' aides and other	15,700	45.1
Total	34,800	100.0

Registered nurses working full time filled 36 percent of all positions (expressed as full-time equivalents), and those working part time filled 2 percent. In the United States as a whole the corresponding figures, it will be recalled, were 40 and 6 percent, respectively. Part-time personnel are especially numerous among general-duty nurses. They constitute 20 percent of all general-duty nurses in hospitals in New York City.

COMPARISON BETWEEN VOLUNTARY MUNICIPAL SYSTEMS

Table 7.1 shows the number of persons in the nursing services of voluntary and municipal general-care hospitals in New York City, the respective percentage distributions, and the computed ratios of personnel per 100 patients (the latter expressed as the average daily census).

The proportions of practical nurses to total nursing personnel in the two hospital systems are close. The large difference between the two systems in the proportion of registered nurses is offset by an equal difference, in the opposite direction, in the proportion of nurses' aides.

Personnel Ratios. The two ratios of total nursing personnel per 100 patients are close—108 in voluntary hospitals and 104 in

Table 7.1. DISTRIBUTION OF STAFF OF NURSING SERVICES IN
VOLUNTARY AND MUNICIPAL GENERAL-CARE HOS-
PITALS BY CATEGORY OF NURSING PERSONNEL
AND RATIO OF STAFF TO 100 DAILY PATIENTS,
NEW YORK CITY, 1958

| Category of Personnel | Nursing Personnel | | | | Ratio of Personnel to 100 Patients | |
| | Voluntary | | Municipal | | Volun- tary | Munici- pal |
	Number	Percent	Number	Percent		
All nursing personnel	18,560	100.0	12,250	100.0	108	104
Registered nurses	8,325	44.7	3,340	27.3	48	29
General duty	3,900	21.0	1,500	12.3	25	13
Other	4,425	23.7	1,840	15.0	23	16
Auxiliary	10,235	55.3	8,910	72.7	60	75
Practical nurses	2,850	15.4	2,000	16.3	17	17
Nurses' aides	5,350	28.9	6,140	50.1	31	52
Other	2,035	11.0	770	6.3	12	6

SOURCE: American Hospital Association, annual questionnaire.

municipal hospitals. Differences in the types of patient cared for, particularly in duration of stay, are more than enough to justify this small difference in ratios, if all other factors were the same. All other factors are usually not the same, however. Comparisons in staffing ratios should be made with care.

There are certain inherent limitations to such comparisons, since personnel ratios fail to convey information on a number of significant factors, such as: [24]

1. The amount of time spent by nurses on nonnursing duties.

2. The proportion of nurses' time spent with patients and away from patients.

3. The preparation of head nurses for administrative responsibilities.

4. The preparation of nonprofessional personel, especially nurses' aides.

5. Classification and assignment of patients to nursing units according to degree of illness.

6. Facilities and equipment available to promote efficient patient care.

7. The number of "per diem" nursing personnel. A per diem nurse may not be as interested as the permanent employee, since

she usually does not participate in continuing inservice educational programs.

8. The extent of turnover among nursing personnel.

9. Satisfaction on the job.

10. The presence of a program of continuing inservice education to keep the staff informed of new medical and nursing procedures.

11. The over-all administrative policies of the hospital that influence the effectiveness of the nursing service in relation to all other hospital departments, including the medical staff.

12. The volume of services provided to ambulatory patients.

It is possible for the nursing service of a hospital to be superior to that of another, despite an inferiority in the ratio of nurses to patients. This may occur because of better organization and management or because responsibility is exercised over a narrower range of functions. When the disparity in staffing ratios between two hospitals is great, however, there is little question as to which hospital is under most circumstances likely to provide the more effective and adequate nursing care.

In this instance the difference between the two systems in the ratio of registered nurses per 100 patients is large—19. Two thirds of this difference is contributed by general-duty nurses and one third by supervisory or administrative nurses, including head nurses.

The difference between the two systems in the ratio of registered nurses to patients remains essentially unchanged if students in schools of nursing are taken into account. For this purpose a student nurse is counted as equivalent to 30 percent of a full-time graduate nurse.[25]

If special-duty nurses are also considered, the ratio of registered nurses per 100 patients in the voluntary system rises to 71 and in the municipal system to 32. The original difference of 19 has doubled.

Rates of Vacancy. The two hospital systems can also be compared in the proportion of vacant to authorized positions.

There is reason to believe that in a time of shortage the rate of vacancy may understate the actual degree of shortage, because positions difficult to fill may be dropped from the budget; this is even more likely if positions are not vacant but are filled by persons with lower qualifications. Favoring an overstatement of shortage is another tendency, namely, failure to review vacancies from time to time. It may be that changes in staffing patterns made in an emergency assume a permanent character.

For municipal hospitals it is possible to calculate vacancy rates for registered nurses according to two methods: (1) the percentage of vacant positions to the total number authorized; and (2) the percentage that the sum of vacant positions and positions filled by persons with lower qualifications constitutes of the total number authorized. The computed rates (percent) of vacancy for the general-care hospitals in New York City are as follows:

Category of Registered Nurse	Voluntary Hospitals	Municipal Hospitals	
		Method 1	Method 2
Total	11	18	52
General duty	18	29	70
Other (administrative)	5	7	7

The vacancy rates for voluntary hospitals correspond to those calculated under Method 1 for municipal hospitals.

According to Method 2 less than one half of the authorized registered nurse positions in municipal hospitals are filled by registered nurses. This compares with a figure of 60 percent ten years ago.

The high vacancy rates shown for the municipal hospital system are not so unreasonable as they may seem, if cognizance is taken of the salaries paid to practical nurses and to general-duty registered nurses. When the ratio of the former to the latter is around 90 percent, as it has been in recent years in municipal hospitals, there is good reason to wish to hire personnel with higher training in preference to personnel with less training. An administrator's views on the extent of the shortage of registered nurses are necessarily affected by his estimate of the net cost of replacing auxiliary personnel with registered nurses, if the latter were to become available.

Between 1954 and 1958 the rate of vacancy in voluntary general-care hospitals declined from 21 to 11 percent. The decline applied to both general-duty and administrative nurses. In municipal hospitals the vacancy rate declined for administrative nurses but increased for general-duty nurses. Since the municipal system makes the greater use of auxiliary personnel, it must provide more supervision and give a high priority to the staffing of administrative positions.

DISTRIBUTION OF HOSPITALS BY RATIO OF
REGISTERED NURSES TO PATIENTS

A comparison between aggregates can be misleading, since large hospitals exert a predominant influence on the data. Another limitation of aggregates is that they obscure variations among hospitals.

It was therefore decided to analyze the ratios of registered nurses to patients for the 98 voluntary and municipal general-care hospitals for which data were available. It is reasonable to focus on registered nurses for two reasons: (1) it is easier to fill auxiliary nursing positions, particularly with untrained personnel; and (2) requirements for registered nurses are less affected by differences in the range of functions performed by nursing departments, such as dietary or housekeeping functions.

Comparisons between the Two Hospital Systems. The 98 hospitals—81 voluntary and 17 municipal—are distributed by the ratio of registered nurses per 100 patients in Table 7.2. Municipal hospitals are clustered in the class intervals at the lower end of the

Table 7.2. DISTRIBUTION OF VOLUNTARY AND MUNICIPAL GEN-
ERAL-CARE HOSPITALS BY RATIO OF REGISTERED
NURSES TO 100 DAILY PATIENTS,
NEW YORK CITY, 1958

Registered Nurses per 100 Daily Patients	Voluntary		Municipal	
	Number of Hospitals	Percent	Number of Hospitals	Percent
15.0–24.9	7	8.6	5	29.4
25.0–34.9	16	19.8	6	35.3
35.0–44.9	21	25.9	4	23.5
45.0–54.9	14	17.3	2	11.8
55.0–64.9	14	17.3	0	0
65.0 and higher	9	11.1	0	0
Total	81	100.0	17	100.0

SOURCE: American Hospital Association, annual questionnaire.

distribution, whereas voluntary hospitals are distributed throughout the six class intervals.

Certain summary statistics throw further light on the two frequency distributions.

Statistic	Registered Nurses per 100 Patients	
	Voluntary Hospitals	Municipal Hospitals
Mean (arithmetic average)	48	29
Median (50th percentile or midvalue)	40	29
1st quartile (75th percentile)	57	40
3rd quartile (25th percentile)	33	23
Range in ratios	15–106	17–51

All percentiles are arranged in descending order from the highest ratio to the lowest (the 75th percentile is 25 percentage points from the top).

The above statistics show that:

1. The range in ratios is much wider in the voluntary system than in the municipal.

2. In the voluntary system the larger hospitals tend to have the higher ratios of registered nurses to patients, as evidenced by the excess of the mean over the median. Larger hospitals tend to be teaching hospitals.

3. There is no tendency for higher ratios in large hospitals in the municipal system. Indeed, when the ratios of registered nurses to patients in the municipal system are studied separately for university and nonuniversity hospitals, no such association is found. If anything, nonuniversity hospitals have slightly higher ratios.

Similar statistics can be computed for the distributions of ratios of registered nurses per 100 patients after student nurses and special nurses are taken into account. They follow:

Statistic	Registered Nurses per 100 Patients	
	Voluntary Hospitals	Municipal Hospitals
Mean (arithmetic average)	71	32
Median (50th percentile or midvalue)	52	34
1st quartile (75th percentile)	71	40
3rd quartile (25th percentile)	37	28
Range in ratios	21–132	17–62

The difference between mean and median for voluntary hospitals is now 19, compared with 8 previously. The relatively high ratios in large hospitals, the chief recipients of services from student nurses and private-duty nurses, have become still higher.

In municipal hospitals the difference between mean and median is now negative. The small hospitals have made the greater gains as a result of the introduction of students' services and special nurses into the personnel to patient ratios.

Comparison with Standards. Municipal hospitals have lower ratios of registered nurses to patients than voluntary hospitals, on the average and in most instances. It is possible to go somewhat beyond this conclusion, though not to the point of comparing actual staffing patterns with some optimum standard.

Standards currently employed to estimate staffing requirements for the bedside care of patients can be traced back to a study of 14 hospitals made in 1938 by the National League for Nursing Education. Subsequent adjustments pertain to the proportion of registered nurses to total nursing personnel and to the staffing of other positions in the nursing service. The Department of Hospitals calculates nursing staff requirements hospital by hospital in systematic fashion; [26] it is the results of these calculations that constitute the number of positions authorized, from which vacancies are counted.

According to these formulas the number of registered nurses required in municipal general-care hospitals in 1958 was 7,050. In relation to patients, the required ratio of registered nurses was 59 per 100. None of the municipal hospitals approached this ratio, while 17 of 81 voluntary hospitals met it prior to counting students and private-duty nurses, and 34 did after counting them.

Possibly a standard of staffing developed for municipal hospitals is too high for voluntary hospitals, as the latter have a lower ratio of services for ambulatory patients to inpatient services. On the other hand, voluntary hospitals have a more active inpatient load, with fewer patients accommodated in large wards (and these tend to economize on nursing care).

If voluntary hospitals in New York City had been able to fill all their budgeted vacancies in 1958, as reported to the American Hospital Association, they would have had a ratio of 54 registered nurses per 100 patients. This standard of demand for registered nurses is perhaps more realistic for still another reason, namely, that voluntary hospitals pay practical nurses only 75 percent of the salary paid to registered staff nurses. Without student nurses and private-duty or special nurses, the standard was met by 24 voluntary hospitals and no municipal hospital; with student nurses and private-duty nurses counted, the standard was met by 48 voluntary hospitals and 2 municipal hospitals.

Some leeway should be allowed for variations in the staffing requirements of individual hospitals. If this is arbitrarily set at 20 percent of the standard, the resulting minimum ratio is 43 registered nurses per 100 patients. This standard is met by 44 voluntary hospitals and 3 municipal hospitals, prior to counting students and private-duty or special nurses, and by 55 voluntary and 4 municipal hospitals, after counting them. Among the four municipal hospitals none has a university affiliation.

The above comparisons with standard ratios can be summarized.

Ratio of Registered Nurses per 100 Patients	*Number of Hospitals Exceeding Specified Standard Ratio*			
	Without Students and Private-Duty Nurses		*With Students and Private-Duty Nurses*	
	Voluntary	*Municipal*	*Voluntary*	*Municipal*
59	17	0	34	0
54	24	0	48	2
43	44	3	55	4

Ranking of Hospitals. Perhaps the simplest way to compare the staffing ratios in the two hospital systems is to arrange all 98 hospitals in descending rank order and to distribute them in four equal groups (quartiles).

Quartile	*Total*	*Voluntary*	*Municipal*
First	24	24	0
Second	25	22	3
Third	25	20	5
Fourth	24	15	9
Total	98	81	17

If the ratios of registered nurses to patients were the same in the two hospital systems, one might expect 20 or 21 voluntary hospitals and 4 or 5 municipal hospitals in each quartile. In fact, no municipal hospital was found in the top quartile and one half of the municipal hospitals fell in the fourth quartile. Even so, the majority of the hospitals in the fourth quartile are under voluntary control.

Special Problems of Municipal Hospitals

Certain aspects of the current nursing situation pertain to both hospital systems, but to an unequal degree. Problems associated with the use of relatively large numbers of auxiliary personnel, relatively thin staffing during evening and night shifts, and large numbers of authorized registered nurse positions vacant (either filled by auxiliary personnel or not filled at all) press more heavily on municipal hospitals. Problems of using part-time personnel to best advantage impinge more heavily on voluntary hospitals. With increasing specialization in certain nursing duties, the task of hiring or replacing key personnel is becoming more difficult for both systems. Sometimes the lack of one or two such individuals may prevent the operation of an existing service or establishment of a new one.

Municipal hospitals suffer from certain special disadvantages. In the past these were somewhat compensated for by special advantages. For example, ten years ago their work week was shorter than in private hospitals. The City hospitals abandoned the burdensome split shift long before the others.[27] The City paid pensions long before voluntary hospitals instituted retirement benefits. Today the City's pension arrangements are still more liberal than those of voluntary hospitals,[28] but they are no longer unique.

Stated salaries for beginning positions are higher in municipal than in voluntary hospitals.[29] There are however, certain perquisites, such as gratuities and subsidized apartments (outside the nurses' residence), that some voluntary hospitals offer and municipal hospitals do not. The most important difference is this: a voluntary hospital can—and does—hire a nurse at any step in the salary range for her grade, whereas the City's personnel policies require that nurses, like others, be hired at the bottom step of the salary range (see Chapter 9). The City of New York is less flexible than the federal government, which authorizes Veterans

Administration hospitals to exercise local discretion in hiring applicants at one or more steps above the minimum salary, without risk of reversal by higher authority.

Working conditions at municipal hospitals are frequently inferior to those in voluntary hospitals, although the length of the work week is the same and the vacation allowance for new employees is more generous in municipal hospitals. In its report on the survey of Kings County Hospital Center in 1952, the Hospital Council discussed at length the adverse working conditions, pointing to overcrowding, poor plant maintenance, and frequent lack of supplies.[30]

Since then the situation with respect to crowding has improved in most municipal hospitals, if not in all. The condition of physical plant is better in new hospitals, but not in the old ones. As for supplies, there is no change.

The fact remains that there are municipal hospitals with new plant, not crowded, and good to excellent medical staff that are unable to attract nurses in sufficient numbers. One factor may be the high proportion of auxiliary nursing personnel in municipal hospitals, since this increases the burden of management and supervision.

Perhaps more important in some of the new hospitals is isolation from convenient transportation and lack of small apartments in the neighborhood at moderate rentals. Sometimes the hospital is in a double-fare zone. It would be in order for the Department of Hospitals to try to arrange improved bus transportation to certain of its hospitals. Likewise, the Department might explore ways of acquiring or building and, if necessary, subsidizing the rentals on apartments for nurses. These apartments should not be in nurses' residences.

Coverage of the nursing service at night and evenings is very thin. Fifteen years ago a substantial number of nurses in this country were rotated through three shifts.[31] Under conditions of shortage mandatory rotation is not realistic.

In municipal hospitals, for which information is available, the evening shift has 19 percent of all general-duty nurses and the night shift 16 percent. More revealing perhaps is the ratio of practical nurses to registered nurses on general duty. The ratios are 1.1 to 1 on the day shift, 2 to 1 on the evening shift, and 2.4 to 1 on the night shift.

The realities underlying this statistical picture are well conveyed in the reports of the City Hospital Visiting Committee. For example, at one hospital:

There has been a steady decrease in the total number of professional nurses available for bedside care, particularly on the afternoon and night tours of duty. On these two tours, one staff nurse is usually responsible for the supervision of about five to six wards. . . . Practical nurses are now being given more responsibility, such as the management of ward units.

It is getting more difficult to persuade professional nurses in the operating room to work on afternoon and night tours of duty. Technicians are assigned to these tours but the services of professional nurses are also required.[82]

Municipal hospitals pay a shift differential of $20 a month in the evening and $10 at night. In 1957 these differentials were lower than those paid in private hospitals.[33]

The City of New York does not pay for overtime work, whereas many voluntary hospitals do.[34] Municipal hospitals can only grant compensatory time off for overtime hours spent on the nurse's regular job.

Some nurses prefer remuneration to compensatory time. It would be advantageous for the City to allow the Department of Hospitals to pay for authorized overtime either in cash or with time off, at the employee's option.

Some voluntary hospitals recruit nurses abroad and hire foreign-trained nurses in this country prior to their registration in New York State. The Department of Hospitals has refrained from recruiting nurses in other countries and has hired few foreign-trained nurses prior to registration. Recently the Department announced that it plans to sponsor and offer employment to qualified nurses from other countries when they apply.

Hospital Schools of Nursing

The role of the hospital school of nursing is worth elaborating, with special reference to the local scene.

Over the past decade enrollment in hospital schools of nursing in this country has remained reasonably constant,[35] with some indication of a small decline in the past few years. In New York City the trend has been gradually upward, after a precipitous drop in enrollment that accompanied termination of the Cadet Nurse Program after the war.

Hospital schools of nursing used to be the sole source of supply of registered nurses for all fields of nursing. A school of nursing formerly was a source of income to its hospital, in the sense that it was cheaper to use the services of student nurses than to hire graduates to render equivalent services. As late as the middle 1940s a study of the finances of hospital schools of nursing in this country found that in the aggregate income exceeded cost by 5 percent.[36]

Today hospital schools are still the predominant source of supply of nurses, but they no longer bring in revenue. The justification for a hospital's operating a school is the need to staff its own general duty nursing positions. A good nursing school has become a source of net cost to its hospital.

There may be some question about the amount of net loss incurred. Five elements enter into the equation: (1) direct expenses of the school; (2) the allocated portion of the hospital's overhead expenses; (3) the cost of room and board for students; (4) tuition and fees received from students; and (5) the value of students' services. The last is the most controversial item and much research and experimentation have been conducted in recent years on methods of measuring it. The chief alternatives developed are replacement cost and students' ability and usability. Despite technical differences in the method of measurement, a number of recent studies point to a net loss of $1,000 to $1,500 per student per year.[37] (Appendix 7.B.)

Last year the Department of Hospitals was able to retain 83 percent of its graduates (including graduates of the Lincoln School of Nursing, which is under a separate voluntary board and is in the process of closing). Among voluntary hospitals there is considerable variation in the proportion of graduates retained, ranging from 50 to 75 percent and higher. In both groups of hospitals it is reported that significant numbers of the new recruits leave after six months or a year.

Possibly one reason for early departure is the large proportion of nonresidents in the nursing schools in New York City. Ten years ago the proportion of female high school graduates in New York City who entered nursing school was only one half as high as the proportion in upstate New York.[38] The local schools of nursing attract a large proportion of students from other parts of the state and from outside the state. In 1957 one third of the 5,250 students in hospital schools of nursing in New York City came from outside the local region [39] (defined as the five boroughs plus Nassau and Suffolk counties on Long Island and Westchester and Rockland counties).

Of the six municipal hospital schools five were fully accredited by the National League of Nursing. One was too new in 1958 for consideration, as it had not yet graduated a class. Among the 23 voluntary hospital schools, 17 had full accreditation and 6 had temporary accreditation.[40]

The ratio of student nurses to registered nurses was approximately the same in the two hospital systems—45 per 100. In the voluntary system a hospital with a school of nursing tends to have a higher ratio of registered nurses to patients than a hospital without a school of nursing, but in the municipal hospital system there is no such association. Thus, every voluntary hospital with a school of nursing falls in the first or second quartile of hospitals ranked according to the ratio of staff to patients. Conversely, only two municipal hospitals with a nursing school are in the first or second quartile, whereas four are in the third or fourth quartile.

This does not mean that its own school of nursing contributes to the staffing of a voluntary hospital and not to that of a municipal hospital. As has been shown, the municipal hospital system is at least as effective and perhaps, on an over-all basis, more effective than the voluntary hospital system in recruiting a high proportion of its graduates for employment during the first year after graduation. The other factors previously mentioned that bear on the retention of new graduates and on recruiting from the outside appear to exert the greater impact.

Private-Duty or Special Nurses in Hospitals

In the work week nearest September 30, 1958, there were 3,800 private-duty or special nurses reported by hospitals in New

York City. This was 300 more than in 1957, which, in turn, exceeded the figure for 1954. Even so, the registries are unable to fill all requests for such nurses, particularly for evenings and nights.

This upward trend is surprising in view of the decline in private-duty nurses that has been projected by various students of nursing and that is widely believed to be taking place. In fact, the number of private-duty nurses in the United States has declined from 80,000 in 1920 [41] to 70,000 in 1958,[42] but as a proportion of all active nurses they have declined a great deal more. The ratio of private-duty nurses (working in homes or in hospitals) to registered nurses employed (and paid) by hospitals has changed from 6 to 1 in 1920, to 1 to 1 in 1938,[43] and 1 to 4 in 1958.[44] Today the majority of private-duty nurses work in hospitals.

There were 2,800 private-duty nurses in voluntary hospitals in New York City in 1958. A large number of these nurses worked in a small number of hospitals, with one fourth of all hospitals reporting two thirds of the nurses. There are hospitals in which the number of private-duty nurses exceeds the number of registered nurses on general duty.

As a group private-duty nurses in New York City are getting older.[45] They tend to be older than nurses in other fields, and some may be unable to handle the arduous work of staff nursing on the floor. Although private-duty nursing is not frequently chosen as a career, the convenient hours and time schedule ultimately prove attractive to some nurses.[46]

It is estimated that in 1958 approximately $25 million was spent for private-duty nursing in hospitals in New York City, $18 million in voluntary hospitals and $7 million in proprietary hospitals. A small proportion of the total was incurred for ward patients, perhaps $1 to $2 million. The remainder was paid by patients, mostly without assistance from insurance plans. In some voluntary hospitals expenditures for private duty nurses approach 50 percent of the hospital's own expenditures for nursing service.

When the medical condition of the patient requires special nursing and the latter is prescribed, it should be covered by insurance. A number of major purchasers of hospital care, including the City's Handicapped Children's program, Medicare (for dependents of the military), and many Blue Cross plans, now pay for private-duty nursing, subject to certain safeguards. In the summer of 1958 it was reported that 26 Blue Cross plans did or were about to include private-duty nursing in benefits under extended coverage provisions of their contracts.[47] Twenty-one of these plans provide benefits in the hospital or at home, whereas five limit coverage to the hospital. The major medical insurance plan for employees of New York State covers private-duty nursing, subject to a deductible clause.

Despite the inability of registries to fill requests, efforts to further the efficient use of private-duty nurses in hospitals by grouping patients and assigning one nurse or two or more patients have been confined to a few hospitals and have enjoyed limited success. As a result, private-duty nursing in the hospital costs the patient more than $50 a day. It would be advantageous to the community's interest if representatives of nurses, hospitals, and major purchasers of care would consult together in an effort to promote the more efficient use of private-duty nurses in hospitals.

Summary

1. Beginning with World War II there has been a "shortage" of registered nurses in hospitals in this country, in the sense that at prevailing salaries the number that would be hired exceeds the number available for employment. The shortage is the result of a more rapid increase in demand than in supply.

2. Adjustments to the shortage have taken a number of forms, including the transfer of certain functions from the nursing department to other departments of the hospital, employment of increasing numbers of part-time registered nurses, and, most important, employment of increasing numbers of auxiliary nursing personnel, including practical nurses. These adjustments have created problems of management and supervision.

3. In New York City in the mid-1950s the number of registered nurses rose in voluntary hospitals and declined in municipal

hospitals. In the latter the slow decline has been coupled with increasing activity in several hospitals, which calls for additional, not fewer, nurses.

4. In the general-care hospitals in New York City there were 35,000 persons staffing the nursing services in 1958, composed of 38 percent registered nurses, 17 percent practical nurses, and 45 percent nurses' aides and others. The proportion of registered nurses is lower than in the country as a whole.

5. The ratios of total nursing personnel per 100 patients (average daily census) are close in the two major hospital systems in New York City. The differences are a higher ratio of registered nurses in the voluntary system and a higher ratio of nurses' aides in the municipal system. The difference in the ratio of registered nurses to patients is widened if student nurses and private-duty nurses are counted.

6. The distribution of hospitals by the ratio of registered nurses to patients shows that the differences in aggregates between the two systems reflect differences among the large majority of members. In the voluntary system the larger nursing services and services in teaching hospitals have the higher ratios of registered nurses to patients. This is not true in the municipal system. In the latter system, unlike the voluntary, hospitals with schools of nursing do not have higher ratios of registered nurses to patients than hospitals without schools.

7. There are no generally accepted standards for optimum staffing of a nursing service that can be applied without reference to the qualifications and experience of the staff and the organization of the service. However, application of alternate criteria shows that a much larger proportion of voluntary hospitals than of municipal hospitals meet a specified standard.

8. A number of suggestions are made to help overcome the special disadvantages hampering the municipal hospital system. These include: authority to hire nurses at a salary above the minimum set for the position; authority to pay for overtime; raising the differentials for evening and night tours; arrangements for improved bus transportation to certain hospitals; and acquisition of apartments for nurses at moderate rental, including subsidization by the City, if necessary.

9. The hospital school of nursing has become a source of net cost to the hospital rather than of net income, as in the past. The main justification of such a school today is the availability of its graduates to staff the sponsoring hospital's nursing service, at least for the first year after graduation.

10. There has been an increase in the number of private-duty nurses in hospitals in New York City. It is estimated that expenditures for private-duty nursing in these hospitals amount to $25 million a year—$18 million in voluntary hospitals and $7 million in proprietary hospitals. Most of these expenditures are paid by patients. When medically indicated, private-duty nursing in hospitals should be covered as a benefit by voluntary health insurance plans. Efforts should also be exerted to make more efficient use of private-duty nurses in hospitals.

Appendix 7.A

COUNTING NURSING PERSONNEL AND STUDENTS
IN SCHOOLS OF NURSING IN HOSPITALS
IN NEW YORK CITY

NUMBER OF NURSES

1958. The data for the key year 1958 derive from the annual questionnaire submitted by hospitals to the American Hospital Association, copies of which were made available to the Hospital Council by the New York State Hospital Association. The data are intended to reflect staffing in the payroll period closest to September 30.

The data for municipal hospitals were complete as submitted. For voluntary hospitals several questionnaires were missing in 1958, and data from the questionnaires filed in 1957 were substituted. Only two thirds of the proprietary hospitals submitted personnel information, and the remaining one third were estimated in relation to bed capacity.

1957. The procedure was the same as in 1958.

1954. All data for this year derive from *A Survey of Nursing Personnel Resources in Hospitals in New York State.*[48] They are intended to refer to the staffing of inpatient services in general hospitals; in this instance general appears to stand for general care.

Earlier Years: Voluntary Hospitals. For the year 1938 data are taken from the annual published report of the United Hospital Fund of New York. Data for 1940–48 are unpublished, taken from the files of the New York State Hospital Study. Data for 1953 are also from the United Hospital Fund.[49]

Earlier Years: Municipal Hospitals. Data are taken from the annual reports of the Department of Hospitals. In several instances numbers were calculated from percentages and percentage changes given in the published reports. Data from the files of the New York State Hospital Study could not be used, because authorized positions were frequently reported in place of filled positions.

NUMBER OF STUDENTS IN SCHOOLS OF NURSING

1957. For the key year 1957 the data are taken from an unpublished table furnished by the University of the State of New York.[50]

Trends. For voluntary hospitals data for the 1940s are taken from the files of the New York State Hospital Study. For 1953 and later years they are available from a United Hospital Fund report.[51] Students in schools for practical nurses were excluded.

For municipal hospitals data are taken from the annual reports of the Department, supplemented by unpublished information provided by the Department's Director of Nursing Education and Nursing Service.

Appendix 7.B

COST OF A NURSING SCHOOL TO A HOSPITAL

There are many indications that the net cost of nursing education to the hospital has increased. One set of indications is the opinions expressed by hospital administrators who conduct such schools. They point to the reduced hours of service rendered by students, on the one hand, and the higher costs of instruction due to raised standards, on the other hand. Another set of indications is found in the literature.

Five elements determine the net cost of a school of nursing to a hospital:

1. The direct expenditures of the school
2. The indirect expenditures allocated to the school
3. The cost of providing room and board for the students
4. The hospital's income from students' tuition and fees
5. The value of the services rendered by students

In an analysis of the costs of nursing education from society's standpoint item 3 should be neglected. Item 4 duplicates item 1 in part and should be disregarded. Item 5 serves to offset a sixth—missing—component, that is, earnings foregone by students.

For the purpose at hand the equation is this:

Net cost to the hospital = Σ (4,5) $-$ Σ (1,2,3).

Item 2 is usually questionable, but it is not of major importance. Item 5 has caused the most controversy and work. There are no studies available of this item for hospitals in New York City.

However, several studies of costs of hospital schools of nursing have recently been performed elsewhere. These are assembled in Table 7.3.

Table 7.3. ANNUAL COST AND INCOME PER HOSPITAL STUDENT NURSE (IN DOLLARS)

Item	United Hospital Fund Member General Hospitals, 1957	Newport Hospital, 1957	Connecticut Hospitals, 1957	Illinois Hospitals, 1958	Cook County Hospitals, 1958
1. Direct cost, school	725	735	750	1,162	1,148
2. Allocated cost, school	n.a.	313	} 1,550	268	276
3. Cost of room and board	1,107	954		1,190	1,230
4. Tuition and fees	105	112	150	189	186
5. Value of student's services	n.a.	969	1,050	811	922
Net cost, school	n.a.	921	1,100	1,620	1,546

SOURCE: United Hospital Fund member general hospitals—United Hospital Fund of New York, *Sundry Financial and Statistical Information Relating to Hospitals in New York City, December 31, 1957* (New York, 1958), for room and board; its *Analysis of Direct Departmental Expenses, Supplement 1, Financial Statistical Analysis, Year 1957* (New York 1958), for direct cost; and unpublished information, for tuition and fees.

Newport Hospital, R.I.—William K. Turner, "Financing Nursing Education—an Unfair Burden for 1,100 Hospitals," *Hospitals*, XXXIII, No. 19 (October 1, 1959), 42.

Connecticut hospitals—*ibid.*, pp. 43–44.

Illinois and Cook County hospitals—Illinois Hospital Association, *Report on 1958 School of Nursing Cost Study*, I (Chicago, 1959), p. 3.

The corresponding items for voluntary hospitals in New York City are shown, when available.

It seems that the cost figures developed elsewhere do not depart greatly from the corresponding items in New York City.

8 CONDITION OF PLANT AND EXPENDITURES FOR CONSTRUCTION

In this chapter the condition of physical plant in the three hospital ownership groups is compared and the capability of the owners to improve and expand such plant is assessed in light of past achievement. The first part of the chapter deals with changes in the suitability of buildings with patients' beds, size of hospital, and size of patients' accommodations. The second part deals with expenditures for construction. Comparisons are made between New York City and the United States in the distribution of capital expenditures by hospital ownership and by source of funds.

Suitability of Plant

Medicine of high quality is known to have been practiced in wartime under extremely adverse front line conditions and in temporary shelters. Even then it was preferred, if possible, to postpone definitive treatment until the patient reached a fixed facility behind the lines. Under peacetime conditions a well-designed, well-constructed, well-equipped, and well-maintained plant makes an important contribution to the provision of safe and good hospital care. Historically, the determination of the volume, location, and quality of physical facilities has been the core of community planning for hospital care.

Evaluation of physical plant is a time-consuming and painstaking process that must include field work. Self-reporting by hospitals according to stated criteria is not likely to yield uniform data.

The comparison of plant between voluntary and municipal hospitals presented here rests mainly on its suitability for long-range planning, as defined below. Nothing was to be gained by comparing the two hospital systems in range of facilities, such as laboratory, x-ray, or recovery room, because in New York City nearly every hospital has a wide range of facilities.

Criteria of Suitability. Criteria of suitability for a hospital building have evolved over the years. When the *Master Plan for Hospitals and Related Facilities for New York City* was prepared in the mid-1940s, an unsuitable building for patients was essentially one that was not of fire-resistive construction. In a few instances small buildings incapable of expansion or not originally built as hospitals were also classified as unsuitable. Although age was not directly employed as a basis of classification, it was sometimes regarded as an indication of obsolescence.[1]

Today a non-fire-resistive building is still classified as unsuitable. Criteria for measuring the degree of fire resistiveness have become explicit and definite. For example, according to one set of standards structures are expected to have a two-hour fire rating or better.[2] When a building is classified as fire resistive, it may still be unsuitable for other reasons, which are subsumed under the concept of major inadequacy.

Reliability of Bed Count. The volume of services a hospital can render to inpatients is conveyed by its bed capacity. This is the number of beds a hospital was designed for.[3] A change in bed capacity should reflect a structural change of permanent character, not a temporary or emergency shifting of beds.

Except in hospitals that have received a Hill-Burton grant (explained later in this chapter), the counting of bed capacity in voluntary and municipal hospitals remains within the discretion of the individual hospital. It can change its bed count at will, because it need not apply uniform standards. Under existing circumstances a comparison of bed capacities between hospital systems is not as meaningful as it should—and can—be made by measurement.[4]

Recently the Hospital Council of Greater New York began a

survey, designed to measure hospital bed capacity according to uniform criteria of space, as developed by the United States Public Health Service, and according to uniform instructions for including and excluding certain areas, as developed by the New York State Joint Hospital Survey and Planning Commission (now the Division of Hospital Review and Planning of the State Department of Health). A leeway of 10 percent was allowed.[5]

Preliminary findings show that there is considerable variation among hospitals in the size of the difference between the number of beds routinely reported by a hospital and that determined by the survey. In a few hospitals the result of the survey was a small upward adjustment in bed capacity, but in most instances the adjustment was downward. The latter ranged widely, from a reduction of 2 percent to one as high as 40 percent. The apparent overstatement of bed capacity appears to be greater in voluntary than in municipal hospitals. It may be that the overstatement will prove to be greater in unsuitable buildings than in suitable ones.

The hospitals initially surveyed are not a representative sample of the hospitals in New York City. It is premature to anticipate the adjustment in total bed count that would result from a complete survey. The need for caution in comparing reported bed figures between hospital systems or from year to year is, however, obvious.

TOTAL HOSPITAL BEDS IN SUITABLE BUILDINGS, *1945* AND *1958*

The number of beds in a hospital is usually taken as an index of size with respect to all services, not only for inpatients. The concept of the hospital bed is analogous to that of the division slice in the military, that is, the bed stands also for the various supporting and associated facilities.

The year 1945 is the first for which complete data were developed on the number of beds in suitable and unsuitable patients' buildings; this was done in connection with the preparation of the *Master Plan*. Table 8.1 shows the distribution of all hospital beds in New York City by ownership at the end of 1945 and 1958. Nearly one half of the increase of 5,300 beds was contributed by municipal hospitals. The increase in beds in suitable buildings was 9,900, far above that in total beds. The difference

Table 8.1. DISTRIBUTION OF TOTAL BED CAPACITY * BY
HOSPITAL OWNERSHIP, NEW YORK CITY,
1945 AND 1958

Ownership	1945		1958		Increase, 1945–58	
	Number	Percent	Number	Percent	Number	Percent
All hospitals	42,754	100.0	48,056	100.0	5,302	100.0
Voluntary	23,175	54.2	24,885	51.8	1,710	32.2
Municipal	15,876	37.1	18,415	38.3	2,539	47.9
Proprietary	3,703	8.7	4,756	9.9	1,053	19.9

* Excludes beds in public-home infirmary and nursing-home units of hospitals.
SOURCE: Hospital Council of Greater New York.

is accounted for by the decline of 4,600 beds in unsuitable buildings. Municipal hospitals contributed nearly one half of the increase in beds in suitable buildings. Voluntary hospitals contributed a larger proportion of the increase in beds in suitable
buildings than in total beds, and the converse was true of proprietary hospitals.

Table 8.2. DISTRIBUTION OF TOTAL BED CAPACITY * IN SUIT-
ABLE BUILDINGS BY HOSPITAL OWNERSHIP,
NEW YORK CITY, 1945 AND 1958

Ownership	1945		1958		Increase, 1945–58	
	Number	Percent	Number	Percent	Number	Percent
All hospitals	30,306	100.0	40,223	100.0	9,917	100.0
Voluntary	16,617	54.8	20,502	51.0	3,885	39.2
Municipal	11,316	37.4	16,094	40.0	4,778	48.2
Proprietary	2,373	7.8	3,627	9.0	1,254	12.6

* Excludes beds in public-home infirmary and nursing-home units of hospitals.
SOURCE: Hospital Council of Greater New York.

It is possible to classify the beds in unsuitable buildings in
1945 and in 1958 by cause of unsuitability. Three designations
are employed: non-fire-resistive, obsolete, and "not built as a hospital." These categories are mutually exclusive in the data
presented below, with non-fire-resistiveness receiving priority in
classification over "not built as a hospital" and the latter over
obsolescence.

There were 12,450 beds in unsuitable buildings in 1945, of
which one fifth were obsolete. In 1958 there were 7,830 beds in
unsuitable buildings, of which one fourth were obsolete. The
1945 data reflect, however, a retroactive, rather than contem-

porary, evaluation of plant. They incorporate the findings of later surveys of physical plant by the Hospital Council, which in some instances yielded results substantially different from the original evaluations.

Table 8.3 distributes three bed totals by reason of unsuitability. Column *1* for 1945 shows the bed figures according to the original classification and column *2* for 1945 shows them in light of subsequent reclassification. Column *3* is for the year 1958.

Table 8.3. DISTRIBUTION OF TOTAL BED CAPACITY * IN UNSUITABLE HOSPITAL BUILDINGS BY REASON OF UNSUITABILITY, NEW YORK CITY, 1945 AND 1958

| | 1945 | | | | | |
| | (1) Original Classification | | (2) Retroactive Classification | | (3) 1958 | |
Reason for Unsuitability	Number	Percent	Number	Percent	Number	Percent
All hospitals	10,183	100.0	12,448	100.0	7,833	100.0
Non-fire-resistive	9,393	92.3	9,610	77.2	5,485	70.0
Not built as hospital	227	2.2	366	2.9	340	4.4
Obsolete	563	5.5	2,472	19.9	2,008	25.6

* Excludes beds in public-home infirmary and nursing-home units of hospitals.
SOURCE: Hospital Council of Greater New York.

Obsolescence has gained in importance as a reason for classifying hospital buildings as unsuitable. This is not the result of increased obsolescence of plant but is largely due to a change in criteria. In 1945, as plants were then evaluated, 560 beds, or 6 percent of all unsuitable beds, were in obsolescent buildings. In 1958, under modern criteria of evaluation, 2,000 beds, or one quarter of all unsuitable beds, were in obsolescent buildings. When the modern criteria are applied retroactively to 1945, the number of beds in obsolescent buildings at that time rises to 2,470.

What are the modern criteria of obsolescence? In 1956 the Hospital Council had occasion to apply stated criteria in uniform fashion to one large group of voluntary hospitals, the member hospitals of the United Hospital Fund. Patients' buildings were classified as having a major inadequacy if their defective conditions could only be corrected at excessive cost, that is, a cost equal to or larger than that of equivalent new construction. When structures not built as hospitals are excluded, the classification of major inadequacy comprises buildings with partly open stairwells or elevator shafts, buildings with narrow bays, narrow corridors, small rooms, and small elevators, buildings for patients located at a distance from the main hospital, and buildings with small, inefficient nursing units of 10 or 12 patient beds on a floor. Several hospitals have succeeded in eliminating all or some of these faults in old buildings through extensive reconstruction.[6]

Ancillary facilities were assessed from the standpoint both of adequacy (space) and obsolescence (status of equipment).

GENERAL-CARE BEDS IN SUITABLE BUILDINGS, *1945* AND *1958*

General-care beds accounted for 3,600 of the increase of 5,300 in total beds, or two thirds. Sixty percent of the increase was contributed by voluntary hospitals and 18 percent by municipal hospitals. These proportions are much higher for voluntary hospitals and lower for municipal hospitals than those shown in Table 8.1 for total hospitals beds.

Table 8.4. DISTRIBUTION OF GENERAL-CARE BED CAPACITY BY HOSPITAL OWNERSHIP, NEW YORK CITY, 1945 AND 1958

	1945		1958		Increase, 1945–58	
Ownership	Number	Percent	Number	Percent	Number	Percent
All hospitals	33,180	100.0	36,766	100.0	3,586	100.0
Voluntary	19,584	59.0	21,723	59.1	2,139	59.7
Municipal	10,176	30.7	10,816	29.4	640	17.8
Proprietary	3,420	10.3	4,227	11.5	807	22.5

SOURCE: Hospital Council of Greater New York.

The increase in general-care beds in suitable buildings was 6,650, or 3,050 more than in total general-care beds. The latter is equal to the number of general-care beds in unsuitable buildings that were eliminated. (On the basis of other studies conducted by the Hospital Council, it is clear that more than 1,000 beds in suitable buildings must also have been displaced in the process of construction and reconstruction.[7] This sometimes happens when old buildings are converted to use as ancillary facilities.)

The distribution of the increase by hospital ownership reverses that in Table 8.2 for all hospital beds. In general care voluntary

Table 8.5. DISTRIBUTION OF GENERAL-CARE BED CAPACITY IN SUITABLE BUILDINGS BY HOSPITAL OWNERSHIP, NEW YORK CITY, 1945 AND 1958

	1945		1958		Increase, 1945–58	
Ownership	Number	Percent	Number	Percent	Number	Percent
All hospitals	24,079	100.0	30,722	100.0	6,643	100.0
Voluntary	14,388	59.7	17,634	57.4	3,246	48.9
Municipal	7,318	30.4	9,725	31.7	2,407	36.2
Proprietary	2,373	9.9	3,363	10.9	990	14.9

SOURCE: Hospital Council of Greater New York.

hospitals play the larger role. Even so, they failed to maintain the proportion of all general-care beds in suitable plant that they held in 1945.

The proportion of general-care beds in suitable buildings improved in each hospital system. The greatest improvement occurred in municipal hospitals and the smallest in voluntary hospitals. Over-all, the proportion of general-care beds in unsuitable buildings declined from 30 to 16 percent.

Table 8.6. PROPORTION OF GENERAL-CARE BED CAPACITY IN SUITABLE BUILDINGS BY HOSPITAL OWNERSHIP, NEW YORK CITY, 1945 AND 1958

Ownership	1945 (Percent)	1958 (Percent)
All hospitals	70.5	83.6
Voluntary	73.5	81.2
Municipal	72.0	89.8
Proprietary	69.3	79.5

SOURCE: Tables 8.4 and 8.5.

According to Table 8.6, nine tenths of all general-care beds in municipal hospitals in 1958 were in suitable buildings. This figure understates the volume of new construction still needed because the criterion of plant evaluation here employed is essentially that of fire resistiveness. Similarly, the proprietary hospitals' proportion of beds in suitable buildings may be lower than shown, because their plants have not yet been evaluated according to the modern criteria of obsolescence.

LONG-TERM BEDS IN SUITABLE BUILDINGS, 1945 AND 1958

Whereas general-care beds increased by 3,600 between 1945 and 1958, long-term beds (excluding those in nursing-home or public-home infirmary units) increased only by 1,700. There was actually a decline in the voluntary system, resulting from the reclassification by two hospitals of certain beds for the chronically ill to general care.

Table 8.7. DISTRIBUTION OF LONG-TERM BED CAPACITY *
BY HOSPITAL OWNERSHIP, NEW YORK CITY,
1945 AND 1958

Ownership	1945		1958		Change, 1945–58	
	Number	Percent	Number	Percent	Number	Percent
All hospitals	9,574	100.0	11,290	100.0	+1,716	+100.0
Voluntary	3,591	37.5	3,162	28.0	– 429	– 25.0
Municipal	5,700	59.5	7,599	67.3	+1,899	+110.7
Proprietary	283	3.0	529	4.7	+ 246	+ 14.3

* Excludes beds in public-home infirmary and nursing-home units of hospitals.
SOURCE: Hospital Council of Greater New York.

The increase in long-term beds in suitable buildings was almost double the increase in total long term beds. The municipal system was, and is increasingly, predominant in the field of long-term care, even with public-home infirmaries excluded. One half of the total increase in suitable beds in municipal hospitals between 1945 and 1958 was devoted to long-term care, compared with 16 percent in voluntary hospitals and 21 percent in proprietary hospitals.

Table 8.8. DISTRIBUTION OF LONG-TERM BED CAPACITY * IN
SUITABLE BUILDINGS BY HOSPITAL OWNERSHIP,
NEW YORK CITY, 1945 AND 1958

Ownership	1945		1958		Increase, 1945–58	
	Number	Percent	Number	Percent	Number	Percent
All hospitals	6,227	100.0	9,501	100.0	3,274	100.0
Voluntary	2,229	35.8	2,868	30.2	639	19.5
Municipal	3,998	64.2	6,369	67.0	2,371	72.4
Proprietary	0	0	264	2.8	264	8.1

* Excludes beds in public-home infirmary and nursing-home units of hospitals.
SOURCE: Hospital Council of Greater New York.

MINIMUM SIZE OF GENERAL HOSPITAL

The *Master Plan for Hospitals and Related Facilities* states: "There is little justification for the establishment of general hospitals of less than 200 beds in New York City." [8] In designating participating hospitals in the *Master Plan*, the Hospital Council later extended the principle to existing institutions.

In 1957 the Hospital Council inquired into the progress achieved in carrying out the recommendations of the *Master Plan*.[9] Table 8.9 for December, 1943, and December, 1956, shows changes in the numbers of hospitals and of beds by size of hospital. Between 1943 and 1956 the total number of general-care hospitals in New York City declined by 9, but the number of hospitals with fewer than 200 beds declined by 21. More than one half of all general-care hospitals in New York City were still below this size.

Table 8.9. DISTRIBUTION OF ALL GENERAL-CARE HOSPITALS AND THEIR BED CAPACITIES BY SIZE OF HOSPITAL, NEW YORK CITY, 1943 AND 1956

Size of Hospital (Number of Beds)	Number of Hospitals			Number of Beds		
	1943	*1956*	*Change*	*1943*	*1956*	*Change*
All hospitals	*149*	*140*	*– 9*	*34,963*	*41,618*	*+ 6,655*
0– 99	56	40	– 16	2,887	2,391	– 496
100–199	41	36	– 5	5,945	5,228	– 717
200–399	32	37	+ 5	8,856	10,102	+ 1,246
400 and over	20	27	+ 7	17,275	23,897	+ 6,622

SOURCE: Hospital Council of Greater New York.

The total number of beds in general-care hospitals—all their beds, including those for long-term patients—increased by 6,650, whereas the number of beds in hospitals with fewer than 200 beds decreased by 1,200. As a result, the proportion of beds in the smaller hospitals fell from 25 to 18 percent.

Municipal general-care hospitals are of moderate or large size. Their average (mean) bed capacity was 830 beds in 1943 and 880 in 1956. Voluntary general-care hospitals in New York City have tended to be smaller on the average, and proprietary hospitals still smaller. Between 1943 and 1956 the average bed capacity of voluntary hospitals rose from 230 to 280 beds and of proprietary hospitals from 70 to 106. It is interesting that all of the net decline in bed capacity in hospitals with fewer than 100 beds occurred in proprietary hospitals. By contrast, the net decline of 700 beds in the next size group was the resultant of a decline of 1,750 beds in voluntary hospitals and an increase of 1,050 beds in proprietary hospitals.

A distribution of hospitals by size in each ownership group shows that in 1956 almost all proprietary hospitals and 34 of 79 voluntary hospitals had fewer than 200 beds. The 7,600 beds located in hospitals with fewer than 200 beds are divided almost equally between voluntary and proprietary hospitals.

Table 8.10. DISTRIBUTION OF VOLUNTARY, MUNICIPAL, AND PROPRIETARY GENERAL-CARE HOSPITALS AND THEIR BED CAPACITIES BY SIZE OF HOSPITAL, NEW YORK CITY, 1956

Size of Hospital (*Number of Beds*)	*Voluntary*		*Municipal*		*Proprietary*	
	Number	*Percent*	*Number*	*Percent*	*Number*	*Percent*
Hospitals						
Total	79	100.0	17	100.0	44	100.0
0– 99	17	21.5	0	0	23	52.3
100–199	17	21.5	1	5.9	18	40.9
200–399	30	38.0	5	29.4	2	4.5
400 and over	15	19.0	11	64.7	1	2.3
Bed capacity						
Total	21,982	100.0	14,974	100.0	4,662	100.0
0–99	1,190	5.4	0	0	1,201	25.7
100–199	2,641	12.1	166	1.1	2,421	51.9
200–399	8,216	37.4	1,366	9.1	520	11.2
400 and over	9,935	45.1	13,442	89.8	520	11.2

SOURCE: Hospital Council of Greater New York.

FLEXIBILITY IN USE OF HOSPITAL ACCOMMODATIONS

The *Master Plan* provides for "complete flexibility" in use between ward and semiprivate accommodations. It states: "Physical facilities for both of these groups may be identical." [10] Under this principle the Hospital Council has recommended that patients' rooms in voluntary hospitals should be built for four beds or fewer.

Unpublished data are available comparing the number of rooms by size of accommodation in voluntary general-care hospitals in 1946 and in 1954. Although complete information is not available for subsequent years, it is known that progress toward the elimination of large wards has continued.

In 1954, 756 of the single rooms were not reported as private rooms. Presumably they were used for semiprivate and ward patients in need of privacy or isolation. Between 1946 and 1954

Table 8.11. DISTRIBUTION OF BEDS IN VOLUNTARY GENERAL-CARE HOSPITALS BY SIZE OF ACCOMMODATION, NEW YORK CITY, 1946 AND 1954

Room Size (Number of Beds)	Number of Beds in Each Room Size			Cumulative Number of Beds in Each Room Size and All Those Below It		
	1946	1954	Change 1946–54	1946	1954	Change 1946–54
1	3,879	3,892	+ 13	3,879	3,892	+ 13
2	3,268	4,634	+ 1,366	7,147	8,526	+ 1,379
3	1,098	1,344	+ 246	8,245	9,870	+ 1,625
4	2,056	3,580	+ 1,524	10,301	13,450	+ 3,149
5	1,075	855	– 220	11,376	14,305	+ 2,929
6	852	894	+ 42	12,228	15,199	+ 2,971
7	273	392	+ 119	12,501	15,591	+ 3,090
8	576	568	– 8	13,077	16,159	+ 3,082
9 and over	6,405	5,211	– 1,194	19,482	21,370	+ 1,888
Total beds	19,482	21,370	+ 1,888			

SOURCE: New York State Public Works Planning Commission Joint Hospital Board, Hospital Schedule of Information, 1946, in possession of Hospital Council of Greater New York; and Hospital Council, annual inventory.

the number of large wards—nine beds or more—declined from 456 to 348. The average number of beds in the remaining wards increased slightly, from 14 to 15. Total beds in these hospitals increased by 1,900. This was accomplished mainly by an increase of 2,900 beds in two- and four-bed rooms and by an offsetting decline of 1,200 beds in large wards.

In the postwar period new construction in municipal hospitals has emphasized four- and six-bed rooms. The aim of flexibility here is not to meet changing economic conditions, as in voluntary hospitals, but to raise the rate of occupancy by reducing rigidity in the use of rooms resulting from segregation of patients by sex and by clinical service.

Expenditures for Hospital Construction

One way in which a hospital or group of hospitals demonstrates vitality is through improving and expanding physical facilities. Today capital improvement requires large sums of money. Completely new hospital construction costs about $25,000 per bed or $36 per square foot.[11] Construction or reconstruction in an existing building may cost more or less than this amount, depending on the type of work involved.

Estimates of expenditures for hospital construction by owner-ship group were developed for the period 1945–56. The resulting totals were checked against an independent set of estimates, and the discrepancy between the two aggregates for the entire period came to 2 percent (see Appendix 8.A).

The annual estimates of expenditures by each hospital owner-ship group are presented in Table 8.16. The analysis is limited to voluntary, municipal, and proprietary hospitals, except when it is desirable to introduce state and federal hospitals, in order to obtain comparability between the city and the country as a whole. For convenience, the analysis deals with data for intervals of four years.

Table 8.12 shows that the three hospital ownership groups differed in the timing of expenditures for hospital construction in the postwar period. In the first period proprietary hospitals spent 22 percent of their total postwar expenditures for construc-tion, whereas voluntary hospitals spent less than 10 percent. In the third period proprietary hospitals spent approximately the same proportion of their postwar total as in the first, but voluntary hospitals spent 42 percent of theirs.

Table 8.12. DISTRIBUTION OF EXPENDITURES FOR CONSTRUC-TION BY FOUR-YEAR PERIODS AND BY HOSPITAL OWNERSHIP, NEW YORK CITY, 1945–56 (IN THOUSANDS OF DOLLARS)

Time	Voluntary		Municipal		Proprietary	
Interval	Amount	Percent	Amount	Percent	Amount	Percent
Total	162,803	100.0	225,062	100.0	19,284	100.0
1945–48	14,317	8.8	31,245	14.0	4,160	21.6
1949–52	80,936	49.7	129,944	57.6	10,746	55.7
1953–56	67,550	41.5	63,873	28.4	4,378	22.7

SOURCE: Table 8.16.

Table 8.16 shows that the peak effort by municipal hospitals was made in the early 1950s. Proprietary hospitals reached peak expenditures about the same time or slightly earlier. Voluntary hospitals show a sustained effort. Beginning in 1949 their expendi-tures fluctuate considerably, but the trend line is constant. It should be added for the period after 1956, from general knowledge of activity in hospital construction in New York City, that voluntary hospitals are still maintaining a sustained effort; municipal hospitals are entering another period of major expenditures; and proprietary hospitals, after a period of relative inactivity, are building new institutions at a rapid rate.

For each group of hospitals certain factors help to explain the pattern of expenditures for construction. When the war ended proprietary hospitals were able to get under way fairly quickly, because they are owned by single proprietors or partners or small groups of stockholders and presumably can quickly reach a decision to build. Mortgage money was more readily available to hospitals operated for profit than to nonprofit hospitals. In addition, cost per bed is lower than in the voluntary or municipal system because area per bed tends to be smaller and the ratio of space for ancillary services to space for nursing units is also lower. An undertaking of a given size requires less money under proprietary auspices than it would under other auspices. Moreover, the typical proprietary undertaking tends to be small and requires a small investment. Finally, proprietary hospitals rely more than voluntary or municipal hospitals on converting existing buildings into hospitals, and this again is cheaper than building new hospitals, though less adequate. (Incidentally, the cost of purchasing an existing building is not reflected in expenditures for construction, so that the data in this chapter tend to understate postwar capital investment in proprietary hospitals.)

Both the amount and timing of capital expenditures in the municipal system are affected by the expenditure of $150 million from a special bond issue outside of the City's debt limit. When this bond issue was approved in 1949, the City of New York had already appropriated $44 million for capital purposes during the postwar period. Altogether, the City appropriated $236 million for capital purposes ($225 million in Table 8.12, plus $11 million for the purchase of land and acquisition of existing plants) between 1945 and 1956. Of this, $42 million came from funds subject to the debt limit that were appropriated after the exempt funds had been committed.

In voluntary hospitals decisions to build are decentralized, as they are in the proprietary group, and fluctuations in construction expenditures tend to be random. Most voluntary hospitals in New York City rely on an appeal to the community for all or some of their capital funds. Such an appeal takes time to initiate, develop, and complete. The availability of federal grants under the Hill-Burton program has perhaps contributed a stabilizing influence, particularly in marginal cases where the decision to build was a difficult one.

RELATIVE IMPORTANCE OF THREE OWNERSHIP GROUPS

The relative importance of the three hospital ownership groups in expenditures for construction has varied from period to period. Table 8.13 shows expenditures for 1945–56 and also for an earlier period, 1920–44. The data for 1920–44 are unpublished estimates that the Hospital Council prepared in 1948 for the New York State Hospital Study. The latter show all expenditures for a project in the year of completion of construction rather than in the year of contract award. In splicing these data with those for 1945–56 care was taken to avoid duplication.

Table 8.13. DISTRIBUTION OF EXPENDITURES FOR CONSTRUCTION IN SELECTED TIME INTERVALS BY HOSPITAL OWNERSHIP, NEW YORK CITY, 1920–56 (IN THOUSANDS OF DOLLARS)

Time Interval	Total		Voluntary		Municipal		Proprietary	
	Amount	Per-cent	Amount	Per-cent	Amount	Per-cent	Amount	Per-cent
1920–29	83,049	100.0	60,575	73.0	13,509	16.2	8,965	10.8
1930–34	47,121	100.0	31,648	67.2	14,373	30.5	1,100	2.3
1935–44	55,511	100.0	22,543	40.6	31,698	57.1	1,270	2.3
Total: 1920–44	185,681	100.0	114,766	61.8	59,580	32.1	11,335	6.1
1945–48	49,722	100.0	14,317	28.8	31,245	62.8	4,160	8.4
1949–52	221,626	100.0	80,936	36.5	129,944	58.7	10,746	4.8
1953–56	135,801	100.0	67,550	49.8	63,873	47.0	4,378	3.2
Total: 1945–56	407,149	100.0	162,803	40.0	225,062	55.3	19,284	4.7

SOURCE: Hospital Council of Greater New York and Table 8.16.

Construction activity by proprietary hospitals achieved its greatest importance immediately after the two wars. It was least important during the depression and World War II.

Voluntary hospitals no longer have the major share of capital expenditures, as they once did. The role of municipal hospitals has increased. However, their capital expenditures fluctuate more than those of voluntary hospitals.

The dollar amounts should not be taken at face value. The cost of hospital construction tripled between 1920 and 1956, according to the New York City Construction Cost Index published by the City's Department of Public Works.[12] When money expenditures are deflated by this index, expenditures in constant dollars come to roughly the same totals in the two periods, 1920–44 and 1945–56. The average annual rate of expenditure was, therefore, twice as great in the latter—shorter—period. It should be noted that in the depression and war years hospital construction expenditures were minimal.

APPRAISAL OF ACCOMPLISHMENTS AND ASSESSMENT OF NEED

Index of Accomplishment. For a number of reasons it is difficult to compare the accomplishments of the three hospital systems through their expenditures for construction. These reasons are (1) differences in cost of construction at the time of expenditures; (2) differences among the systems in size; (3) differences in the proportion of expenditures devoted to plant rehabilitation or improvement of plant, compared with new construction; and (4) differences in types of facility built—inpatient buildings or outpatient departments, laboratories, and so forth.

For this report a single index of plant renewal was developed, by converting all expenditures for improvement into equivalents of expenditures for new beds. The number of new bed equivalents was computed by dividing for each year the amount spent for hospital construction by the then current cost per bed (see Appendix 8.B).

The proportion of present plant "renewed" during the postwar period follows for each hospital system:

Ownership	*Percent "Renewed"*
Voluntary	33
Municipal	57
Proprietary	35

Whereas voluntary and proprietary hospitals "renewed" one third of their plant during the postwar period, municipal hospitals "renewed" more than one half of theirs. This considerable achievement was made possible by the special bond issue of $150 million.

Replacement, Rehabilitation, and Maintenance of Plant. The index of plant renewal is an indication of expenditure activity during a specified period and is not an index of the quality of plant. Certain observations regarding the condition of physical plant in voluntary and municipal hospitals follow.

In a survey of the member hospitals of the United Hospital Fund in 1956, the Hospital Council found that $180 million were needed to bring the facilities into satisfactory condition, prior to any provision for expansion in program. By then these hospitals had spent $150 million for capital purposes during the postwar period. Slightly more than one half of the $180 million was needed to replace hospitals unsuitable for long-range planning, either due to non-fire-resistive construction or to major and irremediable inadequacies in design. Nearly one half of the total was needed to raise to a satisfactory condition buildings that were —and are today—classified as suitable for long-range planning in accordance with modern standards. The latter comes to 18 percent of the cost of replacing these beds and is an indication of the extent of obsolescence in suitable buildings.

In municipal hospitals there remain only three major projects to replace hospitals with buildings classified as unsuitable. These have been scheduled in the City's Capital Budget or Capital Program for the next five years at a total cost of $135 million. Neither the Budget nor Program constitutes a commitment to spend money for building.[13] It would appear from surveys that the Hospital Council has made in the past year that several hospitals with buildings currently classified as suitable will also require replacement within the decade, if they continue in use.

One of the major problems facing municipal hospitals is inadequacy of plant maintenance. The range in quality of maintenance is wide, but only one or two hospitals have very good maintenance, whereas the majority have poor maintenance. Even new buildings exhibit premature deterioration.

The Hospital Council's observations on the municipal hospitals agree substantially with the findings of the City Administrator in a recent report.[14] He cites a number of deficiencies, among which are the following: need of paint in older buildings and of protective coating for certain materials in new buildings; absence of a preventive maintenance program in all but three institutions; a backlog of needed repair and maintenance jobs throughout the system; and faults in plumbing, heating, and ventilating systems. The principal finding is that widespread deterioration and obsolescence of plant exist as a result of unsatisfactory maintenance policies.

COMPARISON OF NEW YORK CITY WITH UNITED STATES

Data recently prepared by the United States Public Health Service permit comparisons of expenditures for hospital construction between New York City and the nation.

Expenditures for Hospital Construction, United States, 1948–57. The new nation-wide figures show higher expenditures than are usually reported, because the value of construction put in place has been augmented by other costs associated with building. Movable equipment is excluded.

Table 8.14 compares expenditures for hospital construction in New York City and in the nation by hospital ownership. The data for New York City have been consolidated to conform to the detail published for the United States.

Table 8.14. DISTRIBUTION OF EXPENDITURES FOR CONSTRUC-
TION BY HOSPITAL OWNERSHIP, NEW YORK
CITY, 1945–56, AND UNITED STATES, 1948–57
(IN MILLIONS OF DOLLARS)

	New York City		United States	
Ownership	*Amount*	*Percent*	*Amount*	*Percent*
Total	490	100.0	8,480	100.0
Private (voluntary and proprietary)	182	37.2	3,990	47.1
Public	308	62.8	4,490	52.9
Federal	43	8.8	950	11.2
State and local	265	54.0	3,540	41.7

SOURCE: Hospital Council of Greater New York; U.S. Public Health Service, Division of Hospital and Medical Facilities, *Principles for Planning the Future Hospital System* (Washington, D.C., 1959), p. 221.

From the standpoint of hospital ownership, the largest difference between New York City and the United States is in the relative importance of State and local government hospitals. New

York City is higher by 12 percentage points. Correspondingly, the United States is 10 percentage points higher in the expenditures of private hospitals (voluntary plus proprietary).

Expenditures by private hospitals in the United States cannot be separated into voluntary and proprietary, but an approximate division can be made between State and local hospitals. (This is done by projecting the distribution of beds among levels of government, as formerly reported by the American Medical Association in the annual "Hospital Service" issues of its *Journal,* and the growth in assets in mental hospitals, as reported annually by the American Hospital Association in the "Guide Issue" of *Hospitals.*) It is estimated that 45 percent of the construction expenditures reported by State and local government hospitals were incurred by the States; on this basis the State hospitals' share of total construction expenditures in the United States is 19 percent and that of local hospitals 23 percent. The latter is only one half the share of the construction expenditures of municipal hospitals in New York City, 46 percent.

Differences between the distributions of expenditures for construction by hospital ownership and by source of funds are attributable to the impact of federal construction grants under the Hill-Burton program and, less often, of associated grants by the states.

Table 8.15 compares expenditures for hospital construction by source of funds. The largest difference is in state and local tax funds, with New York City 16 percentage points higher. For local tax funds alone the difference is 27 percentage points—19 percent for the United States and 45.5 percent for New York City. The next largest difference is in federal funds—20 percent in the country as a whole compared with 11 in New York City. The smallest difference is in private funds—7 percentage points in favor of the United States. In this context private funds include philanthropic contributions.

For the member hospitals of the United Hospital Fund unpublished data show that philanthropic contributions to plant fund amounted to $60 million during the period 1949–56, or 44 percent of the estimated expenditures for construction, $136 million. The proportion of philanthropic contributions to con-

Table 8.15. DISTRIBUTION OF EXPENDITURES FOR CONSTRUC-
TION BY SOURCE OF FUNDS, NEW YORK CITY,
1945–56, AND UNITED STATES, 1948–57
(IN MILLIONS OF DOLLARS)

Source of Funds	New York City		United States	
	Amount	Percent	Amount	Percent
Total	490	100.0	8,480	100.0
Private *	172	35.1	3,565	42.1
Tax funds	318	64.9	4,915	57.9
Federal	55	11.2	1,690	19.9
State and local	263	53.7	3,225	38.0

* Includes income from philanthropy, mortgages, loans, net earnings of hospitals, etc.
SOURCE: Table 8.14, adjusted.

struction expenditures was 34 percent in the period 1949–52 and 58 percent in the period 1953–56. Income from philanthropy for operating purposes is not counted here, even where it was not needed to offset an operating deficit.

In the nation philanthropic funds amounted to one half of all private hospital construction until 1956. Although continuing to increase in amount, philanthropic funds were two fifths of private hospital construction in 1957 and 1958.[15] All of these proportions are too high, because the denominator includes only the value of construction put in place, prior to other costs associated with building. When these are considered, the proportion of philanthropy to total expenditures is reduced by 7 percentage points.

Relative Importance of Hill-Burton Grants. Shortly after World War II Congress enacted the Hospital Survey and Construction Act, known as the Hill-Burton Program. The objective was to assist nonprofit hospitals—both governmental, other than Federal, and voluntary—in building facilities according to a long range plan.

During the period 1948–57 Hill-Burton grants in the United States amounted to $740 million. Since the total cost of the projects aided was $2,300 million, federal participation came to 32 percent.[16] In several states there was additional assistance from the state government that amounted to another $95 million, or 4 percent of the cost of the projects aided. In New York City Hill-Burton grants amounted to approximately $12 million between the activation of the program and 1957. The total cost of the aided projects was approximately $58 million, and the proportion of federal participation in them was 20 percent.[17]

There are several reasons for this sizable difference between New York City and the nation in the degree of federal participation: (1) New York State is a high income state and receives a smaller grant per capita under the Hill-Burton formula than do states with low incomes; [18] (2) New York City is an urban area, and the Hill-Burton program was enacted to promote construction of hospitals in rural areas and of hospitals in cities that serve rural areas; (3) the degree of federal participation in an individual project is limited to one third in New York State but ranges between one third and two thirds in other states; and (4) standards of construction and building costs are comparatively high in New York City, so that any effort to limit the sum allocated to a given type of facility (such as psychiatry) in order to free funds for other types of facility tends to reduce the rate of federal participation in each category.

In relation to total nonfederal expenditures for hospital construction, Hill-Burton grants constitute 10 percent of the total in the United States and less than 3 percent in New York City. In view of the limited amount of Hill-Burton funds available here, the program has been directed toward a small number of high priority targets, both with respect to type of program and to the geographic distribution of hospital facilities. Early in the program a high priority was assigned to centers for premature infants and, more recently, to psychiatric units in general hospitals. Rehabilitation centers receive grants under their own category of funds. Geographically, a high priority was initially given to the rapidly growing borough of Queens, which was notably short of hospital beds in the late 1940s. In later years Queens shared the area priority with Staten Island and, more recently, with Brooklyn.

Both experience in administering the Hill-Burton program and field interviews indicate that in certain parts of the city it is extremely difficult or almost impossible to raise money for hospital construction by appeal to the community. In four of the boroughs, other than Manhattan, a Hill-Burton grant may make the difference between a hospital's building and not building.

If voluntary hospitals are to build and meet their community obligations in every part of the city, most of them will require some assistance from a central source, whether it be a sectarian federation, a denominational conference, or a government program. A joint appeal for philanthropic contributions for construction and development would be highly desirable.

Frequently, in order to demonstrate its ability to build—indeed, its very eligibility to receive a federal grant—a hospital assumes a heavy burden of debt. The Columbia University study of Blue Cross plans in New York State reports an increase in the amount of capital debt owed by short-term voluntary hospitals in the New York City area from $14.5 million in 1947 to $23.0 million in 1957.[19] The United Hospital Fund reports for its members general hospitals that mortgages outstanding plus notes and accounts payable by Plant Fund rose from $12 million in 1947 to $20 million in 1954 and subsequently declined to $15 million in 1958.[20] It is possible that there has been a greater increase in capital debt in the suburbs than in New York City.

In the future, capital replacement, if not totally new construction, is likely to be financed in part by income from patients. When the new Blue Cross reimbursement formula was adopted, a payment for depreciation was included for those hospitals that agreed to set it aside in a special fund. Since the daily allowance for depreciation is geared to patient-day cost, it contains a factor of built in protection against inflation in construction costs.

Summary

1. Counts of bed capacity, as reported by hospitals, do not reflect uniform criteria. Preliminary findings of a Hospital Council survey suggest that bed capacity in this city may be overstated.

2. Between 1945 and 1958 total hospital beds in New York City increased by 5,300. With the elimination of 4,600 beds in unsuitable buildings, beds in suitable buildings increased by 9,900. Municipal hospitals accounted for almost one half of the increase.

3. Obsolescence has gained in importance relative to non-fire-resistiveness as a reason for classifying patients' buildings as unsuitable.

4. In 1959 four fifths of the general-care beds in voluntary hospitals and in proprietary hospitals were in buildings classified as suitable. In municipal hospitals nine tenths were suitable.

5. Although some progress has been made in reducing the number of small hospitals in New York City, more than one half of its general-care hospitals, with nearly one fifth of all beds, have fewer than 200 beds. These institutions are divided almost equally between the voluntary and proprietary systems.

6. Progress is reported toward the elimination of large wards in patients' accommodations.

7. Between 1945 and 1956 almost $500 million were spent for hospital construction in New York City. More than $400 million represent expenditures by voluntary, municipal, and proprietary hospitals.

8. The period 1945–56 witnessed the emergence and consolidation of the role of the municipal system as an important factor in hospital construction during periods other than a depression. Voluntary hospitals once incurred almost three fourths of all construction expenditures in New York City; in the recent four year period 1953–56 their share was one half. Construction by proprietary hospitals was most important immediately after the two wars.

9. It is estimated that during the postwar era municipal hospitals "renewed" more than one half of their physical plant, and voluntary and proprietary hospitals "renewed" approximately one third of theirs.

10. The need for capital funds goes beyond replacement of beds in unsuitable buildings. The index of obsolescence in suitable buildings for one group of voluntary hospitals is estimated at almost one fifth. In most municipal hospitals the quality of plant maintenance is known to be poor, frequently resulting in premature obsolescence.

11. The foremost difference between New York City and the United States in the distribution of construction expenditures by ownership is in the larger role played here by local government. At 46 percent of the 1945–56 expenditures for hospital construction in the city, New York's municipal hospitals are twice as important as local government hospitals in the nation.

12. In recent years philanthropic contributions for construction were more important in New York City than in the nation—over one half of private hospital construction compared to one third.

13. In the United States Hill-Burton grants amounted to $740 million between 1948 and 1957. They constituted 32 percent of construction expenditures in aided projects and 10 percent of total expenditures, other than in federal hospitals. In addition, associated grants by several states amounted to $95 million, or 4 percent of expenditures in aided projects and 1 percent of total expenditures.

14. In New York City Hill-Burton grants amounted to $12 million by 1957. They constitute 20 percent of expenditures in aided projects and less than 3 percent of total expenditures, other than in federal hospitals. In view of the limited funds available, the program has been pointed toward selected high priority targets, both with respect to type of program and to the geographic distribution of hospital facilities.

15. In four boroughs of New York City other than Manhattan, a Hill-Burton grant frequently makes the difference between a hospital's building and not building. Assistance from some central source would be desirable.

16. Earnings from patients are likely to play an increasing role in financing future hospital construction.

Appendix 8.A

ESTIMATE OF EXPENDITURES FOR HOSPITAL
CONSTRUCTION, NEW YORK CITY,
1945–56

The annual estimates for the several hospital ownership groups were derived as follows:

VOLUNTARY HOSPITALS

Separate estimates were prepared for the United Hospital Fund member hospitals and for hospitals that are not members of the Fund.

United Hospital Fund Member Hospitals. Unpublished data were furnished by the Fund on the value of additions to buildings and equipment. The timing of these figures was adjusted in those instances in which data were available to the date of contract letting, in order to bring them into closer conformity to the timing of the Dodge data (see below).

Other Voluntary Hospitals. Estimates were prepared on the basis of information in the Hospital Council's files for individual hospitals.

MUNICIPAL HOSPITALS

Project by project appropriations, as made by the New York City Board of Estimate, were furnished by the Department of Public Works of the City of New York. Appropriations involving the purchase of land or the acquisition of existing hospital plants were excluded. In the Capital Budget of the City an appropriation is tantamount to the award of a contract.

PROPRIETARY HOSPITALS

Changes in beds, both total and suitable, were studied year by year for each institution. Cost figures were available for a number of proprietary hospitals, and these were applied to the estimated increase in bed count.

STATE HOSPITALS

Expenditures by the State in New York City reflect expenditures by the Department of Mental Hygiene. The Department furnished detailed worksheets on capital expenditures for each of its institutions located within city limits.

FEDERAL HOSPITALS

These are exclusively expenditures by the Veterans Administration hospitals. The managers of the three hospitals in the city and the central office in Washington cooperated in furnishing the requested information. Other civilian federal hospitals are omitted, because they had only minor changes in physical plant.

Fortunately, it was possible to check the sum of the several components against an independently derived total. This total is based on data on the value of hospital construction contracts let in New York City, furnished by the F. W. Dodge Corporation. These were adjusted upward by allowances for equipment and other costs, such as architectural services. The allowances used here were 10 percent of project cost for equipment and 6 percent for other costs, based on major projects contracted for in New York City under the Hill-Burton program between June 1, 1952 and June 1, 1957.[21] These adjustments are consistent with estimates given in other sources, such as *Design and Construction of General Hospitals* and *Preliminary Cost Estimates for Health Facilities,* issued by the United States Public Health Service.

Table 8.16. EXPENDITURES FOR HOSPITAL CONSTRUCTION, NEW YORK CITY, 1945–56 (IN THOUSANDS OF DOLLARS)

Year	Total	Voluntary	Municipal	Proprietary	State	Federal
1945	2,874	478	1,669	727	0	0
1946	7,018	1,799	2,616	2,603	0	0
1947	37,967	5,610	14,265	125	0	17,967
1948	20,141	6,430	12,695	705	311	0
1949	36,651	15,692	16,565	2,755	0	1,639
1950	44,238	21,820	20,131	2,113	174	0
1951	82,622	9,744	48,710	2,743	386	21,039
1952	81,985	33,680	44,538	3,135	632	0
1953	67,018	15,863	25,992	2,435	20,346	2,382
1954	31,654	17,885	12,657	713	399	0
1955	43,712	11,737	16,074	965	14,936	0
1956	34,449	22,065	9,150	265	2,969	0
Total: 1945–56	490,329	162,803	225,062	19,284	40,153	43,027

SOURCE: Hospital Council of Greater New York.

The Dodge data, original and adjusted, are shown in Table 8.17.

Table 8.17. VALUE OF HOSPITAL CONSTRUCTION CONTRACTS LET IN NEW YORK CITY, ORIGINAL DATA BY F. W. DODGE CORPORATION AND DATA ADJUSTED FOR VALUE OF EQUIPMENT AND ARCHITECTS' SERVICES, 1945–56 (IN THOUSANDS OF DOLLARS)

Year	Dodge Data	Adjusted
1945	1,916	2,281
1946	7,206	8,579
1947	26,250	31,250
1948	38,484	45,814
1949	47,358	56,379
1950	8,190	9,750
1951	83,886	99,864
1952	51,243	61,004
1953	56,885	67,720
1954	12,498	14,879
1955	17,933	21,349
1956	47,845	56,958
Total: 1945–56	399,694	475,827

SOURCE: Letter from F. W. Dodge Corporation to Herbert E. Klarman, May 16, 1958.

The adjusted total in Table 8.17 is $476 million, compared with $490 million in Table 8.16. It is believed that $4 million of the $490 million are not likely to be reflected in Dodge contracts; these comprise annual expenditures of less than $100,000 in State mental hospitals and most of the expenditures of the City of New York through the Department of Hospitals for general modernization and rehabilitation of existing plant. The statistical discrepancy is $10 million, or approximately 2 percent.

Appendix 8.B

INDEX OF PLANT RENEWAL

In examining a time series on hospital construction expenditures, it is difficult to get a sense of the accomplishments of one system in relation to the accomplishments of another. The reason is that a number of variables intrude into the comparison.

Among these variables are:

1. The size of each hospital system. A given amount of expenditures may be large for one hospital system and small for another, depending on the size of each.

2. The distribution of expenditures by type of facility. One hospital system may concentrate on building ancillary facilities, whereas the other concentrates on buildings for inpatients.

3. The distribution of expenditures between rehabilitation of plant and new construction. One system may be removing a great deal of obsolescence by rehabilitating existing buildings, whereas the other is purchasing additional beds in new, suitable buildings.

4. The timing of expenditures. The cost of hospital construction has risen. A given sum of money purchased more new building in the late 1940s than in the middle 1950s.

5. The cost per bed. At a given time one hospital system may have more elaborate (or more adequate) requirements for space and equipment than another hospital system.

The Index of Plant Renewal, as employed in this report, is an attempt to measure past achievement in improving physical plant. It attempts to solve the problems posed above, as follows:

All construction expenditures are treated *as if* they were incurred for building new beds. A new outpatient department is equated to x beds on the basis of their relative costs of construction. This takes care of problems 2 and 3 above.

Expenditures in a given year are divided by cost per bed in the same year, in order to meet problem 4. Since construction cost per bed is not available annually, the equivalent result was achieved by deflating each year's expenditures by the corresponding value of the index of hospital construction prices. In effect, this step converts expenditures in current dollars into expenditures in constant dollars.

A cost per bed was estimated for each hospital system: $27,500 in the municipal, $25,000 in the voluntary, and $15,000 in the proprietary. This overcomes problem 5.

Finally, to meet problem 1, the sum of the numbers of new bed equivalents purchased each year, computed by dividing expenditures in a year by the then cost per bed, is divided by the current bed capacity of each hospital system. The latter is taken to represent the size of each system.

9 PROBLEMS IN HOSPITAL MANAGEMENT

The ideal model of hospital management is tripartite: [1] the board of trustees sets goals for the institution and defines broad policies; the administration carries out these policies from day to day and performs coordinating functions; and the medical staff renders medical care of adequate quality, thereby meeting the responsibilities to the community assumed by the board of trustees. In actuality the ideal model is frequently modified, so that the pattern by which a hospital is managed is highly variable. The management pattern is particularly influenced by the hospital's ownership. Selected aspects of the three elements of hospital management are dealt with in the three sections comprising this chapter.

No attempt is made to deal with the management problems of proprietary hospitals. Although there is some discussion of voluntary hospitals in New York City, the major emphasis rests on municipal hospitals. The reasons are three: (1) centralized ownership creates a homogeneous, if not a single, set of problems that can be encompassed in a broad study; (2) there is a need for early action to improve the management of municipal hospitals; and (3) the problems of the voluntary system are varied and not so amenable to analysis.

The Policy Making Group

BOARDS OF TRUSTEES OF VOLUNTARY HOSPITALS

The activities of boards of trustees of voluntary hospitals are not known, and much discussion pertaining to boards of trustees refers to the ideal model. A recent pilot study of 18 hospitals in upstate New York found considerable differences among boards in the areas of hospital management emphasized and in the division of labor between trustees and hospital administration.[2]

Unfortunately, it was not feasible to survey the role of the boards of trustees of voluntary hospitals in New York City, on whose leadership the future development of voluntary hospitals is heavily dependent. From observation and experience it is known that in some hospitals the board is a tower of strength and in others a source of weakness. More knowledge than is now available about the characteristics and behavior of strong boards is a prerequisite to any major effort to strengthen and rebuild ineffective boards. Such knowledge would also be useful in evaluating the merits of more modest proposals, such as establishing in New York City branch hospitals under a single board of trustees or assigning newly elected trustees to serve an apprenticeship with an experienced and effective board in another hospital.

It was feasible to assemble and analyze certain data on the composition of boards of trustees of most voluntary hospitals in New York City and on attendance at board meetings, the latter serving as one index of trustee participation in hospital affairs. These data are taken from reports routinely filed by member institutions with the Greater New York Fund.

Table 9.1 distributes 46 voluntary hospitals by size of board. (Excluded are the boards of Catholic hospitals, whose form of organization differs from that of other voluntary hospitals.) The number of board members varies between 15 and 60 according to authorization and between 9 and 60 in actuality. An average

Table 9.1. NUMBER OF VOLUNTARY HOSPITALS WITH SPECIFIED SIZE OF BOARD, AUTHORIZED AND ACTUAL, NEW YORK CITY, 1957

Size of Board (Number of Members)	Number of Hospitals with Specified Size of Board	
	Authorized	Actual
0– 9	0	1
10–19	3	6
20–29	14	17
30–39	9	11
40–49	9	7
50 and over (through 60)	11	4
	46	46

SOURCE: The Greater New York Fund.

(mean) size of 31 board members in New York City compares with a nation-wide figure of 14 reported by the American Hospital Association in 1951.[3]

Analysis of attendance at board meetings in relation to the actual size of boards shows that the larger the board, the larger the average attendance. The proportion of members attending meetings is almost constant, in the neighborhood of 55 to 60 percent. All but 8 of the 46 boards of trustees meet eight to twelve times a year. One meets more often and 7 less often. The typical number of meetings held during the year is ten. There appears to be no relationship, one way or another, between the proportion of board members attending meetings and the annual number of meetings.

Seventeen hospitals furnished data on the number of meetings held by their executive committees. Hospitals with less active executive committees, as reflected in the number of times they met during the year, tend to have a higher rate of attendance at meetings of the board than hospitals with more active executive committees.

Neither the size of the board nor average attendance at meetings is related to the size or teaching class of the hospital (as defined in Chapter 5). Some of the major voluntary hospitals in New York City have high average attendance, but so do some of the smaller and less prominent ones. The converse is also true. The degree of activity and effectiveness of a hospital board of trustees is not encompassed or measured by board attendance.

A striking finding is the disproportionately large role played by trustees listed from Manhattan. The listed address may pertain to the trustee's residence or his office. Although the data based on the trustee's listed address do not necessarily signify the absence of ties with another borough, they do so in fact. More detailed data for 11 voluntary hospitals outside Manhattan show that the data derived from listed addresses understate the role of the home borough by three to four board members on the average, but typically only by one or two.

The data based on the trustees' listed addresses show that Manhattan furnished 88 percent of the trustees in Manhattan hospitals and 40 percent of the trustees in hospitals located in the other four boroughs. The proportion of trustees from Manhattan is particularly high in hospitals affiliated with one central federation. In other hospitals outside Manhattan the number of trustees from the home borough is sometimes small or a bare majority. Among 11 voluntary hospitals in Brooklyn without central ties, 3 hospitals draw less than a majority of their board members from Brooklyn, and another 5 draw less than 60 percent of their board from Brooklyn.

Few voluntary hospitals have physicians on the board of trustees; when they do, these are frequently retired practitioners. Most voluntary hospitals have a joint conference committee of the board and medical staff to deal with problems of medical care and medical staff organization. The legal doctrine, which is worth nothing, is that "the board of trustees is responsible for the quality of medical care given patients in the hospital and therefore has the duty and responsibility of appointment of the [medical] staff and for making of reasonable rules and regulations for the control of the professional work of the hospital." [4] A trustee who is an active practitioner may be involved in a conflict of interest.

Trustee-physician relations in the hospital resemble trustee-faculty relations in the university. On the latter score a group of trustees recently urged self-restraint, as follows: "The legal supremacy of trustees and their final authority to act as they wish is unquestioned, but the most experienced trustees are themselves constantly warning their newer colleagues that overactivity in certain areas—particularly in the area of education itself—is as great a sin against the modern spirit of trusteeship as is neglect." [5]

The physician exerts a great deal of authority in the hospital. He is influential in determining the amount of expenditures, yet bears little of the responsibility. As one student of hospital affairs suggests: "It may well be that the voluntary hospitals, with their desire to facilitate the work of physicians, have gone too far in releasing them from an important share of the responsibility for making the hospital itself operate at optimum." [6]

BOARD OF HOSPITALS OF THE CITY OF NEW YORK

The municipal system has lay advisory boards appointed and functioning at each hospital. With the exception of the board of Sydenham Hospital, which is a continuation of the board of this hospital when it was under voluntary ownership, none of the others has ever exercised policy-making functions, with ultimate responsibility for the institution's medical and fiscal affairs. Rather, these advisory boards are intended to convey a neighborhood's interest in the hospital located in its midst and to support the hospital's case before higher officials of the City government.

Beginning in 1929, when the Department of Hospitals was organized, authority for operating municipal hospitals was vested in the Commissioner of Hospitals. In 1950 the Board of Hospitals was established, as an outgrowth of the Mayor's committee to study the allocation of $150 million from exempt funds for hospital construction. It consists of five physicians and five laymen appointed by the Mayor, with the Commissioner of Hospitals serving as chairman.

The Board of Hospitals was given the power and duty to develop long range programs for the Department of Hospitals and to approve the estimates for the Capital Budget prepared by the Commissioner. The Board was also empowered to approve his estimates for the Expense Budget and to devise methods for increasing efficiency of operation in municipal hospitals. Finally, the Board of Hospitals was to establish and promote "the highest possible standards" for the care of the sick in municipal and proprietary hospitals and in voluntary hospitals in receipt of public funds.[7] With specific reference to proprietary institutions for the sick, the Board was authorized to promulgate a Hospital Code, prescribing, with the force of law, the rules and regulations governing their licensure.

Since its establishment the Board of Hospitals has prepared and adopted new codes for proprietary hospitals and nursing homes in New York City. It has been active in the administration of the municipal system, both through detailed budgetary review and otherwise. Most recently the Board of Hospitals has worked on problems of staffing municipal hospitals, especially those without medical school affiliation. Although its activities in all these fields have indirectly affected the quality of care, it has taken no action bearing on this directly and has, therefore, not affected the operation of voluntary hospitals.

Budgetary Controls and Personnel Administration

Every hospital has an administrator, of course. One obvious difference is that the administrator of a voluntary hospital faces the problem of achieving a balance among several sources of income, whereas the administrator of a municipal hospital does not. In fact, the differences in administration between municipal and voluntary hospitals in New York City go much further and are surprisingly wide on the expenditure side.

AUTONOMY AND FLEXIBILITY IN VOLUNTARY HOSPITALS

Among voluntary hospitals the individual institution, even when a member of a sectarian federation, enjoys autonomy in developing and pursuing its personnel and fiscal policies. Considerable exchange of information among hospitals takes place through surveys conducted by the Greater New York Hospital Association and United Hospital Fund of New York, and more frequently informal exchanges take place over the telephone and at meetings. Nevertheless, each hospital regards itself as ultimately responsible for its own course of action and feels free to follow it.

Most voluntary hospitals in New York City have a budget. The budget of a hospital is peculiarly its own and reflects its special circumstances. After approval by the board of trustees, it becomes a flexible plan for spending in the coming year and can serve as a vehicle for management control. Thus, although not every voluntary hospital has a formal buget and although not every hospital with a budget employs it as a tool of management, many hospitals do both and no hospital that wishes to adopt these practices is precluded from so doing.

CENTRALIZED CONTROL IN MUNICIPAL HOSPITALS

In the municipal system the administrator of an institution has little control over the amount spent and no discretion as to its distribution by program or by object of expenditure. True, in recent years the City government has moved toward a system of program budgeting under which expenditures are related to the volume of services rendered and costs per unit of service are calculated and compared. The program budget has, however, not replaced the traditional line-item budget but has been superimposed on it. Under the line-item budget significant control over expenditures in each City agency continues to be exercised by the Director of the Budget.

The basis for the control exercised by the Budget Director is the accrual system, and the instrument of control is fashioned in the preamble to the City's Expense Budget ("The Terms and Conditions of the Budget"). Accruals apply only to the personnel service lines of the Budget; for certain positions enumerated in the Budget all or a portion of salaries are to remain unspent (that is, to accrue). The amount appropriated to a department is less than the sum of the amounts shown in all the lines listed in the Budget by the amount of required accruals. This is true on the very day the Budget is adopted.

Of course, a certain amount of savings is to be expected from vacancies associated with normal attrition and job turnover, employee leave without pay, and replacement of older with new employees in lower salary grades. Under the accrual system, however, the accumulated amount of savings must reach a stated sum by the end of the year. To assure this the Budget Director is empowered to pass on the filling of all job vacancies.[8]

The Budget Director may grant approval for filling vacancies job by job or through a blanket certificate for certain types of occupation in specified salary grades. In the former case delay in granting a certificate of approval is typical. A certificate expires in sixty days, so that failure to fill the job in time means another round of application and delay.

A majority of positions in the Department of Hospitals are covered by a blanket certificate; this means that the individual hospital can hire nurses without reference to the Budget Director, provided it has the requisite spaces or vacancies. A blanket certificate is given to an emergency department and is renewable every three months. A vacancy does not, however, exist as long as the incumbent is on terminal leave. Terminal leave is prolonged by adding compensatory time off to accumulated annual leave and, sometimes, also sick leave. In one City agency (the Fire Department) provision was recently made for lump-sum terminal payments, so that a man leaving the department may be replaced immediately.

The accrual system is a device for limiting City expenditures. It was instituted in the depression, when the bankers who marketed the City's securities found it necessary to impose certain restrictions on the City administration before agreeing to continue to support its credit. They sought—and obtained—closer supervision over its expenditures.

Over the years the amount of required accruals in the Expense Budget has increased, and the tactic of delay in authorizing the filling of old jobs was extended to new jobs in new programs. In the Department of Hospitals the amount of accruals has reached sizable proportions, and more recently a savings feature was added. The latter is based on the assumption that increased expenditures for certain programs, such as public-home infirmaries, are to yield immediate savings in other expenditures, such as general hospitals.

In the Expense Budget for fiscal year 1960 the Department of Hospitals had a Schedule (line-item) total of $175.5 million; this was offset by $14.6 million of accruals and $5.5 million of savings, to yield a Code (appropriation) total of $155.4 million. The offsets constituted 13.7 percent of the Department's authorized personnel service budget.[9]

With rare exceptions all positions are filled at the bottom step of the salary range of a given title. In a competitive labor market this can result in a serious disadvantage to City agencies, since voluntary hospitals seldom fill positions in scarce occupations, such as nursing, at the starting salary. The practical effect is that in hiring new employees the City cannot reward experience that falls short of meriting a promotion. If it is found that the starting salary of a position does not attract applicants, then all persons occupying that position must be allowed the extra salary steps above the minimum required for recruitments.

Municipal hospitals also lack flexibility in assigning personnel to cover services twenty-four hours a day and seven days a week, as required in a hospital. Voluntary hospitals have raised shift differentials for evening and night duty, and some pursue flexible policies. One hospital pays a nurse a differential during the entire period that she participates in the rotation scheme, not only when she is on duty in the less desirable tours. The City pays a monthly differential of $10 nights and $20 evenings while the staff nurse serves in these tours. Here and there the medical boards of municipal hospitals have found it necessary to supplement the City's shift differentials in order to persuade persons to volunteer for the less attractive tours; under conditions of shortage in the labor market rotation of shifts cannot be made mandatory. Unofficial supplementary stipends have limited effectiveness, since they are selective in application and cannot be counted upon to continue.

Municipal hospitals have also encountered dissatisfaction among personnel because raises in pay are given to all City employees in a certain grade, without reference to the special problems created for an individual department. Several years ago the lower grades of nursing personnel—practical nurses and nurses' aides—were reevaluated under the City's Career and Salary Plan and received a pay raise. Registered nurses did not. Even prior to this raise the salary ratio of practical nurses to registered staff nurses was significantly higher in municipal than in voluntary hospitals (see Chapter 7). Following the raise it was often the case that a practical nurse who had received several annual increments was earning more money than a registered nurse. It took considerable effort and time by many interested parties to correct the situation by winning a job reevaluation and a higher grade for registered staff nurses.

Efficient operation of municipal hospitals is hindered by the provision that the Director of the Budget must approve requisitions for equipment listed in the Expense Budget. This takes time. The Budget Director may also at his discretion request justification anew, even though justification preceded the item's inclusion in the Budget.

Small expenditures that are not specifically provided for in the Expense Budget and are not foreseeable entail a great deal of paper work and much waiting. The latter has a particularly deleterious effect on plant maintenance, because of the high degree of centralization in engineering and supply services. The Department of Hospitals can authorize an expenditure up to $25 in response to a telephone call, provided that funds exist for the specific Code to which that item is chargeable.

Medical superintendents of some municipal hospitals have petty cash funds on which they can draw, either from bequests or income from bequests previously made to the hospital, or from contributions by the hospital's social service auxiliary or medical board, or from earnings from vending machines operated on the premises. These miscellaneous sources of income are not always used to the full. It is also true that their availability is not always correlated with need and willingness to use.

A small petty cash fund should be maintained at each hospital, to be used at the discretion of the medical superintendent. It is important that small needs be attended to promptly at the local level without reference to headquarters, so that they will not become major problems. In the Hospital Council's survey of Kings County Hospital Center in 1952, a petty cash fund of $200 a month was recommended.[10]

It is recognized that municipal hospitals are an integral part of the government of the City of New York and cannot be operated under special rules of their own. Nevertheless, it will be recalled that the movement to adopt a program budget was predicated on the expectation that it would result in improved management, owing to the delegation of control over expenditures to the several City departments under conditions of accountability. It is important that the Department of Hospitals assume full responsibility, including financial, for the operation of its own institutions, and that the individual superintendent be held responsible and accountable for the operation of his institution.

No doubt conditions will occasionally arise that call for additional savings beyond those projected in the Budget. Such occasions should be kept to a minimum. When they occur, it should be the responsibility of the Department to allocate the required savings among its institutions. It then becomes the responsibility of each administrator to decide where and how to effect his portion of the savings.

Such a linking of authority and responsibility is essential for improving efficiency of operation and raising the level of care. It can also serve to attract to the municipal system capable and qualified administrators from other City departments and outside the government, as the opportunities and challenges of municipal hospital administration increase.

DECENTRALIZED CONTROL IN VETERANS ADMINISTRATION

It is not a new idea that a government hospital, which is a member of a system, can have both authority and responsibility for its expenditures. Indeed, this is currently the practice in the Veterans Administration. Although many aspects of operation and management are not comparable between municipal and Veterans Administration hospitals, the level of maintenance of physical plant alone would seem to demonstrate the advantages of the latter.

There was a time when Veterans Administration hospitals were subject to line-item supervision; this method of budgetary control was abandoned many years ago. Today Veterans Administration hospitals operate without a prescribed table of organization and without a personnel ceiling. The latter was abandoned after the Korean War, when the personnel shortage eased. Congress had found the management of personnel in the Veterans Administration too demanding a task, and decided to rely on appropriations as its chief instrument of control.

Today the manager (administrator) of a Veterans Administration hospital has considerable discretion in spending his annual allotment. He is also held to a high degree of accountability after spending it.

Prior to the beginning of a new fiscal year he is advised of the total sum allotted to his hospital. The manager then prepares an operating plan showing the pattern of expenditures he intends to follow, quarter by quarter. He lists the number of positions he expects to fill in each personnel category and puts down the amount of money involved; and he puts down so much for blood, so much for supplies, and so forth. He has no discretion over certain items, such as travel expense or medical research, which are limited by Congress. Certain other items, such as education and training, are controlled by administrative action at headquarters. However, in most expenditures the manager has leeway. His written plan is subject to review by the area office and by central headquarters, which can raise questions and make recommendations. The manager is expected to consider these suggestions, but he is not compelled to adopt them.

The operating plan, as finally approved, is regarded as a statement of intent. It is expected that the manager will adhere to it within reasonable limits, but not line by line. He may shift funds to meet changing circumstances and may, for example, purchase equipment costing $1,000 or $2,000 on his own decision. For larger expenditures, particularly those that entail structural alterations, he does need approval from headquarters. Much of this can be arranged informally by telephone, subject to confirmation in writing.

It is assumed, as is true in all spheres of the federal government, that the manager's conduct is subject to the Anti-Deficiency Act. In effect, this law provides that an official cannot spend money that has not been allocated to him unless he can establish that the expenditure was necessitated by danger to human life or limb.

Local Veterans Administration officials, as well as those at headquarters, consider the present arrangement workable, although by no means perfect. There is a constant flow of questions directed at the hospital from the area office in Boston and from headquarters in Washington. Frequent comparisons are made between one institution and others in cost of service and in level of performance, and comments are invited to justify differences. Occasionally funds may be withdrawn suddenly; when that occurs, it is left to the manager to decide how to adapt himself to the reduced income. The degree of accountability is high, and it is understood that the manager's job and prospects of promotion depend on his performance.

One official of the Veterans Administration stated:

There are problems in the financial management of our system, but . . . these problems would occur with either a decentralized or a centralized system—recruitment difficulties, price increases, changing patterns of need for resources, and obsolescence of plant. . . . These may [not] necessarily be solved simply, but . . . their resolution is enhanced by putting the requirements fairly up to local management and providing them with the maximum of leeway subject to the total availability of funds, the application of agency policy, and a program of evaluation of performance.[11]

The City of New York would profit by moving toward a similar degree of decentralized authority in operating its hospitals. There is no question here of giving the hospital administrator a blank check. Decentralization in the Veterans Administration has not meant a loss of fiscal control or of the ability to evaluate performance. The degree of discretion allowed should be commensurate with the job to be done. This follows from the assumption that the administrator of a hospital knows more about managing it than the Director of the Budget.

Recruitment of Administrators

Central to the above discussion is the presence of an able administrator. Unfortunately, like all agencies of government, municipal hospitals are now suffering from the steady loss of the stalwarts who entered civil service during the depression. The private practice of medicine is more attractive today than it was in the 1930s and also more remunerative than a salaried position with the City. Voluntary hospitals offer more varied opportunities and higher salaries to physicians interested in administration. These advantages are offset in part by the greater uncertainty of tenure.

The medical superintendent of a municipal hospital is appointed from a civil service list of eligible candidates who have passed both written and oral examinations. For many years this has been a promotion list of persons within the municipal hospital system, that is, deputy medical superintendents who had passed the examination. No examination open to qualified persons from other City departments or from outside the City government has been given since 1951.

Departmental policy requires that the medical superintendent and the deputy medical superintendent be physicians. Unable to attract a sufficient number of young deputy medical superintendents who could pass the examination—the present deputies are older than the superintendents—the Department of Hospitals has recently recruited layment to serve as assistant hospital administrators. This position is comparable to that of deputy in many respects, including salary, but differs significantly in that the assistant administrator is not eligible to become a superintendent. Assistant hospital administrators play an important role in several municipal institutions.

Among voluntary hospitals there is wide variation in the professional background of administrators. In New York City in 1960, 9 of 80 hospitals were headed by nurses, 13 by physicians, and 58 by persons with other training. Five of the 9 nurse administrators were in hospitals with fewer than 100 beds, while 7 of

the 13 physician administrators were in hospitals with 500 or
more beds. Indeed, physicians headed all but 2 of the 9 hospitals
with 500 or more beds. Some voluntary hospitals do not follow
a fixed pattern and hire a physician at one time and a lay administrator at another.

In the nation available data for the year 1952 show a much
higher proportion of nurse administrators than in New York City
(40 percent, compared with 11 percent) and a slightly lower proportion of physician administrators (11 percent, compared with
16 percent). In government hospitals in the United States, the
proportion of physician administrators is 20 percent, which is
higher than in voluntary hospitals in the nation or in New York
City, but far below the latter's figure of 100 percent in municipal
hospitals. In government hospitals with 250 or more beds the
proportion of physician administrators in the United States is 60
percent.[12]

In the Veterans Administration system several major hospital
centers have lay managers. Physician or otherwise, the manager
earns his position and grade not by passing a test but by meeting
the requirements of civil service in terms of his educational background and work record, as evaluated by a board at headquarters.
It is interesting that in all of the federal civil service qualification
for the higher grades is by passing an unassembled examination
that rates the applicant on his education and experience in relation to the requirements of the job.[13]

To make non-physicians eligible for the top management position in municipal hospitals is not to preclude the appointment of
physicians, if available and qualified. The question of the comparative advantages and disadvantages of physicians and laymen as
hospital administrators is still moot, and it may be that the City
would prefer to limit appointments to physicians as long as it is
able to attract them in sufficient numbers. Retention of the existing policy of appointing only medical superintendents may im-
pede recruitment of lay individuals for positions on the second
level of management or even induce the departure of those
already recruited. Whatever choice is made, action is urgently
required to bring individuals with top qualifications in hospital
administration into the municipal system before long.

Finally, to be truly competitive with comparable positions in other hospitals and agencies, salaries will have to be raised. Today there are three grades of medical superintendent in municipal hospitals, with the lowest grade paying $12,000 a year at entry and the highest grade, for administrators of hospital centers, paying $14,400 annually at maximum. These are far below salaries of administrators in voluntary hospitals of comparable or smaller size and below salaries contemplated for full-time directors of clinical service in municipal hospitals (see below). A determination of what is an appropriate salary level should reflect a balancing between the municipal hospital and competing positions of cash income, stability of tenure, retirement benefits, as well as the more elusive nonpecuniary advantages and disadvantages of a job.

It would be useful for some appropriate agency to resume the institutes for the development of executives in municipal hospitals that were pioneered by the Hospital Council in 1953. It is generally believed that these institutes were effective in stimulating and strengthening top and middle management in the municipal system.

Full-Time Chiefs of Clinical Service

It has been proposed to the City administration that in selected municipal hospitals not staffed by medical schools full-time salaried chiefs be appointed to direct the four basic clinical services—medicine, surgery, pediatrics, and obstetrics-gynecology. The proposal also encompasses hiring chiefs of radiology and laboratory services on a full-time basis at comparable salaries.

In the ancillary services the proposed change would be one of degree. The present salary level would be more than doubled, in order to buy full-time service from men with high qualifications. The change would, however, be of great significance. Today's salaries of $7,000 to $9,000 are not only unrealistic, but the tacit understanding that full-time personnel are not expected to render full-time service is demoralizing and is likely to result in a loosening of organization.

In the clinical services the proposed change is one of kind, since currently all attending physicians on the inpatient services of municipal hospitals without medical school affiliation (with the exception of psychiatrists and physicians serving in public-home infirmary units) are contributing their services as volunteers. The contemplated change would be an even more radical departure from present practice if three or four salaried assistants to the chief were also appointed.

FULL-TIME CLINICAL CHIEFS IN VOLUNTARY HOSPITALS

Among municipal hospitals in New York City only those staffed by medical schools have paid chiefs of clinical service and assistants on a full-time basis. Some have large numbers and some a few. In the voluntary system, however, there are today 12 hospitals not staffed by medical schools that have one or more full-time chiefs of clinical department to administer the service and to direct teaching and research. Eight of these are affiliates of the Federation of Jewish Philanthropies, which has favored this development and promoted it through financial support.

Among these 12 voluntary hospitals 1 is staffed by chiefs on "geographic full time," 9 by chiefs on "institutional full time," and 2 by both types. In this context the terms "geographic full time" and "institutional full time" are employed in the same way as in the Hospital Council's report, *Full-Time System of Medicine*.[14] Both types of physician spend all of their time at the hospital; both may have the privilege of seeing private patients; and both may receive a salary from the hospital. The essential difference is that the income of the institutional full-time physician is effectively limited in one manner or another while that of the geographic full-time person is not. In the absence of services for private patients the concept of geographic full time would appear to be inapplicable to municipal hospitals.

The distribution of the 12 voluntary hospitals by the number of full-time chiefs of clinical service is as follows:

Number of Clinical Chiefs	Number of Voluntary Hospitals
9	1
6	1
4	3
3	4
2	1
1	2
Total number of hospitals with one or more chiefs	12

The 2 hospitals with 1 full-time chief of clinical service are, respectively, a special hospital and a general hospital with heavy emphasis on a specialty.

If these 2 hospitals are excluded from consideration, all remaining 10 have a full-time chief of medicine, 8 have a chief of surgery, and 7 a chief of pediatrics. Next in frequency are chiefs of psychiatry, of whom there are 4—3 in general hospitals and 1 in a special hospital.

ROLE OF FULL-TIME CHIEFS

The movement to appoint chiefs of clinical service is a reflection of the increasing complexity of the technology of modern medicine. Every year there are new discoveries and many more applications of these discoveries. The range of services rendered in a hospital is broadening, and the knowledge an individual physician must have is increasing. More investigative work is being carried on in hospitals toward which the intern and resident should be oriented. It is frequently found that supervision and direction by the visiting staff is not workable, since they cannot afford the necessary time.

This point of view is expressed in a recent annual report of a local hospital:

As the scope of our services to patients increased, and our training and research programs developed, it became evident that members of the Attending Staff who had given of their skills and time freely, could not continue to accept the vast responsibility of the larger services. Consequently, in keeping with a trend which has developed throughout the country, the Board of Trustees authorized full-time and geographic full-time positions. . . . These directors administrate for their own services, direct the activities of research, and supervise and participate in the teaching of medical students and in the post-graduate training programs.[15]

Director of Medical Education. This proposal must be viewed in relation to another recent development. *The Essentials of an Approved Internship*, issued by the Council on Medical Education and Hospitals of the American Medical Association, states that appointment of a director of intern education on a full-time or part-time basis may be desirable.[16] Such a director, if appointed, would organize and supervise the hospital's teaching program in a manner that would enhance the effectiveness with which members of the attending staff participate in it.

A recent survey of directors of medical education in 150 non-university hospitals in the United States shows that only 10 percent of them are employed on a full-time basis. However, 60 percent receive some pay, varying from half time to quarter time, whereas 30 percent receive none. Among the last, it is suggested, some probably do not play a really effective role as educational director.[17]

In discussions of the characteristics that make for an effective director of medical education emphasis is usually placed on maturity,[18] competence—professional qualifications comparable to those of a chief of a clinical service [19]—and authority. He should have a seat on the hospital's medical board, with or without a vote.[20]

A director of medical education for the entire hospital, most frequently a specialist in internal medicine, may not be able to contribute much to the conduct of the other services, such as surgery or obstetrics. If so, a guiding hand is indicated for each clinical service. It has been suggested that the head of the teaching program should do some of the teaching, thereby setting a good example. He must not be restricted to the task of coordination.[21]

The above considerations suggest that a full-time chief of a clinical service is likely to be much more effective than a young man who has recently completed residency training and is appointed to serve as a coordinator of medical education. It is recognized, however, that the problem of organizing medical education in hospitals and simultaneously improving the quality of care is undergoing intensive discussion on the basis of considerable experimentation and experience with a variety of approaches. This is a time of rapid transition, which does not permit firm, definitive conclusions.

Appointing full-time chiefs of clinical service is not the same as appointing complete full-time medical staffs. It would be a mistake to lose the contributed services of practicing physicians in municipal hospitals, just as it would be in voluntary hospitals. In the 12 voluntary hospitals with full-time chiefs of clinical service, the task of the chief is viewed as one of organization and leadership, with the aim of facilitating the work of practitioners in the hospital, not of replacing them.

Conclusions for Municipal System. In light of the above discussion the following policies seem reasonable.

1. All municipal hospitals not staffed by universities should move to improve their radiological and laboratory services by appointing chiefs who will give full-time service. Standards for filling these positions should be set at a high level, with a sufficient salary to attract well-qualified applicants. In the ancillary services physician assistants and technicians should be appointed, as indicated by the volume of work.

2. With respect to clinical services, the policy of choice is to appoint chiefs of service, rather than complete full-time staffs. The well-qualified chief may require full-time assistants for his research activities; this is another matter and need not cost the City of New York anything.

3. Even with respect to the chief of a clinical service, there are instances in which the incumbent volunteer is doing all that the full-time person might be expected to do. If so, there is no reason to apply this policy. Rather, the policy should be carried out in those hospitals and in those services where the opportunity to achieve improvement is substantial.

4. Where a decision to hire a full-time chief is made, it should be prosecuted with vigor. For example, pay must be adequate. In the voluntary hospitals previously discussed, the most frequent salary for a full-time chief of a clinical service is $25,000. In some instances it is higher. It would be a waste of money to attempt to pay too low a salary, thereby attracting people with lower qualifications than needed or encouraging part-time work in positions requiring full-time performance.

5. In setting up a system of full-time chiefs of service in hospitals without university affiliation, it is important to open channels of communication with the medical schools. It would be desirable to have a committee of deans advise on the selection of these men, as in the Veterans Administration hospitals.

6. Success in carrying out these or similar proposals while retaining the goodwill and loyalty of the voluntary attending staff depends on enlisting the cooperation and understanding of

the medical boards of municipal hospitals. They must be persuaded that the value of their services can be enhanced under the leadership of full-time chiefs of clinical service and assured that their services are appreciated and will continue to be sought.

A special committee of the Hospital Council has made specific recommendations along these lines.[22]

Summary

1. Boards of trustees are highly important in the management and development of voluntary hospitals, but not enough is known about their activities and characteristics.

2. Data on the boards of 46 voluntary hospitals in New York City show: (a) the average size of board is 31, or approximately twice that in the nation; (b) most boards meet 8 to 12 times a year; (c) average attendance at board meetings is 55 to 60 percent of actual membership; (d) where there is an active executive committee, attendance at board meetings tends to be lower than where the executive committee is less active; and (e) the Borough of Manhattan furnishes a disproportionate number of trustees, not only to its own hospitals but to those located in the other four boroughs.

3. The Board of Hospitals of the City of New York has broad and varied powers and duties. These include long range planning, setting standards of efficiency, and review of items in the two Budgets—Expense and Capital—for the Department of Hospitals. It legislates the Code for proprietary hospitals and nursing homes. It has not yet acted in regard to quality of care, over which it has authority in all three ownership groups.

4. In voluntary hospitals the budget is a flexible instrument to guide expenditures and can be used as an instrument of management control.

5. In municipal hospitals the budget is not within the discretion of the individual institution. Examples are given of the supervening authority of the Director of the Budget and of the City's inflexible rules in hiring personnel. Delay in filling vacancies is a practice essential to achieving stated goals for annual accruals and savings.

6. Both authority and responsibility for operating municipal

hospitals might more appropriately be placed in the hands of the Commissioner of Hospitals for delegation to his medical superintendents. Accruals and savings, if any, should be expressed as a lump sum and not exacted by line item controls.

7. Establishment of petty cash funds out of City moneys is indicated. The figure of $200 a month was suggested in the Hospital Council's survey of Kings County Hospital Center in 1952.

8. The budgeting and spending process of the Veterans Administration hospitals is described as an example of government operation without line item controls and personnel ceilings. The manager of the individual hospital enjoys discretion in spending most of his annual allotment; he is also held to a high degree of accountability after spending it.

9. The City of New York is losing the medical superintendents recruited during the depression. Their replacements are not in sight; indeed, the deputy medical superintendents are older. Recently a number of lay assistant hospital administrators have been recruited, adding strength to the administration of the municipal system. They are not eligible under existing policy to succeed to the top position.

10. The question is raised whether lay administrators should be appointed. It is proposed that (a) the top position be opened to qualified applicants from other City departments and elsewhere; (b) an applicant's qualifications be evaluated on the basis of his education and experience, rather than by testing him in writing and orally; and (c) the salary be raised to a competitive level.

11. In New York City 12 voluntary hospitals not staffed by a medical school have one or more full-time chiefs of clinical service. Eight are affiliated with the Federation of Jewish Philanthropies.

12. Factors underlying this development are noted, chiefly the increasing complexities of medical care, education, research, and administration. It is suggested that the qualities that are sought in full-time or part-time directors of medical education are precisely the qualities possessed by a full-time chief of service. What is required under existing circumstances is leadership, not merely coordination.

13. With specific reference to certain proposals concerning municipal hospitals not affiliated with medical schools, the Hossital Council has recommended that (a) their ancillary services be improved through the appointment of qualified radiologists and pathologists to serve full-time at appropriate salaries; (b) well-qualified chiefs of clinical service be appointed at appropriate salaries, without a staff of full-time assistants; and (c) the volunteer incumbent chiefs of clinical service be retained where they are doing what a full-time person might be expected to do.

10   QUALITY OF CARE

Over the years various mechanisms have been developed that aim to assure the public of an adequate standard of hospital care. Unlike some other parts of the country, New York State depends less on governmental authority and more on voluntary compliance and places substantial reliance on the work of professional accrediting and approving bodies.

This chapter deals with the following: the nature and extent of governmental supervision of hospitals in New York City; accreditation; and methods of appraising quality of care. An appendix on medical research in New York City hospitals appears at the end of the chapter. Approval of teaching programs is mentioned briefly, since it is discussed at length elsewhere (Chapter 6).

Supervision by Government

Although evaluation and approval of hospitals by professional organizations are characteristic of this country, they are usually supported by a floor of supervision by government. In many states government acts by granting or withholding a periodically renewable license. Licensure gained considerable impetus after World War II, under the impetus of the Hill-Burton program.

In New York State general authority for the regulation of hospitals rests with the State Board of Social Welfare, which, in turn, acts through the State Department of Social Welfare or through municipalities. The jurisdiction of the Board of Social Welfare does not extend to federal hospitals, state hospitals, or other psychiatric hospitals (licensed by the State Department of Mental Hygiene).

The Department of Health has special responsibilities and

powers in maternity and newborn care and is concerned with sanitary conditions, food handling, and laboratories in all hospitals. In addition, under the physically handicapped children's program, the City's Department of Health sets standards and evaluates each hospital's program prior to approving it for payment. Its physician consultants regularly review patients' length of stay.

Before a new voluntary hospital can be established in New York State, the Board of Social Welfare must approve its charter. In reviewing an application for a charter, the Board considers a number of factors, including the reputation of the incorporators, adequacy of the proposed program, evidence of financial support, and existence of a community need for the proposed service.[1] When in doubt as to the merits of an application, the Board may grant a charter for a limited period.

Voluntary hospitals in New York City, like hospitals upstate, are inspected periodically by representatives of the State Department of Social Welfare. Essentially, the Department is concerned with the humane treatment of patients and with provisions for the safety, reasonable comfort, and general well being of patients. A full-time staff of registered nurses performs the inspections.

The same inspectors visit municipal hospitals. In both instances approval by the Department of Social Welfare is a prerequisite to reimbursement by the State and the federal government for the care of certain public-charge patients.

The Department of Social Welfare also exercises a degree of regulation over voluntary hospitals by requiring them to submit plans for new buildings or major alterations for review by the Department's architects. To avoid needless duplication, projects receiving Hill-Burton grants are reviewed by the architect of the State Hill-Burton agency under delegation of authority from the Department of Social Welfare.

Proprietary hospitals in New York City are licensed and regularly supervised by the Department of Hospitals. The State recognizes the activities of the municipal agency in this area and visits proprietary hospitals only for special purposes, such as inspection for eligibility to receive payment from Blue Cross, supervision of birth records, and inquiry into questionable conditions.

For a proprietary hospital to receive a license, which may be issued for one year or less, it must comply with the provisions of the Code formulated by the City's Board of Hospitals. The Code specifies minimum requirements for space, facilities, certain types of personnel, and ownership.[2] Once the requirements of the Code are met, the Department has until recently deemed it mandatory to issue the license. Unlike the Board of Social Welfare, the Department of Hospitals does not take into account the community's need for a new facility. Licensure is prerequisite to a hospital's eligibility to receive payment from Blue Cross.

It may be questioned whether a government department that has as its primary mission the operation of a large hospital system should be expected to supervise another group of hospitals. Unless a major reorganization of agencies takes place under which many of the regulatory, coordinating, and planning tasks now performed by the State will be regrouped, consideration should be given to transferring supervision of proprietary hospitals in New York City to another interested department of the City that does not operate institutions and has had regulatory experience. It might then be feasible to bring the municipal and voluntary hospitals within the same regulatory framework, under delegation from the State.

A proposal has recently been advanced that inspections should be performed by a team. The team, to consist of clinicians, experts in management and finance, nurses, dietitians, and social workers, would spend several days at an institution and appraise the institution as a whole. Team members would be drawn from panels of individuals whose major affiliations are outside the regulatory agency. This proposal merits serious consideration.

A recent development in New York State, as well as in some other states, is the enhanced role played by the Superintendent of Insurance. Charged by statute with reviewing the level of Blue Cross premiums, he is becoming concerned with the level of hospital cost and with the factors that are conducive to the economical operation of hospitals and consistent with adequate quality of care. Thus, the Superintendent of Insurance has become interested in community planning of hospital facilities, regionalization of services, and the collection and analysis of uniform financial and statistical data.

Accreditation and Approval for Graduate Training

Both accreditation and approval for training are granted by agencies representing the professions engaged in providing medical and hospital care. Accreditation directly, and approval for training more incidentally, is intended to assure the public that the quality of care in a hospital is adequate.

ACCREDITATION

The Joint Commission on Accreditation of Hospitals, established in 1952, took over the standardization program that had been conducted by the American College of Surgeons since 1918. The Commission is composed of representatives of the American College of Surgeons, American College of Physicians, American Hospital Association, and American Medical Association.

The standards promulgated by the Joint Commission "are considered necessary to insure the quality of medical care in hospitals which [it] can faithfully recommend to the public." [3] These are divided into basic principles and methods of procedure. They deal with the construction and arrangement of physical plant to insure the safety of patients; facilities, including laboratory and radiology; medical records; responsibilities and modes of organization of the governing board; medical staff responsibilities, qualifications for membership, and organization; adequacy of nursing personnel, particularly professional. The standards are interpreted and applied to the individual hospital during a one-day or two-day visit by an inspecting physician.

In New York City all but 8 voluntary hospitals are accredited, as are all but 2 municipal hospitals. Among proprietary hospitals only a minority are accredited: there were 2 in 1952, 3 in 1954, and 9 in 1957, 1958, and 1959. In 1960 there was a spurt, and by the end of the year 13 out of 45 proprietary hospitals were accredited. (Announcement by Associated Hospital Service that accreditation status was to be considered in approving a hospital for payment by Blue Cross undoubtedly provided the impetus for hospitals to seek accreditation.)

The published list of accredited hospitals does not distinguish between accreditation for three years and that for one year. The former is full accreditation and signifies that the hospital meets the standards set by the Joint Commission. One year accreditation is also accreditation but signifies that the hospital was close to the borderline of not passing and must improve in the two subsequent surveys or it will lose accreditation.

There is no public information on the extent of one year accreditation, if any, among voluntary and proprietary hospitals. For municipal hospitals there is information from the Department of Hospitals for 1959, namely, that, when one hospital lost accreditation, three others were changed from three-year to one-year accreditation, and one improved sufficiently to be given three-year accreditation in place of one-year. Among the demoted three was a hospital closely affiliated with a medical school and it subsequently regained full accreditation.

In general, it is worth noting, deficiencies are better known in municipal hospitals than in voluntary, because municipal hospitals are larger and come under close public scrutiny. It would be unwise to assume that every hospital with a voluntary charter is a superior institution. The range in quality of care is wide in each hospital system, and accreditation assures only a floor of adequacy, not an optimum. As a result of medical advances, the range in quality may be widening.

APPROVAL FOR INTERN AND RESIDENCY TRAINING

Approval of a hospital for intern or residency training is extended by the Council on Medical Education and Hospitals of the American Medical Association. The proposed teaching program is evaluated for its potential as a training opportunity, without reference to the number of programs already approved and the probable supply of candidates to staff them.

The distribution of hospitals in New York City by teaching status is given elsewhere (Chapter 6). Suffice it to note here that, owing to the inability of some hospitals to attract graduates of American (United States and Canadian) medical schools, approval can no longer be taken to signify the presence of an active and stimulating program, which, in turn, would be conducive to good care of patients.

The percentage of autopsies to deaths in the hospital is re-garded by medical authorities as an index of the staff's interest in teaching and, therefore, of quality of care.

Appraising the Quality of Medical Care

A serious evaluation of the roles of the two major hospital systems in New York City must face the question of the adequacy of the care given to patients. All other questions are almost sub-sidiary.

It was not possible in this study to appraise quality of care directly. The following discussion suggests how such an appraisal might be made and the resources required for doing it.

CRITERIA FOR MEASUREMENT

Ultimately the quality of care rendered in a hospital should be judged by its effect on the health and well-being of patients. This appears to be a simple criterion. The difficulty lies in measuring the effect on patients.

There are too many instances in which a direct correlation cannot be established between what a physician does or prescribes and the health of his patient. Where a direct correlation can be demonstrated, as in immunization against diphtheria in childhood or vaccination against smallpox, the carrying-out of the procedure or failure to do so is a sufficient measure of the quality of care. Where a direct correlation cannot be demonstrated, the best pro-cedure is to ascertain whether there was prompt and adequate provision of appropriate diagnostic and therapeutic services, in accordance with the best current concepts and practices.[4] In the present state of knowledge this is the method of choice for ap-praising quality of care in an institution and for comparing it among institutions.[5]

It is sometimes possible to compare the health status of two or more population groups, each of them the recipient of medical care through different auspices or types of organization.[6] This method is not usually appropriate to a comparison between hos-pitals or hospital systems, because the population served by one hospital or hospital system is not known and cannot be isolated from that served by another hospital or hospital system.

In view of the difficulty of appraising the quality of care in terms of the effect on patients, some physicians find it preferable to rely on inferences drawn from the conditions under which medical care is given.

Availability of Resources. The reasoning is that, if a hospital has modern buildings and equipment and a well-trained medical staff and other personnel, it is likely to provide good care; and conversely, it is likely to provide poor care if available resources are deficient. Sometimes all of the conditions surrounding the provision of medical care are reduced to a single key factor: the professional qualifications—knowledge, experience, and ability— and integrity of the physician.[7]

It would seem logical to assume that the physician, if he is the key to quality of care, would practice at substantially the same level in all hospitals in which he holds staff appointments. It would also follow that hospitals with many attending physicians in common would render the same quality of care. Each of these propositions is yet to be tested.

Capability is not, however, synonymous with actual performance. A poorly qualified staff cannot do good work. It is also true that a good doctor would try to do good work under almost any conditions but may be hampered by unsatisfactory conditions. Provision of proper facilities and equipment to a well-trained staff, as recommended by accrediting and approving bodies, makes it easier to practice high quality of medical care. The potential for good care may be realized routinely or only under special, exceptional circumstances.[8] Much depends on the leadership exercised by the chief of service.

Hospitals have been compared by listing and counting the range of services offered. This procedure is not a useful guide to quality of care for two reasons. In the first place, in New York City it is difficult to distinguish among hospitals in terms of basic facilities, since almost every hospital has a complete, or nearly complete, range. Second, the fact is that a hospital with a limited range of facilities may provide excellent care. Indeed, the provision of elaborate diagnostic and therapeutic equipment without a staff competent to use them can be dangerous for the patient.

Importance of Teaching. There is broad agreement that the presence of a teaching program in a hospital enhances the quality of its medical care. A recent report states: "The most effective medical care is provided when the staff is under the greatest stimulus to excel. The opportunity to teach is the greatest stimulus to professional growth." [9]

A hospital without an approved program for training interns or residents can, however, render high quality care to its patients, provided the chiefs of service and attending staff recognize that a physician's education is never completed. The medical leadership of the institution must imbue the staff with the constant desire to learn. Without a spirit of inquiry, self-criticism, and a desire to learn among the medical staff, even a hospital approved for intern and residency training is not likely to provide care of good quality; and a hospital without formal and regular teaching programs and without these attributes in its staff will almost certainly fail to do so.

There is no similar consensus as to the importance of medical research in a hospital for the quality of care (see Appendix 10.A).

RELIANCE ON MEDICAL RECORD

In the evaluation of the quality of care actually provided in a hospital, it has been customary to place heavy reliance on the medical record.

Ratios or Indexes. From the medical record it is possible to develop gross measures of performance in a hospital, such as death rates, consultation rates, proportion of patients discharged as recovered, and so forth. These rates are matched against standard indexes, and a judgment is made that the quality of care is adequate or inadequate.

Comparison of the rates for a given hospital with standard rates is now questioned as a method of appraising the quality of care. It has been criticized as illogical and incorrect [10] and incomplete.[11] With specific reference to the death rate, it has been pointed out that the great majority of hospital patients are discharged alive and are treated with the aim of relieving pain, preventing disability, and restoring function.[12]

Internal Medical Audit. Perhaps one half of the hospitals in this country regularly have a medical audit.[13] Most audits are conducted by the medical staff of the hospital.

Among internal audits perhaps the most systematic and best reported is that developed jointly by the Commission on Professional and Hospital Activities and the American College of Surgeons. It has two components: (1) a system of professional service accounting; and (2) an evaluation of selected records by each hospital's medical staff.

For the first the medical record librarian prepares an abstract of the medical record of every patient discharged from the hospital. This form is coded, its contents are punched on cards, and the cards are then processed by machine. The resulting tabulations provide routine hospital statistics, medical record room indexes, and comparative analyses of practices among hospitals.

The second component is an intensive evaluation of a sample of records, up to 10 percent of a particular diagnostic category. The evaluation is performed by one or more members of the hospital's medical staff specializing in the particular area under study and is recorded on a special form adapted to processing by machine.

A case review schedule or check sheet has been devised on which the reviewing physician records his opinions concerning all significant aspects of hospital care. These are grouped under the headings of hospitalization, diagnostic workup, and treatment. Under this procedure hospitalization has three aspects: necessity for admission, promptness of admission, and adequacy of length of stay. Responsibility for inadequacies, if any, is attributed to the medical profession, the hospital, the patient, and so forth. The diagnostic work-up embraces a history, physical examination, consultations, laboratory and x-ray services, and other diagnostic aids. Under treatment the check sheet deals with medications and other forms of therapy, complications, and deaths. For patients undergoing surgery the justification for the operation is established. These forms are processed by a statistical service center, and the report from the center juxtaposes the physician's opinions regarding the care given to a particular patient and the facts regarding the care actually rendered.

The medical staff of each hospital is expected to establish its own standards for evaluating the quality of care. This method, therefore, assumes the basic competence of physicians in a hospital. By developing its own standards the medical staff of a hospital is said to receive the maximum educational benefit from the audit. The standards are intended to reflect current medical thinking, thereby avoiding rigid criteria imposed from the outside and a freezing of medical practices.

Experience with this program has shown that maximum benefit is derived when the medical staff of one hospital participating in a medical audit can compare its results in caring for patients with a given disease with the results obtained in other hospitals. Patients with the same medical condition are, therefore, studied simultaneously in every hospital participating in the medical audit program. Over a long enough period of time this type of medical audit aims to cover the entire range of conditions cared for in a hospital.[14]

External Medical Audit. The external audit, conducted by an outside expert, is not so common. One of its leading exponents maintains that few hospital staffs have the degree of detachment necessary to evaluate the quality of care rendered to their patients.[15]

The external audit best reported in the literature is described as a systematic analysis of a sample of case records for accuracy of diagnosis and appropriateness of treatment. Statements in the medical record are verified in so far as possible by a postoperative pathological diagnosis, preoperative laboratory or x-ray diagnosis, documentation, or consultation. Uniform criteria are employed, written down with care, to judge the results in each hospital. The measure of quality in a hospital is the degree to which the proportion of cases conforming with the stated criteria approaches the standard degree of compliance, as ascertained from practices in one or more teaching hospitals that are noted for medical care of good quality.[16]

The auditor regards as acceptable a level of conformity to criteria well below 100 percent, thereby making implicit allowance for differences in clinical judgment. This is perhaps equivalent to the view that the quality of care cannot be measured for a single patient but only for a group. The precise formulation of this approach is: What is the probability that among a group of patients with defined characteristics a specified proportion will have received care of desired quality?

The appropriate selection of diagnostic procedures is considered more important than completeness. As one physician-administrator, formerly a medical educator, has said: "Completeness or inclusion [of services] does not necessarily constitute excellence. . . . Discriminating selection of information, deliberation, deduction, and astuteness are more significant in the qualitative care of a patient." [17]

The major objections to the external audit are three: (1) few individuals can perform it; (2) the method cannot handle evaluation of the whole hospital, since for many diseases objective criteria for diagnosis and treatment are lacking; and (3) the method yields little or no educational effect, for lack of staff participation.

Despite these objections, the external audit is acknowledged even by its critics as the method of choice when measurement of quality of care, rather than continuous improvement, is the primary aim. The external audit may also be regarded as preferable when the quality of care in a hospital is being questioned. [18]

USES AND LIMITATIONS OF MEDICAL RECORD

Some physicians rely on the medical record as the basis for appraising quality of care, because they see no feasible alternative. Direct observation of the patient by a physician other than the one caring for him is too costly. [19] Other physicians regard the medical record as the best possible source of information on what did and did not take place in the course of a patient's stay in the hospital. In addition, a complete medical record is essential in maintaining continuity of care when more than one physician is involved.

It has been said that the completeness of the medical record is in itself the best index of the quality of medical care. One such statement was made at the Beverly Hospital seminar on graduate

medical education: "It is pretty hard to have a poor teaching program [and poor medical care] and turn out first-class clinical
records, with good histories, good physical examinations, good
progress notes, and good discharge summary notes. If those are
present, you can almost discard all the rest of the criteria." [20]

The adequacy of the medical record for evaluating the quality
of care has also been questioned. In the first place, some doubt
its inherent accuracy, for a doctor may write his notes several
days or weeks after the event, sometimes completing several records at a time. The medical record's completeness has also been
questioned,[21] but there is evidence that failure to record may be
correlated with deficiencies in treatment.[22] Finally, and perhaps
most important, it has been noted that the medical record fails
to disclose certain elusive but nonetheless important aspects of the
doctor-patient relationship, an interaction between two personal-
ities.

A recent report on measuring the quality of medical care concludes that (1) an appraisal of the medical records in a hospital
can be an effective means of improving medical records and (2)
evaluation of medical care through the study of medical records
is more concerned with improving care and education than with
measuring quality.[23] It is perhaps not practicable to appraise the
quality of care without reference to the medical record. Although
a good medical record is indispensable,[24] the record alone is insufficient and should be supplemented with personal observation
and professional judgment by competent physicians.

OBSERVATION AND PERSONAL JUDGMENT

Observation can be performed by physicians informally. For
example, physicians in two local medical schools who supervise the
family care programs carried out by clinical clerks (third or fourth
year medical students) report that they have had occasion to care
for patients discharged from several municipal hospitals. Almost
invariably they find that patients fare poorly in municipal hospitals without medical school affiliation and do well in hospitals
with medical school affiliation. They agree that these impressions
have not been confirmed by systematic studies.

More systematic are judgments made by physician observers

from the outside who participate in ward rounds during which every patient is seen individually, his condition reviewed, and necessary measures instituted, continued, or changed, as indicated. The consultants appraise their colleagues in medicine, surgery, or other specialty according to their knowledge of how similar patients are cared for by leading physicians in good hospitals. This type of appraisal is usually made according to criteria that are not explicitly stated and are perhaps imperfectly understood.

A further refinement would be to make the criteria of judgment more explicit, so that the results might be reproduceable by different persons. Reproduceability of results cannot be assured because even experienced physicians have a significant degree of observed variation. Physicians with similar qualifications and backgrounds have been known to disagree in their appraisal of the quality of care even when working with carefully defined criteria.[25] In one study of the quality of care, diagnosis and treatment of patients were discussed with physicians after a review of the course of treatment described in the medical record. This method of study has been applied to medical group practice but not to hospitals.[26]

CONCLUDING COMMENTS

During staff interviews the suggestion was encountered that ultimately it will be necessary to go beyond the quality of medical care to the quality of hospital care, which includes services rendered by personnel other than physicians. In many illnesses tender and loving care of nurses is just as important as the care rendered by the physician. It would also be desirable to move on to a concept of appraising the end results of care, to take into account the patient's retention or restoration of function. This implies routine follow-up of patients some time after discharge, as was contemplated many years ago when measurement of quality of care was first proposed.[27] Consideration of the cost of care and of alternative modes of treatment may also be relevant.

The views recently expressed by the special medical advisory group of the Veterans Administration, as cited in a recent report seem apt: "While good medicine could perhaps be evaluated, it cannot be measured by application of any presently available yardstick, but can only be judged by one who is well versed in the medical profession." [28]

Appraising Quality of Care in Local Hospitals

Much has been said recently regarding the poor quality of care in municipal hospitals without medical school affiliation. These hospitals are clearly operating under certain disadvantages, such as house staff educated in foreign medical schools, poorly maintained plant and equipment, insufficient number of registered nurses for three shifts a day seven days a week, and attending staff in the process of attrition. Voluntary unaffiliated hospitals share some of these deficiencies, and even major teaching hospitals in both systems have difficulty in attracting attending staff in certain specialties.

The attending staff is commonly held to be the most important single factor in the quality of medical care. In interviews it was stated that for certain types of patient the medical care was as good in unaffiliated municipal hospitals as in medical school hospitals. This is particularly true for a patient admitted in the daytime, when members of the attending staff are present.

In municipal hospitals that serve as community hospitals, in the absence of a voluntary hospital in the neighborhood, the standards of care can be said to be the best available to that community. These standards are frequently more than adequate for certain types of patient and not adequate for others. It is nothing new that community hospitals are at a disadvantage in caring for patients with unusually difficult diagnostic or treatment problems.

The conditions under which medical care is provided may be difficult in municipal unaffiliated hospitals. These conditions do not, however, preclude physicians from working to the limits of their capabilities. Conversely, where the objective surrounding conditions are good, the incentives to quality performance day by day may conceivably be lacking.

It is not an appraisal of potentialities that is important, but an evaluation of the actual care given. It would be appropriate for the New York Academy of Medicine to take the lead in a major effort to appraise and compare the quality of care in hospitals in New York City—voluntary, municipal, and proprietary. The

Board of Hospitals is vested with broad duties and powers in this field (see Chapter 9) and would undoubtedly wish to cooperate and participate.

For lack of funds investigators have been unable to employ personal observation to appraise the quality of care. In view of the large and increasing expenditures for hospital care, an appropriation as high as $1 million for an appraisal of the quality of care in New York City hospitals would be only one fifth of one percent of total expenditures in New York City in one year, currently estimated at $500 million (see Chapter 12).

Alternative approaches to the appraisal of quality of care might be applied to a sample of hospitals, representative of their ownership groups, size classes, and teaching status. The methods employed should embrace the best elements of the medical audit by means of the medical record and observation and professional judgment by outside experts, with the several elements used in combination or separately. Consideration might be given to adding to the evaluation team persons other than physicians, particularly nurses and social workers, to appraise nonmedical aspects of the care of patients. The decisive factor in a successful outcome would undoubtedly be the knowledge, experience, and judgment of the leaders of the team.

Beyond the immediate objective of appraising the quality of care actually rendered in individual institutions and making comparisons among them, there is reason to expect other useful results. Among them would be recommendations for improvement, where needed, reassurance that the quality of care is adequate, if it is, and new knowledge concerning the advantages and limitations of the several methods. This undertaking could also provide a base-line for future efforts by the hospitals' own medical staffs to improve the quality of care.

Summary

1. Although evaluation and approval by voluntary professional organizations is characteristic of the hospital scene in this country, there is also an underlying floor of supervision by government. In New York State authority for regulating hospitals rests with the State Board of Social Welfare, which exercises its au-

thority by delegation to the State Department of Social Welfare and to municipalities.

2. The question is raised whether a City department with the primary mission of operating a large hospital system should be expected to supervise another hospital system.

3. A proposal is described to have inspections performed by teams of physicians and other personnel, recruited from outside the regulatory agency.

4. Attention is invited to the increasingly important role played by the Superintendent of Insurance.

5. One index of a hospital's potential for providing good care is accreditation. In New York City all but 8 voluntary hospitals and all but 2 municipal hospitals are accredited. Among proprietary hospitals, 9 were accredited in 1957, 1958, and 1959, an increase of 6 from 1954. By the end of 1960, 13 proprietary hospitals were accredited.

6. The published list of accredited hospitals does not distinguish between three-year and one-year accreditation. The latter signifies that the inspector found the hospital on the borderline. To maintain accreditation, it must improve.

7. Approval of a hospital for graduate training, which can be granted only subsequent to accreditation, has been taken to signify the provision of good care as a concomitant of teaching. The failure of many hospitals to attract graduates of American (United States and Canadian) medical schools has impaired the value of approval as an index of quality.

8. The ideal way to appraise quality of medical care would be to observe and judge the effect of specific measures on the patient's health. That cannot be done in many instances.

9. One solution is to appraise quality on the basis of the conditions surrounding the provision of care, including available resources. Of key importance is the medical staff.

10. There are objections to inferring actual performance from capability. On the one hand, there is no assurance that potentialities will be realized day by day, rather than on special occasions. On the other hand, qualified persons working under adverse conditions are not precluded from reaching the limits of their capabilities.

11. Most physicians who wish to appraise the quality of care actually rendered rely heavily on the medical record. Both internal and external audits do this. A major and systematic example of each type of audit is described.

12. It is important that the medical record be supplemented by personal observation and professional judgment. This need is appreciated by many investigators, who have been hampered by lack of funds.

13. In view of the large and rising expenditures for hospital care, which now approximate $500 million in New York City, an appropriation of $1 million to appraise the quality of care in local hospitals would not be unwarranted.

14. It would be appropriate for the New York Academy of Medicine to take the lead in such an enterprise. The Board of Hospitals, with its broad duties and powers in this field, would undoubtedly wish to participate.

15. The study might employ alternative approaches to appraising quality of care in a sample of hospitals, representative of their ownership groups, size classes, and teaching status.

Appendix 10.A

MEDICAL RESEARCH IN HOSPITALS

The importance of research in medicine and the basic sciences is widely recognized. How far hospitals that are not staffed by medical schools can go in these fields depends primarily on the interest and ability of their medical staffs and on the funds available for research. In the past such institutions have made notable contributions to medical knowledge.[29]

Anything that promotes an atmosphere of active and purposeful inquiry into the diagnostic and treatment problems of the sick is apt to have a constructive effect on the type of medicine practiced in an institution. The carrying-on of research (or, at least, the existence of the research point of view) creates such a stimulus. It is doubtful, however, whether a sustained research effort can be maintained in institutions dependent exclusively upon the part-time contributed services of clinicians.

A major study of medical research in this country concluded that in almost all instances hospitals performing research have been able to attract financial support. Lack of funds has seldom been decisive in excluding research from a hospital.[30] It is unlikely that availability of funds would be a decisive limiting factor in the future.

Data are available that throw some light on research activity in New York City hospitals outside the medical school framework. For the first time expenditures for medical research in the hospital setting have been compiled; that is, research conducted in hospitals but not necessarily paid for by hospital funds. The survey was conducted jointly by the National Institutes of Health (NIH) and the American Hospital Association for fiscal year 1958. Although the data for the country as a whole have not yet been published, NIH furnished the Hospital Council with the data for New York City.

Expenditures for research in hospitals in New York City that submitted reports amounted to $19.2 million. This figure falls short of the total, as 4 of the 6 hospitals whose medical staffs are appointed on nomination of medical schools are not included.

Voluntary, municipal, and proprietary hospitals whose staffs are not appointed by medical schools accounted for $3.85 million of the expenditures reported. On the basis of supplementary data, including postcard inquiries, a more nearly complete total for these institutions is $4.2 million. This sum constitutes more than one but less than two percent of the total expenditures of these hospitals. Table 10.1 shows the distribution of total research expenditures by hospital ownership.

Table 10.1. DISTRIBUTION BY HOSPITAL OWNERSHIP OF MEDI-
CAL RESEARCH EXPENDITURES IN NON-MEDICAL-
SCHOOL HOSPITALS, NEW YORK CITY,
FISCAL YEAR 1958

Ownership	Number of Hospitals	Amount (in Thousands of Dollars)	Percent
All hospitals	44	4,225	100.0
Voluntary	33	4,020	95.1
Municipal	10	155	3.7
Proprietary	1	50	1.2

SOURCE: National Institutes of Health, survey of hospital research.

As previously stated, there are no data on research expenditures in hospitals for earlier years. Data on trends in research grants by NIH, which have become an increasingly important fraction of all medical research expenditures, are, however, available. The predominant role of voluntary hospitals goes back at least a decade.

The year 1957 witnessed a sharp increase in research grants to voluntary hospitals not staffed by medical schools, when they rose from $0.5 million to $1 million. Previously annual increases in research grants to institutions in New York City had flowed chiefly to medical

Table 10.2. DISTRIBUTION BY HOSPITAL OWNERSHIP OF NIH
RESEARCH GRANTS TO NON-MEDICAL-SCHOOL
HOSPITALS, NEW YORK CITY, FISCAL YEARS
1951 AND 1956–59 (IN THOUSANDS OF DOLLARS)

Ownership	1951	1956	1957	1958	1959
All hospitals	313	511	1,032	1,391	2,419
Voluntary	310	511	1,014	1,364	2,335
Municipal	3	0	3	12	69
Proprietary	0	0	15	15	15

SOURCE: National Institutes of Health, *Public Health Service Grants and Awards,*
Part I (Washington, D.C., 1951, 1956–59).

schools and their hospitals and to research institutes. Since then voluntary hospitals not staffed by medical schools have registered a substantial gain in the amount of research grants received. Even so, in 1958 NIH grants accounted for only one third of their expenditures for medical research.

The amount of all NIH grants to institutions in New York City increased sixfold between fiscal years 1951 and 1959, as shown in Table 10.3. Voluntary hospitals not staffed by medical schools are receiving an increasing proportion of all NIH grants coming into New York City and seem to be assuming increasing importance in medical research. Of total expenditures for medical research in voluntary hospitals not staffed by medical schools, four fifths took place in the 12 hospitals with full-time chiefs in one or more clinical services (see Chapter 9). These hospitals are receiving an increasing proportion of the funds flowing into New York City. They received 76 percent of the grants to voluntary hospitals not staffed by medical schools in 1957, 81 percent in 1958, and 83 percent in 1959.

Table 10.3. PROPORTION OF TOTAL NIH RESEARCH GRANTS
RECEIVED BY VOLUNTARY HOSPITALS NOT STAFFED
BY MEDICAL SCHOOLS, NEW YORK CITY,
FISCAL YEARS 1951 AND 1956–59

Year	Total Amount (in Thousands of Dollars)	Percent Non-Medical-School Voluntary Hospitals to Total
1951	2,467,000	12.5
1956	5,176,000	9.9
1957	9,829,000	10.3
1958	11,771,000	11.6
1959	15,690,000	14.9

SOURCE: National Institutes of Health, *Public Health Service Grants and Awards,*
Part I (Washington, D.C., 1951, 1956–59).

Compared with the country as a whole, New York City's proportion of total NIH research funds, recently 12 percent, has been declining. The decline may be associated with an increase in the number of institutions in this country receiving NIH grants.

Summary

1. There is no consensus on the essentiality of medical research for improving the care of patients in a hospital.

2. Availability of funds has not been in the past, and is not likely to be in the future, the limiting factor in conducting medical research in hospitals.

3. In New York City research expenditures in the hospital setting in 1958 exceeded by several million the reported figure of $19.2 million. It is estimated that $4.2 million was spent in hospitals not staffed by medical schools; 95 percent of this amount was spent in voluntary hospitals.

4. Voluntary hospitals not staffed by medical schools are attracting an increasing share of the federal research grants coming into New York City. These grants constituted one third of the research expenditures of these hospitals in 1958.

5. Four fifths of research expenditures in voluntary hospitals not staffed by medical schools occur in hospitals with full-time chiefs of clinical service. This proportion appears to be rising.

11 AFFILIATION, REGIONALIZATION, AND COORDINATION

It is helpful to review briefly the principal findings on hospital staffing, facilities, organization, and quality of care. These findings underlie the following discussion of actions that might be taken by hospitals jointly and of separate actions that might be expected to have an important effect on others.

The attending staffs in municipal hospitals without medical school affiliation are undergoing a process of attrition. In 9 of 11 general hospitals the size of staff has declined since 1948. Difficulty in attracting physicians is demonstrated by the need to pay more of them for work in the outpatient department. Persistent differences exist between municipal and voluntary hospitals without medical school affiliation in the characteristics of attending staff. There are no comparable differences between municipal and voluntary hospitals with medical school affiliation (see Chapter 5).

Twelve voluntary hospitals in New York City not staffed by medical schools have instituted a system of full-time chiefs of clinical service, whereas all municipal nonuniversity hospitals continue to rely on their volunteer attending staffs to supervise patient care, medical education, and research. The laboratory and radiology services of the latter suffer from the absence of full-time chiefs and other personnel; salary is so inadequate that part-time service in what is supposed to be a full-time position is tacitly and widely assumed and tolerated (see Chapter 9).

As for teaching programs, all but one of the municipal general hospitals are approved by the Council on Medical Education and Hospitals of the American Medical Association for internship training and for residency training in two or more fields. A large number of voluntary hospitals are not approved for either type of training and employ paid house physicians. However, municipal hospitals not staffed by medical schools have almost uniformly failed to recruit graduates of American (United States and Canadian) medical schools, whereas a considerable number of voluntary hospitals not staffed by medical schools but with more limited forms of affiliation have been successful in so doing. To a lesser degree the inability to attract graduates of American medical schools to house staff is also displayed by two of the four municipal general hospitals staffed by medical schools (see Chapter 6).

There is a wide difference between the two hospital systems in staffing the nursing service, particularly with registered nurses. The difference in staffing ratios is widened if cognizance is taken of the large number of special duty nurses in some voluntary hospitals. Municipal hospitals are experiencing increasing tightness in staffing their registered nurse positions, both because of gradual attrition and expanding need (see Chapter 7).

Municipal hospitals in New York City face a serious problem in replacing their medical superintendents, many of whom entered the system during the depression of the 1930s. There is a greater than normal separation of authority and responsibility for expenditures and personnel in municipal hospitals, with authority lodged chiefly in the office of the Bureau of the Budget (see Chapter 9).

Municipal hospitals have accomplished a much greater degree of physical plant "renewal" during the postwar period than voluntary hospitals. This superior achievement is somewhat offset by poor quality of plant maintenance (see Chapter 8).

When all these findings are considered, as well as differences in the scale of medical research, it would seem that the ability of municipal unaffiliated hospitals to render care of high quality is below that of comparable voluntary hospitals. Capability is not a conclusive index of performance, however, since individuals and organizations may not live up to it. It is important that the quality of care actually provided in the two hospital systems, particularly in the unaffiliated hospitals, be evaluated and compared (see Chapter 10).

The gradual attrition of the attending staffs of municipal unaffiliated hospitals means that their relative disadvantages are in the process of being aggravated. Measures to arrest and, if possible, to reverse the course of events are, therefore, in order.

Among the proposals advanced in the preceding chapters, certain ones can be carried out in one hospital or group of hospitals because they do not impinge on the operations of others. Included are appointment of full-time chiefs of clinical service under appropriate circumstances; a pay differential for interns and residents between municipal unaffiliated and affiliated hospitals; larger differentials for nurses participating in a three-shift rotation scheme; improved maintenance of municipal hospital plant; vesting greater authority in the administrators of municipal hospitals; and appraisal of the quality of care.

In addition, certain proposals are now pending that cannot be carried out by a single hospital or by one group of hospitals, because their implementation would impinge on the operations of others. Among these proposals, which are discussed in the succeeding sections of this chapter, are close affiliations between municipal unaffiliated hospitals and medical schools or voluntary major teaching hospitals, regionalization of hospital services, and establishment of services for private and semiprivate patients in municipal hospitals.

Affiliation among Institutions

Affiliation among medical institutions can take many forms. It may be limited to a relationship between a clinical department in one hospital and its counterpart in another, or it may apply to entire institutions. It may be limited to rotation of student nurses, interns, or residents, or it can involve exchange of attending staff as well. It can extend to the flow of patients, as in regional patterns of organization (see below). It may be an arrangement among three hospitals of equal size and strength that agree to share in offering a three-year residency program in a specialty, or it may be an arrangement whereby a larger and stronger institution tries to help a weaker one. The stronger institution may be a medical school or a hospital. The weaker institution may be a general hospital or a facility for the care of long-term patients, such as a hospital for the chronically ill, a nursing home, or a home for the aged.

There is nothing new about the idea of affiliation or the arrangements for carrying it out. Affiliation exists today among a large number of hospitals in New York City, usually for graduate medical training. Most frequently a single department of a hospital is involved.

There are 11 municipal general hospitals that are not staffed by a medical school or on nomination by its faculty. Of this number, 6 have some degree of association (weaker than affiliation) with a medical school, and 5 do not. Among the 6 hospitals, 3 may be classified as having nominal or inactive associations, and 3 as active in one or more clinical departments. Among the 5 with no medical school association, 1 has an association with a voluntary teaching hospital. The presence or absence of some degree of association with a medical school does not seem to make any difference in a hospital's ability to recruit attending staff or house staff.

Under proposals now outstanding it is intended that the scope of affiliation be broader and more intensive than in the past. The thought is that a stronger institution, either a medical school or a voluntary hospital with a broad teaching program, would take a municipal nonuniversity hospital under its wing and assist in staffing its services. Chiefly involved are the attending staff and interns and residents. Before such an arrangement can be effectuated, the laboratory and radiology services of the municipal hospital must be improved by enlarging space, acquiring new equipment, hiring additional technicians, and providing full-time supervision by physicians.[1]

Affiliation of the scope envisioned now exists between 8 municipal hospitals (4 general, 2 cancer, and 2 long-term), on the one hand, and the 6 medical schools in New York City and 1 voluntary hospital, on the other hand. While one medical school is responsible for staffing approximately 3,000 beds in the municipal hospital system, another is responsible for less than 300.

Experience with existing and past arrangements suggests that certain obstacles must be overcome for broad and intensive affiliations to succeed. These obstacles can be grouped under three headings: absence of mutual advantage, distance, and lack of depth in staff.

ABSENCE OF MUTUAL ADVANTAGE

Although all parties to an affiliation arrangement may be imbued with social purpose and a desire to serve the community, the expression of this purpose and desire is limited by the needs of their own institutions.

It is evident why a weak hospital should welcome assistance to upgrade it, especially if the proffered assistance does not entail loss of identity. It is not easy to see what a medical school stands to gain by furnishing such assistance, unless it is seeking additional, or a different type of, clinical material. Although some medical schools do not believe in academic seclusion,[2] others have traditionally eschewed an active community role, focusing their interest and energies on medical research and education. From a financial standpoint affiliation is more likely to bring losses than gains.

Experience in New York City indicates that a medical school will terminate an arrangement, even a recent one, to staff a municipal hospital if its medical staff shows a disinclination to travel. When this arrangement is terminated, it is not possible to return to the situation that prevailed prior to the affiliation, because in the interim the original staff has been dispersed. Experience also indicates that, if recruitment falls short of goals, a university hospital will withdraw residents from rotation among affiliated hospitals, giving priority to its own requirements for house staff.

It would appear that the advantages of affiliating with a municipal nonuniversity hospital might be much greater for a voluntary hospital than for a medical school. The reason is that access to the ward patients of a municipal hospital for teaching purposes creates the prospect of reducing or eliminating the operating deficit of the voluntary hospital. To begin with, the number of public-charge inpatients, for whose care the City's daily payment fails to meet average cost, would be lower than formerly. In addition, the volume of services rendered in the outpatient department, which has become an increasingly important source of financial loss, could be curtailed, since the outpatient department would no longer be needed as a source of patients for the ward services (see Chapters 2 and 14).

One problem that might prove more troublesome for a voluntary hospital than for a medical school attempting to improve the staff of a municipal hospital pertains to the latter's willingness to accept control over staff appointments or nominations to the attending staff. For reasons of prestige and administrative organization, the necessary measure of control may be more acceptable when it comes from a medical school.

DISTANCE

In New York City travel is time-consuming even for short distances and parking space near hospitals is usually at a premium. Although some members of the attending staff will travel from one hospital to another if requested to do so, many will not do so on a regular schedule. It is often observed that a physician will not actively participate in the work of a facility if he cannot walk to it bare-headed and without his overcoat. The problem posed by travel can be mitigated by making use of full-time staff at voluntary hospitals who are perhaps more accountable for their actions in this regard; by building separate staffs or cores of separate staffs at the two institutions; and by offering extra inducements to the attending staff, such as accelerated promotion to men at the assistant or associate attending level and more opportunities to admit private and semiprivate patients to the home hospital.

Perhaps a majority of voluntary hospitals not staffed by medical schools that might be considered suitable sources of assistance in the staffing of municipal hospitals have one or more full-time chiefs of clinical service. However, only one has them in all four basic clinical services.

LACK OF DEPTH IN STAFF

To build duplicate staffs of equal competence at two institutions calls for a depth in attending staff that few hospitals have achieved. No hospital should undertake an affiliation of the scope envisaged unless it can do so creditably and without undue strain on its resources. There should also be reasonable prospects that a stable relationship can be maintained for the foreseeable future.

For one hospital to recruit an attending staff of sufficient size and quality to staff two institutions is merely difficult; for it to recruit such a house staff is virtually impossible.[3] The arithmetic is clear: the number of positions in graduate training programs in hospitals is far beyond the capacity of American medical schools to fill. There is no prospect that this over-all shortage will be overcome, since the decision of the Council of Medical Education and Hospitals in approving a given educational program and the decision of an approved program in setting the number of positions to staff are independent of the total supply of new physicians in this country (see Chapter 6). The existing shortage will continue to affect nonuniversity hospitals primarily, as long as students regard the educational opportunities at university hospitals as more attractive. The individual nonuniversity hospital is not helpless, however, to influence the outcome; it can compete with its peers in quality of training program, level of salary, and quantity and types of amenities offered.

The program of affiliation should be encouraged where it promises to be an effective and lasting relationship. This implies willingness, as well as ability, on the part of the voluntary hospital to discharge the obligations assumed in an affiliation over an extended period of time. As a practical matter, it might be desirable to associate a medical school with one or more voluntary hospitals in staffing a given municipal hospital.

CONTIGUOUS LOCATION

The obstacle to close affiliation posed by distance can, of course, be overcome by eliminating it. Examples of contiguous or adjacent location between affiliated institutions in New York City are James Ewing (municipal) at Memorial (voluntary) and Francis Delafield (municipal) at the Columbia University–Presbyterian Medical Center. Another notable example is Rochester Municipal and Strong Memorial (voluntary) hospitals.

When a municipal hospital affiliated with a voluntary hospital or medical school is slated for replacement because of a deteriorated or obsolete physical plant, it can be relocated on the campus of the voluntary hospital or medical school if the site permits. One consequence of such relocation may be increased travel time for some indigent and medically indigent patients. A balanced judgment must then be made whether high quality care obtained at some distance and inconvenience is preferable to readily accessible medical care of poorer quality. A further advantage of relocation, it has been suggested, is that the presence of a ward service in an adjacent municipal hospital would enable the voluntary hospital to reduce the size of its own ward service.[4]

All other things being equal, a close and effective affiliation is more likely to continue between adjacent institutions than between distant ones. All other things are usually not equal, however. Experience indicates that where the appeal of mutual advantage is sufficiently strong, effective affiliations are maintained between institutions separated by some distance. In such cases, it may be necessary to develop cores of separate medical staffs.

Relocation of municipal hospitals at the sites of voluntary hospitals or medical schools affiliating with them could lead to freezing the size of the municipal general-hospital system at a high level. Conceivably the new level could be higher than the existing one, if each municipal hospital incorporated at its new site its previous bed capacity plus the ward beds about to be eliminated by the voluntary hospital. The amount and proportion of tax funds spent for hospital care would remain high. Moreover, there would be a tendency to maintain a large number of ward beds in voluntary hospitals without municipal hospital affiliation because all other hospitals would continue to rely heavily on ward patients for teaching.

There is the further problem of deciding which one among the voluntary hospitals that wish to attract a municipal hospital to its campus would get one. In areas of the city where one voluntary hospital is preeminent, the decision is easy; here the only problem is that there is no way to assure continued preeminence. In areas where there is no single preeminent voluntary hospital, however, to select one is to deprive all others of the opportunity to help the municipal system and to reduce the size of their ward services.

AN ALTERNATIVE PROPOSAL

If the suggestions made later in this report on City reimbursement of voluntary hospitals were adopted, there would be no financial reasons for voluntary hospitals to wish to reduce or abandon their ward services and to convert vacated ward areas into semiprivate accommodations (see Chapter 21). In the absence of a financial problem, an alternative plan would seem to cope with the other problems more directly.

At this time, and for the foreseeable future, voluntary hospitals appear to have an advantage in recruiting staff. It is the stronger voluntary hospitals, therefore, that should expand facilities. As additional facilities at voluntary hospitals come into operation, unsuitable facilities at municipal unaffiliated hospitals could be closed and suitable ones converted to other use. The new facilities at voluntary hospitals would be built in accordance with an over-all plan and provide for flexible use of accommodations between semiprivate and ward patients. A larger number of the new beds might be used by ward patients initially than subsequently, when the proportion of private payments to hospital income will have increased.

This plan has several advantages. There would be no need for voluntary hospitals to spend money converting space from ward to semiprivate use, since a reduction in municipal beds would result in the transfer of some ward patients to voluntary hospitals. Ward space is not always convertible to semiprivate use at low or reasonable cost. It would be possible for several voluntary hospitals in an area, rather than one, to participate in an expansion of facilities: to include one would not mean excluding all others. Added inconvenience to patients and longer travel time arising from the concentration of ward beds at one hospital would be avoided. Pressure to maintain large ward services at voluntary hospitals excluded from the previous plan would be absent. In the long run it may also be expected that pressure to establish municipal hospitals in areas of the city that do not now have them would be minimized.

This plan implies continuation of a cooperative relationship between the City and voluntary hospitals. Indeed, the degree of cooperation called for would be greater than now exists. It would no longer be possible for voluntary hospitals to transfer patients with the prognosis of a long stay, because ample municipal hospital beds would not be there to receive them. Voluntary hospitals would also face the necessity of providing facilities for patients no longer in need of general hospital care. Conversely, it may be necessary for the City to lend construction money to voluntary hospitals at favorable terms (see Chapter 21). Certainly, the City's rate of payment would have to be made—and kept—adequate.

Regionalization of Hospital Services

Regionalization of hospital services has many meanings and varied applications.[5] In this book it is distinguished from affiliation, as discussed above, on the basis that the latter is an arrangement between two (or perhaps three) institutions whereas regionalization involves many.

In this country regional hospital organization has usually been aimed at bringing the advantages of modern medical care to rural areas. The mechanisms by which this is done are a reciprocal flow of personnel and services from the medical center to the rural hospital and of patients with difficult diagnostic or treatment problems from the rural hospital to the center. In the formal scheme of regionalization a third level, a district hospital, serves as an intermediary.[6] Many of the plans developed by state Hill-Burton agencies are based on the concept of three levels of hospitals, but few have been carried beyond the schematic outline stage.[7]

It would be useful to describe and distinguish the threefold classification of hospitals in the Hospital Council's *Master Plan for Hospitals and Related Facilities for New York City*. In the *Master Plan* hospitals are defined as community, regional, or central in accordance with the scope of their residency training programs. Since an approved training program is conceived to require a certain number of beds, the classification of a hospital bears some relationship to its size. There is also a relationship between the classification of a hospital and the size of population served, at least for some types of care, because it takes a smaller population to yield enough patients for a training program in a specialty like internal medicine than in a specialty like neurology.

In the *Master Plan* the basis for classifying hospitals is the presence of specified residency training programs, and no cognizance is taken of the range of services actually provided. No hospital is precluded from rendering services in a specialty by virtue of the absence of residency training in this specialty.

Suggestions to organize the hospitals in the city along regional lines have had as their principal aim reduction in unnecessary expenditures by avoiding duplication of expensive hospital facilities for which there is only a limited demand. The most frequently cited examples of duplication are too many hospitals with a cobalt bomb for treating cancer patients or too many hospitals performing cardiac surgery.

More recently, owing to the staffing difficulties that confront certain municipal hospitals, it has been proposed that municipal hospitals be reorganized and changed from a group of medically autonomous institutions into an interrelated regional network.[8] Care of patients requiring certain specialty services would be concentrated at university hospitals, whereas emergency and general services would continue to be rendered in community hospitals. This proposal combines the objective of economy, as above, with that of improved quality of care, as in regional schemes of organization elsewhere.

Specifically, it is intended that certain programs of care be located in some hospitals and be excluded from others. Any attempt to do this is bound to meet difficulties. A discussion of some of these difficulties follows.

1. Boards of trustees are rightfully proud of the identities of their hospitals and zealously pursue the objective of doing the best possible job. Frequently doing a good job is equated with doing the entire job. Sometimes the desire to do a good job and a complete one becomes a desire to do a big job. Apart from the question of bigness for its own sake, it should be possible to convince a hospital that it need not be complete in every respect in order to do a good job. There are certain functions and services that are basic to a good hospital, such as diagnostic x-ray, laboratory, operating suite, and emergency department. Beyond that point selective discrimination is a virtue. If boards of trustees are to be persuaded that it is permissible for their hospitals to forego certain facilities and programs, they must be convinced that other hospitals are also foregoing facilities and programs in the community's interest.

2. When a voluntary hospital surrenders a program of care to another hospital, its medical staff stands to lose income from the care of private patients. There is no reason why the physicians

involved should welcome this. Despite a growing feeling that a physician should limit his active staff appointments to no more than two hospitals,[9] it would seem that a regional scheme of hospital organization in a large city cannot be successfully accomplished without the selective granting of duplicate staff appointments to certain physicians, namely, those with special competence in the fields in which programs are to be confined to a small number of hospitals. Duplication of appointments has not been frequently attempted in other regional plans of organization; and, when attempted, it has not been successfully carried out.[10] Several large cities are, however, recognizing the importance of this step in providing good emergency care.[11]

3. When a municipal or voluntary hospital surrenders a program of care, its physicians stand to lose in professional opportunity. They do not like this to happen, and they are in a position to make their wishes felt in those instances in which the facilities required in the excluded program are highly specialized. Where unique facilities are not required, a plan to distribute selected programs of service among hospitals may not work. For example, several years ago an order was issued by the Commissioner of Hospitals directing that candidates for cancer surgery be channeled to the specialty hospitals of the Department. This order has enjoyed less than full success. Selective duplication of staff appointments for physicians may help to overcome their resistance to the redirection or transfer of patients.

4. The selective distribution of programs of care among hospitals is more easily accomplished for services alone than for services combined with research. In clinical research patients with specified characteristics are needed from time to time, though not routinely.

5. The negotiations envisaged under point one above need guidance from an over-all plan for the selective distribution of services among hospitals. Such a plan would be difficult to prepare and would be even more difficult to keep up to date in light of changing conditions. Yesterday's discovery is today's basic and essential tool; a weak hospital today may be a strong one tomorrow or the day after. It is important that regard for efficiency not be allowed to hamper development and growth.

6. Finally, there is the question whether a regional plan of organization is intended to apply separately within each hospital system or cut across the two systems. If it applies separately within each system, the complexities that would arise from having private and semiprivate patients in municipal hospitals can be avoided (see below). Presumably a patient who can afford to pay both hospital and physician would go to the nearest voluntary hospital designated to render the service (provided his physician held an appointment there). However, patients may not understand the arrangement if the municipal hospital designated to render the same service to the sick poor is located at some distance, perhaps in another borough.

Although municipal hospitals in New York City are primarily for the sick poor, under certain circumstances they also care for patients who can afford to pay. Included are emergency admissions (especially patients picked up by the emergency ambulances of municipal hospitals), patients in need of unique municipal facilities not elsewhere available (such as respirator centers or units for persons with cerebral palsy), and premature infants transferred to centers, all of whose beds—voluntary and municipal—are in effect treated as a pool, with the infant admitted to the nearest vacant bed.

Patients with means who are not emergencies may be admitted to municipal hospitals, but this does not happen often. If regionalization were attempted in a number of specialty areas and if both hospital systems were meshed in one or more of them, the question of caring for patients with means seeking admission to a municipal hospital would arise more frequently. It might then be advisable to permit physicians to charge a fee.

In summary, regionalization in a metropolitan center, such as New York City, has obvious appeal. It signifies a reduction in, or elimination of, unnecessary expenditures. It can also serve to improve the quality of care by bringing patients to hospitals where qualified personnel and suitable facilities are concentrated. A number of obstacles must, however, be overcome for regionalization to succeed. Perhaps the most important single step required is to provide duplicate staff appointments to physicians affected by the selective location of specialty programs in certain hospitals.

Also important is the development of an over-all plan for the geographic distribution of specialty services, with provisions for periodic review and for negotiations among hospital representatives at the highest level. In fields of medical care in which it is desirable to mesh the services of the two hospital systems, it may be necessary to permit physicians to charge professional fees to patients with means admitted to municipal hospitals.

Private Services in Municipal Hospitals

There have been a number of proposals to establish facilities for private patients (those who are cared for by their own physician and pay him; semiprivate patients, including those in private wards, are included) in municipal general hospitals. One proposal is aimed at the special problems faced by medical school faculty staffing a university hospital. Another concerns private patient privileges for practicing physicians now lacking them. Still another aims to offer inducements to physicians to spend more time at municipal hospitals.

NEEDS OF FACULTY AT UNIVERSITY HOSPITALS

It is desirable that the full-time faculty of a medical school have access to facilities for private (including semiprivate) patients. This is important, both to expose the faculty and their students to patients from all economic levels and to afford to the middle- and upper-income groups of the population the opportunities enjoyed by the low-income groups to receive medical care from leading physicians. In some institutions income from private patients supplements the salaries of full-time staff. Elsewhere, it may be a source of extra budgetary income for the several clinical departments of the medical school, helping to finance research and teaching.

The Hospital Council has supported the principle of permitting the full-time faculties of medical schools to see private patients.[12] Once this principle is accepted, it is advantageous that the physicians care for their patients in a hospital located at or near the medical school, so that as little time as possible is lost in travel. The policy question is whether the private patients should be cared for at an existing municipal hospital or in a separate university hospital.

At present four municipal general hospitals in New York City are staffed by medical schools. One of the four, Metropolitan, is located some distance away from the medical school and its associated voluntary hospital. In another instance a voluntary hospital is being built on the campus of the medical school that also houses the municipal hospital, Bellevue. At the third, Kings County Hospital Center, steps are being taken to build a university hospital on the medical school campus with State funds. In the fourth instance, Bronx Municipal Hospital Center, a university hospital that will care for private patients is planned as soon as the necessary funds are raised.

The Hospital Council approved both the university hospital that is now being built and the one in process of development in Brooklyn. It has never passed on the desirability of setting aside 100 or 200 beds in a municipal hospital for the medical school faculty to care for private and semiprivate patients. Without prejudging the Hospital Council's response to such a question, the answer would obviously depend on the specific circumstances of the case. Among the factors to be considered are the feasibility of converting space in an existing municipal hospital for use by private and semiprivate patients, adequacy of the available space in the municipal hospital, if convertible, to meet the bed needs of the full-time medical school faculty, the over-all adequacy of beds in the area to meet community needs, and the degree of assurance forthcoming regarding faculty control of research and teaching in the existing hospital.

If beds for private and semiprivate patients were established in a municipal university hospital, it would be necessary to supplement existing arrangements with billing machinery appropriate to private patients and to provide certain amenities that are customarily afforded to private patients, as is done at Sydenham Hospital. Such beds would presumably be reserved for use by the institutional full-time medical faculty only, whose incomes are restricted in one fashion or another.

DIVERSE OBJECTIVES AT NONUNIVERSITY HOSPITALS

At municipal nonuniversity hospitals the proposal to establish facilities for private and semiprivate patients takes two forms. One is designed to afford relief to certain physicians practicing in the community who are excluded from staff appointments at voluntary hospitals, despite their professional qualifications and ethical behavior. The second views private services as potentially benefiting the hospitals, by making it more convenient and worthwhile for the attending staffs to spend time there.

Relief to Certain Physicians without Staff Appointments. The Hospital Council has repeatedly stated that every physician in practice should have a hospital staff appointment and privileges commensurate with his competence. A staff appointment can be conceived of in two parts: the privilege of caring for private and semiprivate patients and the opportunity to participate in teaching (and learning) by caring for patients in the ward and in the outpatient department. The optimum situation is for the two parts of the appointment to be combined at one hospital.

Application of this principle is frequently complicated by the fact that there are no arithmetic rules for calculating the size of attending staff appropriate for a hospital of a given size and for determining who should be its members. The number of physicians per 100 beds will vary with the ratio of ambulatory services provided in a hospital to the volume of inpatient services, the proportion of ward to total beds, and the diagnostic composition of patients, along with other factors influencing the turnover of hospital beds. As to the identity of physicians comprising the staff of a given hospital, geographic propinquity may play a role, but probably not a preponderant one in a city where hospitals and physicians are frequently clustered.

For physicians in group practice application of the broad principle is further complicated by their preference for practicing as a group inside the hospital as well as outside. It then becomes necessary for a hospital to appoint a number of physicians to its staff as a group, rather than one at a time.

Undeniably serious practical difficulties face an individual hospital in trying to apply the principle of a hospital staff appointment for every practicing physician in the community. There are no simple rules for doing this. The presence of difficulties does not, however, impair the validity of the principle in application to the hospital system as a whole. All hospitals together should— and can—provide an adequate number of staff appointments to accommodate all physicians in practice. This principle must not be evaded if the hospital is to discharge its responsibilities to the community (see Chapter 5).

Notwithstanding, establishment of private services in municipal hospitals for the purpose of assuring private patient privileges to practicing physicians is not a practicable solution. The task of the Department of Hospitals is, under existing circumstances, difficult enough. It should not be complicated by considerations extraneous to the discharge of its mission of providing care to the sick poor. Moreover, recommendations for appointment to the staff of a municipal hospital originate with its medical staff, acting through the medical board, just as they do in a voluntary hospital. It would be an unwarranted burden on the Commissioner of Hospitals to assume the risk of overruling the medical boards of municipal hospitals when they fail to recommend for staff appointments physicians who are members of medical groups affiliated with a prepaid health insurance plan, such as HIP.

Increasing Attractiveness of Municipal Hospitals to Attending Staff. A staff appointment at a municipal hospital provides the physician an opportunity to teach in the ward and outpatient department. Except at Sydenham Hospital, which was acquired by the City under special circumstances, a municipal hospital staff appointment is not complete, since the privilege of caring for private patients is lacking.

In the course of interviews the proposal was frequently encountered that facilities be established in municipal hospitals to which members of the attending staff might admit their private and semi-private patients in limited numbers. The claim was that a physician caring for private patients would visit the hospital more frequently and stay longer. In consequence, he would also be available more often and for longer intervals to supervise the care of ward patients.

Flexibility in the operation of hospitals is highly desirable, since it is the best way to reduce the wasteful expenditures that are associated with vacant beds. There is also reason to believe that maintaining ward and private (including semiprivate) services side by side is mutually beneficial. Just as teaching on the ward permeates the private services and improves the quality of medical care practiced there, so can the attitudes of courtesy and considerate treatment generally exhibited toward private patients benefit ward patients. A hospital serving all income groups is also better able to provide continuity of care and can more closely approach the goal of serving as a community health center.

A major difficulty with this proposal is that there is no obvious way to limit the size of the private service in a municipal hospital. The figures most frequently advanced were 20 to 40 beds per hospital, although higher figures—10 to 15 percent of total bed capacity—were also mentioned. The question is whether units of the size specified would be sufficient to accomplish the objective sought. Might there not develop continuing pressures to increase the size of the private (including semiprivate) service, if it were found that frequency of attendance by staff members had not increased sufficiently and, likewise, if it were found that frequency of attendance had increased a great deal? Moreover, as long as the size of the service was severely limited, what rational criteria could govern the rotation of beds among staff members?

In view of the probable difficulty of keeping the size of the private service within bounds the disadvantages of the proposal seem to outweigh its advantages. The foremost disadvantage is that a majority of the community, certainly in the medical profession and in the hospital field, is strongly opposed to the use of tax funds to build facilities for the care of private and semiprivate patients. The established practice in New York City and in other large cities is to limit municipal hospitals to the care of the sick poor, while opening university hospitals under state auspices to patients from all income groups (see Chapter 20). Moreover, municipal hospitals are not accustomed to providing the kinds of amenities that private and semiprivate patients expect and receive elsewhere; private payments to the City Treasury may fall short of expenditures from tax funds in behalf of private patients; and in most municipal hospitals conversion of ward space to use by private and semiprivate patients is either not practical or would entail substantial capital expenditures.

The point was made that private patients admitted to municipal nonuniversity hospitals would pay their way in full and, therefore, be a source of additional revenue to the City. However, if an equivalent number of patients were diverted to voluntary hospitals for ward care and if the City agreed to pay voluntary hospitals at or in relation to cost, the increase in income would be offset by the increase in expenditures.

It has been suggested that physicians might find service in the wards of municipal hospitals more attractive if they were allowed to charge and keep a fee for the care of emergency patients who have medical-care insurance. There are emergency patients admitted to municipal hospitals who have paid for insurance and are entitled to its benefits. There is no reason why such patients should be treated by a physician without charge. This problem is a rather complicated one in the organization and management of a teaching ward service, and different hospitals approach and solve it differently. The individual hospital decides whether or not a personal physician is assigned to a patient who does not have a physician of his own when admitted. It is frequently left to the individual clinical departments to decide on the division of income received from third parties for physicians' services to ward patients. This appears to be an area in which general rules are not useful.

Although a general policy of establishing private services at municipal hospitals would perhaps be unwise, local circumstances may justify establishment of such services in particular institutions. Chief among such circumstances would be the expectation of substantial improvement in medical staff, existence of a local community need for additional private and semiprivate beds that is not being met, and ease of converting ward space to use by private and semiprivate patients.

In addition, it is recognized that, when full-time chiefs of clinical service are appointed in municipal unaffiliated hospitals, it may be both appropriate and desirable to provide facilities to enable them to care for private and semiprivate patients. The reasoning is the same as that advanced in the discussion of full-time faculty at medical school.

TRANSFER OF OWNERSHIP

More acceptable than services for private and semiprivate patients in municipal hospitals may be the lease or sale of one or more newly built municipal nonuniversity hospitals to nonprofit associations for operation as voluntary hospitals, with the attendant advantages of this status. The legal implications of this proposal should be explored.

Equitable Distribution of Patients between Hospital Systems

For the two major hospital systems to continue to function side by side, there must be due regard for established relationships. This is more difficult to maintain under adverse conditions than under favorable ones.

CASE OF DECLINING PATIENT LOAD

Unlike other large purchasers of hospital care, the City of New York is in the unique position of being also an owner of hospitals. In the short run the City may not be in a position to choose between producing and buying a given service. In the longer run, however, it must do so, in view of its strong interest in the efficient use of its own facilities. Nevertheless, the City also has obligations not to impair the working of the hospital system as a whole. These two commitments can sometimes come into conflict, particularly under conditions of a declining patient load.

An excellent example of such a conflict occurred several years ago, after a period of decline in the tuberculosis patient load in New York City. Since government is practically the sole purchaser of care for tuberculosis patients in New York State, its decisions govern the allocation of patients among hospitals. By the spring of 1955 the City of New York had already reduced overcrowding in its own tuberculosis services and had closed hospitals that were peripheral. It was by no means obvious what the next step was.

At first the Department of Hospitals announced that it would cease referring patients to voluntary hospitals as of an early date, except for a small number of patients needed by two teaching services. The interval between the date of announcement and the projected date of termination was short, and the affected voluntary hospitals reacted strongly. After several conversations the original order was rescinded, with the agreement that new patients would be shared among hospitals in proportion to existing bed capacity.

As a long-range solution this plan had serious limitations, being bound to lead to the operation of tuberculosis facilities at low rates of occupancy. Despite the compromise, one voluntary hospital decided that operation of a tuberculosis service on an economical basis was too uncertain a venture and proceeded to close its large tuberculosis service.

Subsequently time was gained for devising an equitable solution by a decision that the Department of Hospitals would absorb the entire decline in patient census by closing the last and largest of its separate tuberculosis hospitals, Sea View. This would be done in stages as the total tuberculosis load declined.

In devising a-long range solution certain factors should receive appropriate weight.

Needs of Teaching. Tuberculosis facilities needed for teaching deserve priority in the referral of patients. The number of patients per service need not be large, since one teaching service has operated with a complement of 20 beds for some time.

Flexibility in Use of Facilities. Facilities located in general hospitals deserve priority over separate facilities for two reasons. In the first place, care of tuberculosis patients enlarges the scope of service rendered by a general hospital and exposes personnel in other services to the care of patients with communicable diseases. Moreover, operation of a tuberculosis service at a general hospital makes for more ready adaptation to changing community needs; this is particularly important in a field with declining utilization. Separate tuberculosis hospitals now in operation should make timely plans to terminate this program, converting the facility to other appropriate uses, where feasible.

Over the years there have been a number of proposals that additional voluntary general hospitals establish tuberculosis units. For various reasons these proposals were not carried out. In view of the declining inpatient load and the associated shifts in methods of inpatient and outpatient care, establishment of new tuberculosis units, with designated beds, at voluntary hospitals can no longer be regarded as a realistic proposal.

Should a hospital wish to establish a tuberculosis service in connection with its chest service for teaching purposes, it should, however, be encouraged to do so. Once a new program is approved by the City, the hospital has the right to expect that patients will continue to be referred as long as high standards are maintained and that the rate of payment will be adequate.

Geographic Distribution. Tuberculosis is a chronic disease. Patients admitted to the hospital may spend several months there. It is desirable, therefore, that the hospital not be too far from the patient's home, so that it is accessible to visitors while the patient is in the hospital and for follow-up visits to the clinic after discharge. Facilities for tuberculosis patients should be located in those parts of the city where the population with a high incidence of tuberculosis is concentrated, subject to the two preceding considerations.

Except for the change in plans for the disposition of Sea View Hospital, the City's decision in the spring of 1955 was compatible with the long-range proposals outlined above. In retrospect the decision suffered from two serious defects: it was unilateral; and the notice of termination was short.

SHARING OF OTHER PROGRAMS

The overlap in mission between voluntary and municipal hospitals in New York City has traditionally extended to certain programs and not to others. As described above, both hospital groups have cared for tuberculosis patients for many years. Both have also operated general-care facilities for the sick poor caring for inpatients, outpatients, and emergency patients. Both groups of hospitals have participated in the emergency ambulance service. In respect to shared programs, municipal hospitals are playing an increasing role and voluntary hospitals a declining one.

Other categories of care have been almost exclusively the province of municipal hospitals. For example, in acute communicable diseases only a negligible fraction of the beds reserved for such patients were—and are today—in voluntary hospitals. As of now, no voluntary general hospital has established facilities for the care of long-term or nursing-home patients. Where long-term and general-care facilities are to be found at the same voluntary hospital, the general care-facilities were developed and added to what was formerly a long-term hospital. Only two voluntary hospitals in New York City operate organized home care programs of consequence. Not until the 1950s did voluntary general hospitals undertake to establish new psychiatric units for patients admitted from the community.

Almost the converse is true of the municipal system. It contains almost all beds for acute communicable diseases. It operates public-home infirmary units in several general hospitals. Most municipal general hospitals operate a home care program. There have been psychiatric units in two general hospitals for many years, and recently two were added at newly built hospitals (see Chapter 2).

The general hospital is not truly general, unless it cares for all types of patient. It would be an impairment of the tradition of partnership for voluntary hospitals to focus exclusively on the care of acutely ill, short-term patients. Length of stay is not a proper criterion for defining the respective roles of voluntary and municipal institutions. Moreover, voluntary hospitals should recognize their responsibility to long-term patients who can afford to pay for their care; else proprietary hospitals will assume it.

Summary

1. Affiliations among hospitals or between hospitals and medical schools are nothing new. They exist today in one form or another. What is new are efforts to make affiliations in New York City broader and more intensive than in the past.

2. The chief obstacles to effective affiliation of the scope envisaged can be grouped under three headings: absence of mutual advantage, distance, and lack of depth in medical staff.

3. An affiliation arrangement deserves support if it promises to be effective and stable over a period of time.

4. It may be desirable to join a medical school and one or more voluntary hospitals in support of a municipal unaffiliated hospital.

5. The ultimate relocation of municipal hospitals, when slated for replacement, at the sites of voluntary hospitals presents difficulties in many instances. Exceptions are areas with one voluntary hospital in a preeminent position and with a relatively low proportion of municipal to total beds.

6. A suggested alternative plan is for several voluntary hos-

pitals to expand their bed capacities while municipal unaffiliated hospitals close. This assumes that the operating deficits of voluntary hospitals, to the extent that they stem from the care of public charges, are eliminated or minimized.

7. Regionalization of hospital services in New York City poses certain special problems. Perhaps the most important single step to make regionalization workable is provision of duplicate staff appointments to physicians in the specialties in which coordination of services is attempted.

8. It would be too burdensome and a distraction from their main mission of serving the sick poor for municipal hospitals to provide private patient privileges to physicians without appointments in voluntary hospitals.

9. Although a general policy to establish services for private and semiprivate patients at municipal hospitals would perhaps be unwise, local circumstances may justify establishment of such services in particular institutions. Chief among such circumstances would be the expectation of substantial improvement in attending staff, existence of a local community need for private and semiprivate beds that is not being met, and ease of converting ward space to use by private and semiprivate patients.

10. Under conditions of a declining patient load it is easy to lose sight of considerations of equity. How the City's policy on the referral of tuberculosis patients was changed in 1955 and then reversed is described as an object lesson. Suggestions are made to give preference to teaching services and to services in general hospitals; and to try to locate beds for tuberculosis patients as closely as possible to patients' homes.

11. Voluntary general hospitals should play a larger role in the future in caring for long-term patients.

Part III. FINANCING HOSPITAL CARE

12   TRENDS IN INCOME, 1934–57

The third section of this book deals with the income and expenditures of hospitals for current purposes. Capital expenditures were discussed in Chapter 8.

The following subjects are discussed in this section: (1) Trends in hospital income by source. There are three major sources of hospital income—private payments, tax funds, and philanthropy. Chapter 12 deals with all hospitals in New York City, Chapter 13 with voluntary hospitals, and Chapter 15 with municipal hospitals. (2) Deficits of voluntary hospitals. Chapter 14 deals with trends in the size and sources of deficit. (3) Relative importance of certain agencies and sources of hospital income. Chapter 16 discusses the role of government in municipal and voluntary hospitals; Chapter 17, the role of Associated Hospital Service, the New York area Blue Cross plan; and Chapter 18, the relative importance of income from philanthropy and its several components. (4) Hospital cost. Chapter 19 deals with trends in cost, discusses some of the underlying forces at work, and attempts to project probable cost in the future. It also compares cost between New York City and other parts of the country and re-calculates various costs according to uniform criteria. (5) Geographic comparisons. Chapter 20 compares the pattern of financing hospital care in New York City with that in the country as a whole and in other large cities in the United States. The emphasis is on provisions for the indigent and medically indigent.

Chapter 21 presents a proposed pattern of financing hospital care in New York City in light of the preceding findings and after an assessment of the financial implications of various proposals.

QUALITY OF FINANCIAL DATA

A brief comment on the quality of the financial data presented in this report, particularly for the key year 1957, may be in order. For the most part they are estimates prepared from materials drawn from many sources. They are believed to be accurate, in the sense that duplications have been avoided or eliminated and total amounts have been allocated as accurately as available data and informed judgment permit.

The goal was to classify hospital income both by hospital ownership and by source of payment, in a manner similar to national income accounting. Although the stated goal has been approached, it has not been achieved. There are two reasons for the shortcomings: (1) the data furnished by various agencies were originally collected for their own needs—administrative, fiduciary, or research; and (2) no single agency in New York City has continuing responsibility for appraising the finances of all hospitals, with the collateral obligation of making known its needs for appropriate information. The second reason is the crucial one.

Among lacks in the financial data are the failure to isolate the hospital-care benefits paid by commercial insurance plans and expenditures on hospital care by employers, including their contribution toward health insurance premiums. Perhaps the chief deficiency lies in the estimates of expenditures and income of proprietary hospitals. These have been projected for the entire group from reports submitted to the American Hospital Association by one half of the members, with one third containing limited financial information and another one sixth giving only information on personnel (which was translated into money terms).

By contrast, the data on Blue Cross payments to New York City hospitals are exact. The attempt to trace income from tax funds to the level of government paying for it has yielded satisfactory approximations.

PROBLEMS DISCUSSED IN THIS CHAPTER

Expenditures for hospital care have increased greatly in the past generation. Some of the factors underlying this massive and persistent increase are discussed elsewhere (see Chapter 19). Hospitals in New York City have not escaped the general trend.

Expenditures by the public (or the income of hospitals) rose from $61 million in 1934 to $422 million in 1957, a sevenfold increase. These figures reflect current operations of voluntary, municipal, and proprietary hospitals in New York City. Expenditures in state and federal hospitals are excluded. (Also excluded in this and subsequent chapters are expenditures for capital purposes.)

There is no reason to believe that the rising trend in hospital expenditures is slackening; indeed, the contrary is more probable. On the basis of firm evidence for the year 1958—when total expenditures in the three hospital systems amounted to $448 million —and preliminary information for 1959, it is projected that in 1960 hospital expenditures in New York City were proceeding at a rate of $500 million a year or higher.

The remainder of this chapter deals with two questions:

1. Who pays for hospital care in New York City? When the income of all hospitals—voluntary, municipal, and proprietary—is added, what proportion is paid by philanthropic sources, by tax funds, and by private payments? How does the current pattern of financing differ from that of a depression year, 1934, and that of an early postwar year, 1948?

2. What share of total hospital income accrues to each of the ownership groups? How does the pattern of 1957 compare with that of 1934 or 1948? The data on hospital facilities and services provide considerable evidence on the respective roles and relative importance of voluntary, municipal, and proprietary hospitals in New York City. Nevertheless, a distribution of total income by hospital ownership is useful, since some services, such as inpatient days and outpatient visits, are not commensurate and can be compared only through use of a common medium, money. Moreover, an inpatient day in a general-care hospital cannot be equated to an inpatient day in a long-term hospital, since the two have different costs. Finally, sources of income and objects of expenditure differ considerably in the three hospital ownership groups, so that financing presents a distinctive set of problems to each.

Who Pays for Hospital Care?

In New York City in 1957 one half of total hospital income was derived from private payments and the other half from a combination of tax funds, philanthropy, and "other" income (defined below). Tax funds alone amounted to $170 million, two-fifths of total income.

Table 12.1. DISTRIBUTION OF INCOME BY SOURCE FOR ALL HOSPITALS, NEW YORK CITY, 1934, 1948, AND 1957 (IN THOUSANDS OF DOLLARS)

	1934		1948		1957	
Source	*Amount*	*Percent*	*Amount*	*Percent*	*Amount*	*Percent*
All sources	60,692	100.0	205,591	100.0	422,243	100.0
Private payments	28,130	46.4	115,472	56.2	212,653	50.4
Tax funds	23,614	38.9	71,334	34.7	169,630	40.1
Philanthropy	8,948	14.7	18,785	9.1	28,970	6.9
Other	0	0	0	0	10,990	2.6

SOURCE: Hospital Council of Greater New York. See Appendixes 12.A, 13.A, 13.B, 15.A, and 18.A.

The item "other" appears only for the year 1957, because certain items of income for research and undergraduate medical education could not be traced to their sources. This problem did not arise in 1934 and 1948, when different records were employed for developing the estimates of hospital income by source.

Between 1934 and 1948 total income increased nearly three and one half times. This rate of increase lagged behind that of private payments but exceeded that of tax funds. Philanthropy, which doubled in amount, lagged still further behind.

In the period 1948–57 total hospital income doubled. Tax funds exceeded this rate of increase, whereas private payments lagged. Philanthropy also lagged, but not so much as in the earlier period. Also to be considered is the item "other" income, most of which probably represents income from tax funds and from philanthropy.

In summary, the average (geometric) rate of increase in the total income of hospitals was approximately the same in the two intervals—8.5–9 percent annually. However, changes in the composition of income followed dissimilar patterns. As a result, the 1957 proportion of private payments to total income fell between the proportions in 1934 and in 1948; the 1957 proportion of tax funds was considerably higher than in 1948 and even slightly higher than in 1934, a depression year; and the 1957 proportion of philanthropy was approximately one half that in 1934 and somewhat lower than in 1948.

SOURCES OF INCOME

Long-Term Hospitals. These changes in the relative importance of the three major sources of income reflect, in part, another change, namely, the expansion of long-term hospitals. Between 1934 and 1957, the income of the long-term hospitals increased more than ten times, while that of all hospitals increased sevenfold.

Table 12.2. DISTRIBUTION OF INCOME BY SOURCE FOR ALL LONG-TERM HOSPITALS, NEW YORK CITY, 1934, 1948, AND 1957 (IN THOUSANDS OF DOLLARS)

	1934		1948		1957	
Source	Amount	Percent	Amount	Percent	Amount	Percent
All sources	5,859	100.0	24,751	100.0	62,723	100.0
Private payments	679	11.6	5,288	21.4	9,374	14.9
Tax funds	5,035	85.9	16,235	65.6	51,318	81.8
Philanthropy	145	2.5	3,228	13.0	1,785	2.9
Other	0	0	0	0	246	0.4

SOURCE: See Table 12.1.

Some of the shifts in percentages displayed in Table 12.2 are more apparent than real, reflecting the reclassification of hospitals and of large units of hospital centers from long-term to general-care, and conversely. Nevertheless, there is no mistaking the tendency for long-term hospitals to receive most of their income from tax funds.

General Care Hospitals. Expansion of long-term hospitals is only a partial explanation for the rising relative importance of tax funds between 1948 and 1957. The proportion of tax funds also increased in general-care hospitals between 1948 and 1957, after a decline between 1934 and 1948.

Since general-care hospitals represent between 85 and 90 percent of the income of all hospitals, they dominate the pattern of financing hospital care. The proportion of private payments to total income in general-care hospitals rose between 1934 and 1948 and declined between 1948 and 1957; the proportion of tax funds,

Table 12.3. DISTRIBUTION OF INCOME BY SOURCE FOR ALL
GENERAL-CARE HOSPITALS, NEW YORK CITY, 1934,
1948, AND 1957 (IN THOUSANDS OF DOLLARS)

	1934		1948		1957	
Source	*Amount*	*Percent*	*Amount*	*Percent*	*Amount*	*Percent*
All sources	*54,833*	*100.0*	*180,840*	*100.0*	*359,520*	*100.0*
Private payments	27,451	50.1	110,184	61.0	203,279	56.5
Tax funds	18,579	33.9	55,099	30.4	118,312	33.0
Philanthropy	8,803	16.0	15,557	8.6	27,185	7.6
Other	0	0	0	0	10,744	2.9

SOURCE: See Table 12.1.

as noted above, declined in the first period and rose in the second;
and the proportion of income from philanthropy dropped
markedly in the first period and declined slightly in the second.
Perhaps there was no decline in the proportion of income from
philanthropy, if account is taken of "other" income in 1957.

Certain differences between general-care hospitals and all hospitals in the pattern of financing are, however, worth noting. The
proportion of private payments to total income is higher in general-care hospitals than in all hospitals, and the proportion of tax
funds is correspondingly lower. Income from philanthropy and
"other" income constitute a slightly higher proportion of total
income in general-care hospitals than in all hospitals. Finally, in
general-care hospitals the 1957 proportion of tax funds to total
income was slightly lower than in 1934, whereas in all hospitals
the 1957 proportion was slightly higher.

ANTICIPATED RESULTS

These findings are amplified in the following chapters. It may
be helpful to anticipate some of the important results of the detailed analyses.

1. An important factor in the increase in private payments
to the general-care hospitals in New York City is the advent of
voluntary health insurance in 1935 and its subsequent growth.
Blue Cross payments, the only source of hospital income from
voluntary health insurance that can be accurately identified, constituted one fourth of total income in 1957, plus or minus two
percentage points.

2. Although the increase in income from tax funds has cor-
responded with an increase in state aid, the City of New York

remains the preponderant source of tax funds in financing hospital care in this city.

3. Income from philanthropy has increased by large amounts. At the same time donors have increasingly tended to earmark their gifts for designated purposes. Certain components of philanthropic income continue to be highly concentrated in a small number of voluntary hospitals.

4. Income from philanthropy and income from tax funds constitute much higher proportions of hospital income in New York City than in other large cities in the United States or in the country as a whole.

Distribution of Income by Hospital Ownership

Together, voluntary and municipal hospitals in New York City received 91 percent of total hospital income in 1957. Although the 1957 share of proprietary hospitals is shown to have been lower than in 1934 and slightly higher than in 1948, too much significance should not be attached to small fluctuations. As previously noted, financial data for proprietary hospitals are the result of a greater degree of approximation in the estimating procedure than the data for voluntary and municipal hospitals.

Table 12.4. DISTRIBUTION OF INCOME BY HOSPITAL OWNERSHIP FOR ALL HOSPITALS, NEW YORK CITY, 1934, 1948, AND 1957 (IN THOUSANDS OF DOLLARS)

	1934		1948		1957	
Ownership	Amount	Percent	Amount	Percent	Amount	Percent
All hospitals	60,692	100.0	205,591	100.0	422,243	100.0
Voluntary	34,732	57.2	122,163	59.4	229,319	54.3
Municipal	19,548	32.2	65,883	32.1	155,499	36.8
Proprietary	6,412	10.6	17,545	8.5	37,425	8.9

SOURCE: See Table 12.1.

Between 1934 and 1948 total income increased nearly three and one half times. The rate of increase in the income of municipal hospitals was the same, and that of voluntary hospitals was higher. In the period 1948–57 total income doubled. Now, the rate of increase in the income of voluntary hospitals lagged behind that of all hospitals, and that of municipal hospitals was higher. In 1957 voluntary hospitals received a smaller proportion

of total income than in 1948 or 1934, whereas municipal hospitals
received a larger one.

LONG-TERM HOSPITALS

The larger share of municipal hospitals in total hospital income in 1957 reflects in part their greater preoccupation with
long-term care. It will be recalled that between 1934 and 1957
long-term hospitals had a higher rate of increase in income than
did general-care hospitals. In the municipal hospital system 30
percent of total income accrues to long-term hospitals and long-
term units of hospital centers. In the voluntary and proprietary
hospital systems long-term hospitals receive only 6 and 5 percent,
respectively, of total income. It is not surprising, therefore, that
municipal hospitals account for three fourths of the income of
long-term hospitals.

Table 12.5. DISTRIBUTION OF INCOME BY HOSPITAL OWNERSHIP
FOR ALL LONG-TERM HOSPITALS, NEW YORK CITY,
1934, 1948, AND 1957 (IN THOUSANDS OF DOLLARS)

	1934		1948		1957	
Ownership	*Amount*	*Percent*	*Amount*	*Percent*	*Amount*	*Percent*
All hospitals	5,859	100.0	24,751	100.0	62,723	100.0
Voluntary	760	13.0	10,174	41.1	14,310	22.8
Municipal	4,473	76.3	13,367	54.0	46,538	74.2
Proprietary	626	10.7	1,210	4.9	1,875	3.0

SOURCE: See Table 12.1.

GENERAL-CARE HOSPITALS

The municipal hospital system also accounts for a rising proportion of total income in the general-care field. This is the result
not of a relative increase in volume of services but of a greater
increase in unit cost (see Chapter 19).

Table 12.6. DISTRIBUTION OF INCOME BY HOSPITAL OWNERSHIP
FOR ALL GENERAL-CARE HOSPITALS, NEW YORK CITY,
1934, 1948, AND 1957 (IN THOUSANDS OF DOLLARS)

	1934		1948		1957	
Ownership	*Amount*	*Percent*	*Amount*	*Percent*	*Amount*	*Percent*
All hospitals	54,833	100.0	180,840	100.0	359,520	100.0
Voluntary	33,972	62.0	111,989	61.9	215,009	59.8
Municipal	15,075	27.5	52,516	29.1	108,961	30.3
Proprietary	5,786	10.5	16,335	9.0	35,550	9.9

SOURCE: See Table 12.1.

The relative importance of the three hospital systems in the general-care field in 1948 and in 1957 can be summarized as follows: if proprietary hospitals' income is given a weight of 1, that of municipal hospitals is 3, and that of voluntary hospitals 6.

Summary

1. Between 1934 and 1957 expenditures for care in voluntary, municipal, and proprietary hospitals in New York City increased from $61 million to $422 million. The corresponding figure in 1958 is $448 million. It is projected that in 1960 hospital expenditures in New York City proceeded at the rate of $500 million or higher.

2. The annual rate of increase in hospital expenditures in New York City has averaged 8.5–9 percent.

3. In 1957 one half of all hospital income derived from private payments and the other half from a combination of tax funds, philanthropy, and "other" income. ("Other" consists of income for research and undergraduate medical education that could not be traced by source.) Tax funds alone constituted 40 percent of total income.

4. Between 1934 and 1948 the proportion of private payments to total income increased and the proportion of tax funds and of philanthropy decreased. Between 1948 and 1957 the proportion of private payments and of philanthropy declined and the proportion of tax funds increased.

5. Although the proportion of income from philanthropy declined in both periods, the rate of decrease was much faster in the first period than in the second. There was perhaps no decline between 1948 and 1957, if account is taken of the item "other" income.

6. In 1957 long-term hospitals in New York City received $63 million. Tax funds contributed more than 80 percent of the total.

7. General-care hospitals received 85 percent of the income of all hospitals in 1957—$359 million. Trends in the relative importance of the three major sources of income—private payments, tax funds, and philanthropy—are broadly similar to those described above for all hospitals. However, private payments constitute a higher proportion of total income in general-care hos-

pitals than in all hospitals, whereas the converse is true of tax funds.

8. When the income of proprietary general-care hospitals is given a weight of 1, that of municipal hospitals is 3, and that of voluntary hospitals is 6.

9. In all hospitals—general-care and long-term combined—the relative importance of municipal hospitals is greater than above and that of voluntary hospitals is smaller. The reason is that a much larger proportion of total resources is devoted to long-term care in municipal hospitals than in voluntary hospitals—30 percent compared with 6 percent.

Appendix 12.A

ESTIMATES OF HOSPITAL INCOME AND
EXPENDITURES, NEW YORK CITY

Sources of income of voluntary and municipal hospitals in 1957 are discussed in detail in the appendixes of subsequent chapters. This appendix describes briefly the data for 1934 and 1948 and the exclusions for 1957.

The estimates for 1934 are taken from the *Hospital Survey for New York*.[1] One adjustment was made in the published data, to further comparability over time. The value of services rendered to municipal hospitals by other departments of the City was deducted.[2] It was decided to reduce the 1934 estimate, rather than to raise the 1948 and 1957 estimates, by the value of such services, for lack of information in the latter year.

The estimates for 1948 are based on data compiled by the New York State Hospital Study, published and unpublished. The published statistics appear in *A Pattern for Hospital Care*.[3] To further comparability, certain adjustments were made. All of the adjustments entailed additions, as follows: (1) contributions to the women's auxiliaries of municipal hospitals by the United Hospital Fund and the Greater New York Fund;[4] (2) the estimated value of cash expenditures incurred in behalf of municipal hospitals by other departments of the City of New York;[5] and (3) interest on long-term debt. For municipal hospitals the last item was derived by multiplying the amount of debt incurred for the Department of Hospitals by the average rate of interest paid by the City on all debt, as reported annually by the Comptroller of the City of New York. Data for the calendar year were obtained by averaging two consecutive fiscal years. The allocation between general-care and long-term hospitals reflects the respective amounts appropriated for construction in preceding years (see Appendix 15.A).

The estimates for the year 1957 are based on numerous sources. Different methods were employed to develop the data for proprietary, municipal, and voluntary hospitals and, within the last group, for member hospitals of the United Hospital Fund and for nonmember hospitals (see Appendixes 13.A, 13.B, 15.A, and 18.A, and p. 342).

The following institutions are not included in the financial data:

1. Rockefeller Institute, voluntary, devoted exclusively to research, which spent almost $1 million in 1957. (This was reported to the Hospital Council by the institution).

2. Farm Colony, municipal, a separate public-home infirmary, which spent almost $1.5 million in 1957.[6]

The four general hospitals operated by the federal government in New York City—three Veterans Administration and one Public Health Service—spent almost $30.5 million in 1957.

13 SOURCES OF INCOME OF VOLUNTARY HOSPITALS

The voluntary, municipal, and proprietary hospitals in New York City differ markedly in their sources of income. At one end of the spectrum are proprietary hospitals, with private payments as their chief, usually sole, source of income. Only one proprietary hospital receives public funds, for giving care to tuberculosis patients. At the other end are municipal hospitals, with tax funds as their preponderant, though not exclusive, source of income. Payment from the patient is accepted if he has the means; in addition, one hospital admits private and semiprivate patients. Voluntary hospitals occupy an intermediate position, deriving much of their income from private payments and a significant part from tax funds. Most voluntary hospitals also receive some support from philanthropy.

However, there is no valid generalization regarding sources of income that applies to every voluntary hospital. The range of variation is wide, so that some voluntary hospitals depend almost exclusively on private payments, in the manner of proprietary hospitals, whereas others rely heavily on a combination of tax funds and income from philanthropy. The distribution of income by source for all voluntary hospitals combined must not be taken as descriptive of a majority of the group.

Knowledge of the trend in sources of income of all voluntary hospitals combined is useful for certain purposes, such as determining who pays for hospital care and through what mechanisms. To evaluate the financial condition of voluntary hospitals and to assess the probable impact of certain changes in public policy, it is important to consider the situation of the not-so-typical hospital. For this, it is necessary to look at the finances of hospitals one at a time, as is done in the later sections of Chapter 14.

Trends in Income for All Hospitals and Long-Term Hospitals

SOURCES OF INCOME, ALL HOSPITALS

Between the years 1934 and 1957 the income of voluntary hospitals in New York City increased from $35 million to $229 million, or more than six and one half times. During the period 1934–48 total income increased three and one half times. Private payments rose at a faster rate, whereas philanthropy and tax funds rose at considerably lower rates. In consequence, the proportion of private payments to total income approached 80 percent in 1948, whereas that of philanthropy declined to 15 percent and that of tax funds to 7 percent. The 1948 proportion of tax funds to total income was one half that in 1934.

Table 13.1. DISTRIBUTION OF INCOME BY SOURCE FOR ALL VOLUNTARY HOSPITALS, NEW YORK CITY, 1934, 1948, AND 1957 (IN THOUSANDS OF DOLLARS)

	1934		1948		1957	
Source	Amount	Percent	Amount	Percent	Amount	Percent
All sources	34,732	100.0	122,163	100.0	229,319	100.0
Private payments	21,382	61.4	95,350	78.0	165,858	72.3
Tax funds	4,583	13.4	8,110	6.7	23,648	10.3
Philanthropy	8,767	25.2	18,703	15.3	28,823	12.6
Other	0	0	0	0	10,990	4.8

SOURCE: Hospital Council of Greater New York. See Appendixes 13.A, 13.B, and 18.A for 1957 data and Appendix 12.A for 1934 and 1948 data.

In the period 1948–57 total income rose by seven eighths. Private payments increased at a slower rate than total income, and tax funds at a much faster rate. Income from philanthropy lagged slightly behind; even so, it still constituted a larger proportion of total income than tax funds did.

SOURCES OF INCOME, LONG-TERM HOSPITALS

The composition of income by source differs in general-care hospitals and in long-term hospitals. Table 13.2 shows data for the latter. The following comments are indicated.

Table 13.2. DISTRIBUTION OF INCOME BY SOURCE FOR VOLUN-
TARY LONG-TERM HOSPITALS, NEW YORK CITY,
1934, 1948, AND 1957 (IN THOUSANDS OF DOLLARS)

	1934		1948		1957	
Source	*Amount*	*Percent*	*Amount*	*Percent*	*Amount*	*Percent*
All sources	760	100.0	10,174	100.0	14,310	100.0
Private payments	27	3.5	4,078	40.1	7,136	49.9
Tax funds	593	78.0	2,873	28.2	5,165	36.1
Philanthropy	140	18.5	3,223	31.7	1,763	12.3
Other	0	0	0	0	246	1.7

SOURCE: See Table 13.1.

1. Total income of voluntary long-term hospitals was, and remains, relatively small. In 1957 it amounted to 6 percent of the income of all voluntary hospitals in New York City.

2. The total amount in 1934—$760,000—is so small that its distribution by source is probably not meaningful.

3. The sharp decline between 1948 and 1957 in the proportion of income from philanthropy to total is spurious. An important factor was the reclassification of a major hospital for patients with chronic diseases into a general hospital.

4. Although the above figures include the income of two hospitals for patients with tuberculosis, which are financed almost exclusively from tax funds, private payments to long-term hospitals still amounted to $7 million in 1957. Only a small part of this is met by benefits from voluntary health insurance plans.

Income of General-Care Hospitals

TRENDS IN INCOME BY MAJOR SOURCE

Between 1934 and 1957 the total income of general-care hospitals in New York City under voluntary control rose more than six times. In 1934, a depression year, private payments constituted 63 percent of total income, philanthropy 25 percent, and tax funds 12 percent. Between 1934 and 1948 total income rose more than three times. Private payments increased much faster, four and one half times. The rate of increase for income from philanthropy and tax funds, especially the latter, lagged behind the rate for total income. As a result, in 1948 private payments constituted 80 percent of total income. Between 1948 and 1957 total income almost doubled. This time the rate of increase for private payments lagged behind the rate for total income, whereas that for tax funds exceeded it. The proportion of income from philanthropy to total declined slightly.

In summary, the proportion of private payments to total income increased in the first period and declined in the second; that of tax funds declined in the first period and increased in the second; and that of income from philanthropy declined in both periods, markedly in the first and slightly in the second.

Although the amount of tax funds increased three and one half times between 1948 and 1957 whereas that of philanthropy failed to double, tax funds were still only two thirds of the income from philanthropy of voluntary general-care hospitals in New York City in 1957.

Table 13.3. DISTRIBUTION OF INCOME BY SOURCE FOR VOLUN-TARY GENERAL-CARE HOSPITALS, NEW YORK CITY, 1934, 1948, AND 1957 (IN THOUSANDS OF DOLLARS)

	1934		1948		1957	
Source	*Amount*	*Percent*	*Amount*	*Percent*	*Amount*	*Percent*
All sources	33,972	100.0	111,989	100.0	215,009	100.0
Private payments	21,355	62.9	91,272	81.5	158,722	73.8
Tax funds	3,990	11.7	5,237	4.7	18,483	8.6
Philanthropy	8,627	25.4	15,480	13.8	27,060	12.6
Other	0	0	0	0	10,744	5.0

SOURCE: See Table 13.1.

SOURCES OF INCOME, 1957, AND MECHANISMS OF PAYMENT

The distribution of income by major source is too broad a classification for understanding the mechanisms of payment. It makes a difference to the patient and the hospital whether private payments derive from hospital insurance benefits or from the patient's own resources at the time of illness. It makes a great difference to the hospital whether income from philanthropy is available for general purposes (including the provision of free care) or is restricted to designated purposes, and whether or not such income is stable in amount and can be relied on to accrue from year to year. There is a difference in impact between tax funds received in payment for services and tax funds received as a subsidy.

For the year 1957 the income of voluntary general-care hospitals has been distributed in considerable detail. For each of the three major sources of income—private payments, tax funds, and philanthropy—component items are listed, their amounts are shown, and percentages are computed.

Private Payments. Private payments are classified into four items. It was not possible to separate payments by commercial insurance plans.

Table 13.4. DISTRIBUTION OF PRIVATE PAYMENTS BY SOURCE
FOR VOLUNTARY GENERAL-CARE HOSPITALS,
NEW YORK CITY, 1957 (IN THOUSANDS OF DOLLARS)

	Private Payments		
Source	Amount	Percent	Percent of Total Income
Total income: 215,010			
All sources	*158,723*	*100.0*	*73.8*
Associated Hospital Service	60,647	38.2	28.2
Workmen's Compensation	4,038	2.5	1.9
Patients	84,801	53.5	39.4
Other private income	9,237	5.8	4.3

SOURCE: See Table 13.1.

Because of the important role played by Blue Cross in financing hospital care in New York City, it is dealt with elsewhere at length (see Chapter 17). The figure shown in this table includes less than $200,000 paid for outpatient services to Blue Cross subscribers.

The amount shown for Workmen's Compensation is an estimate. The bases for deriving the estimate are believed to be sound (see Appendix 13.A).

The item "other private income" is, in effect, operating revenue for services other than care of patients. Included are fees from nursing students and income from the rental of quarters to hospital personnel, from employees' paid cafeterias, and from restaurants and gift shops for visitors.

Income from patients represents all other payments by or in behalf of patients, except those traceable to government. Included are fees from outpatients and other ambulatory patients, amounting to more than $11 million in 1957. Payments by inpatients include supplementary payments by Blue Cross subscribers for hospital services not covered by benefits; contributory payments by public charges, which are deducted from the City's computed obligations to hospitals; indemnity or cash benefits under commercial health insurance plans, which could not be estimated separately; and payments by those who pay their hospital bills out of pocket. Even if income from outpatients is disregarded, direct payments by inpatients are still almost one half of private payments to voluntary general-care hospitals.

Tax Funds. Income from tax funds is classified into six items.

Table 13.5. DISTRIBUTION OF INCOME FROM TAX FUNDS BY PRO-
GRAM OF PAYMENT FOR VOLUNTARY GENERAL-CARE
HOSPITALS, NEW YORK CITY, 1957
(IN THOUSANDS OF DOLLARS)

	Tax Funds		
Program of Payment	*Amount*	*Percent*	*Percent of Total Income*
Total income: 215,010			
All programs	*18,483*	*100.0*	8.6
Public-charge inpatients	16,210	87.7	7.5
Outpatients	533	2.9	0.3
Emergency ambulance service	771	4.2	0.4
Custodians	450	2.4	0.2
Medicare	302	1.6	0.1
Other	217	1.2	0.1

SOURCE: See Table 13.1.

Income from public charge inpatients is by far the largest item, representing 88 percent of income from tax funds. This is a net figure, after deduction of part payments by patients. Part payments amounted to $1.7 million and served as an offset against the City's computed liability of $17.9 million.

In 1957 income from outpatients comprised estimated payments for drugs furnished to recipients of public assistance and moneys matched by the City of New York to expand mental hygiene clinics in hospitals under the program sponsored by the Community Mental Health Board. Payments by the City for visits to the outpatient department did not begin until September, 1958, when reimbursement was authorized for recipients of public assistance.

Voluntary hospitals participating in the emergency ambulance service received a flat sum of $18,000 per authorized ambulance. When the subsidy was raised in the fall of 1958, a sliding scale of payment was introduced, which varies with the hospital's average work load per ambulance.

Payments for custodians or special policemen go back to the early years of the twentieth century, when it was customary for the City to detail policemen to voluntary institutions providing care to public charges. At one time, when there was a crime wave, the Commissioner of Police felt compelled to withdraw the men in order to use them for patrol duty. The agencies involved, having lost this traditional protection, asked the City for help, and the Board of Estimate responded by voting certain moneys to replace the men.

Under existing policies a hospital is voted a stipend for one or more patrolmen at the rate of $2,750 to $3,050 per year. The number of men allowed to an institution is determined by the Office of the Comptroller on the basis of the institution's service to the community, particularly in behalf of the indigent. In the past four years it has not been possible to increase the number of special policemen authorized because of budgetary stringency. The stipend for each position has also remained fixed.

When payments for custodians in voluntary institutions were initiated, the City's daily rate to voluntary hospitals was less than a dollar per patient day. With the increase in the City's daily rate, particularly in recent years, the question arises whether the City's subsidy toward custodians' services in voluntary hospitals should continue.

Medicare is a program of medical care for dependents of the military who do not receive care in a military installation. In the eastern region of the country Blue Cross serves as agent for the Department of Defense. It pays the hospitals' charges for maternity care and service benefit rates for all other types of care, subject to an initial payment by the patient (a so-called deductible), as required by law.

Associated Hospital Service carefully separates Medicare payments to hospitals from payments under its own program. The amount shown here is estimated, since the figures furnished the Hospital Council by Associated Hospital Service pertained to its entire seventeen-county service area. The Medicare program did not hit full stride until mid-1957, and payments in 1958, as reported by the Blue Cross Association, were 50 percent higher than in calendar year 1957.

The item "other" includes the estimated value of surplus products contributed by the federal government and payments to hospitals by the State through the City Department of Health for taking routine chest x-rays of inpatient admissions. The latter was a new program in New York City in 1957; the 1958 figure is 40 percent higher.

The unit of government that pays the hospitals is not necessarily the one that sustains the expense. Some of the payments made by the City of New York are eventually shared among the city, state, and federal governments. In Chapter 16 an attempt is made to identify the ultimate source of tax funds spent on hospital care in New York City.

Mere description of sources of operating income cannot convey the multiplicity and complexity of rate structures that currently prevail in voluntary hospitals in New York City. Every hospital maintains a set of rates for self-paying patients. Usually there is a room rate for each type of accommodation, modified according to the location and size of the room, and one, two, or three sets of charges for a host of ancillary services to be itemized on the patient's bill. A hospital that cares for public-charge inpatients is subject to a set of uniform across-the-board City rates that vary by category of patient and type of program. Every hospital has all-inclusive flat daily rates of its own for semiprivate and non-maternity-ward patients who subscribe to Blue Cross. From Workmen's Compensation it receives a room rate defined by its size class and a list of ancillary service charges that applies to all hospitals. In several voluntary hospitals the rate structure for self-paying patients is inclusive, in which case the daily rate tends to decline on successive days of the patient's stay, until it flattens out after seven, ten, or fourteen days.

The rates paid to voluntary hospitals by Associated Hospital Service and by the City of New York will be discussed in further detail in subsequent chapters on the role of Associated Hospital Service and of government.

Income from Philanthropy. Income from philanthropy accrues in two ways: from contributions and from income on investments. These can, in turn, be further subdivided; the detailed components of philanthropic income are dealt with in a separate chapter (see Chapter 18).

For present purposes it is sufficient to present the amounts of contributions and of income on investments in relation to total income.

Table 13.6. DISTRIBUTION OF INCOME FROM PHILANTHROPY
BY COMPONENT FOR VOLUNTARY GENERAL-CARE
HOSPITALS, NEW YORK CITY, 1957
(IN THOUSANDS OF DOLLARS)

| | Philanthropic Income | | |
Component	Amount	Percent	Percent of Total Income
Total income: 215,010			
All components	27,060	100.0	12.6
Contributions	15,887	58.7	7.4
Income on investments	11,173	41.3	5.2

SOURCE: See Table 13.1.

The data on philanthropy exclude bequests that can be used for current purposes. The reason is that bequests accrue to hospitals in erratic and unpredictable fashion. Nevertheless, it is sometimes possible to anticipate the maturation of a legacy, and, for certain purposes, it would seem appropriate to take the item into account (see the discussion of hospital deficits in Chapter 14).

In Chapter 18 it is shown that in 1957 contributions to hospitals by all central fund raising organizations—chiefly United Hospital Fund, the Greater New York Fund, and Federation of Jewish Philanthropies—constituted almost three tenths of philanthropic income, the same proportion as investment income for general purposes. Next in size are cash contributions from various other sources, including individuals and churches, which constitute one quarter of income from philanthropy, and investment income for designated purposes, which constitute one eighth. Donated services of Sisters are important for Catholic hospitals, although they constitute only 5 percent of all philanthropic income.

Income for Research and Undergraduate Medical Education. The item "other" appears in 1957 for the first time. It represents the sum of two United Hospital Fund accounts, "appropriations from special funds" and "income for research and medical school purposes," after deduction of estimated income on investments for designated purposes (see Appendix 18.A).

Beginning in 1940 there was a marked increase in the sum of these two accounts (before deduction of income on investments for designated purposes). For United Hospital Fund member general hospitals the figures (in thousands of dollars) were as follows:

1940	760
1948	1,918
1957	13,651

Between 1948 and 1957 there was a sevenfold increase, compared with an increase of three and one half times in income from tax funds and lower rates of increase for the other major sources of income. The sum of these two accounts rose from 2.3 percent of total income in 1940 and in 1948 to 7.4 percent in 1957. Undoubtedly these figures reflect the increasing prominence of research in the hospital setting.

Summary

1. In the voluntary hospitals of New York City total income in 1957 amounted to $229 million, having increased from $35 million in 1934 and $122 million in 1948.

2. Between 1934 and 1948 private payments increased faster than total income, while tax funds lagged. Between 1948 and 1957 these trends were reversed. The relative importance of philanthropic income declined markedly in the first interval and slightly in the second. In 1957 "other" income for research and undergraduate medical education, with sources unknown, constituted 5 percent of total income.

3. Voluntary hospitals for the care of long-term patients received 6 percent of the income of all voluntary hospitals in 1957.

In this group of hospitals private payments accounted for one half of total income.

4. Trends in income by source in voluntary general-care hospitals are substantially the same as in all voluntary hospitals. By 1957 private payments accounted for almost three fourths of total income, compared with five eighths in 1934 and more than four fifths in 1948. Philanthropy accounted for one eighth of the total in 1957, having declined from one quarter in 1934. Tax funds and other income accounted for the remaining one eighth in 1957.

5. Despite the marked increase between 1948 and 1957 in the amount of income from tax funds received by voluntary general-care hospitals, they were equal to only two thirds of philanthropic income in 1957.

6. Public charge inpatients accounted for seven eighths of all income from tax funds. Payments for outpatient department visits by recipients of public assistance did not begin until the fall of 1958.

Appendix 13.A

ESTIMATES OF INCOME OF VOLUNTARY
HOSPITALS, 1957

From the standpoint of data collection there are two groups of voluntary hospitals in New York City: members of the United Hospital Fund and others. For the former there is available a great deal of financial information at a central location. For hospitals that are not members of the United Hospital Fund reports are centrally available only for the few that are members of the Greater New York Fund (at the present time there are no such hospitals, since the two memberships are identical).

Since nonmember hospitals are likely to be the institutions that do not receive public funds, they do not file financial statements with the City (Bureau of Charitable Institutions, Office of the Comptroller) or State (Department of Social Welfare). In any event, the Hospital Council of Greater New York is not an official agency with access to financial reports from individual institutions. It was, therefore, decided to approach each of the nonmember hospitals with requests for specific financial information. The response was excellent, with all but one complying.

The estimates of total income (as well as of expenditures) derive, therefore, from the United Hospital Fund for member hospitals and from the hospitals themselves in the case of nonmembers.

For the nonmember hospitals income from philanthropy is presented as reported by them. For the United Hospital Fund members, however, certain adjustments were made, particularly in income on investments. These are described in Appendix 18.A.

Estimates of income trom tax funds are sufficiently complex to justify a separate note (see Appendix 13.B).

Estimates of income from patients were prepared as follows:

Associated Hospital Service payments. Associated Hospital Service of New York furnished data on payments to individual hospitals for inpatient care, enabling the Hospital Council to prepare alternate tabulations at will. The figure on payments for outpatient care was furnished as a total.

Workmen's Compensation payments. This sum is estimated on the basis of two factors. (1) Patient days, as given by tabulations of a sample of voluntary general hospitals, developed by the United Hospital Fund especially for this study (see Chapter 3).[1] Not all hospitals included in the sample are Fund members. (2) Patient day income, as calculated by the United Hospital Fund for a majority of its member hospitals; this is unpublished information developed from time to time.

Patients' payments. This is a residual item, after subtraction of payments by Associated Hospital Service and Workmen's Compensation from private income from or in behalf of patients.

Appendix 13.B

INCOME FROM TAX FUNDS OF VOLUNTARY HOSPITALS, 1957

This Appendix deals with all income from tax funds to voluntary hospitals and with reimbursement to the City by higher levels of government. The latter is more pertinent to Chapter 16, but the derivation and sources are presented here for the sake of continuity of exposition.

DETAIL BY PROGRAM

The data on government payments to voluntary hospitals are taken from a variety of sources. The single source that might have served this purpose, namely, the budget of the Bureau of Charitable Institutions, was inadequate in a number of respects.

1. The budget of the Bureau of Charitable Institutions includes

all institutions paid by the City, whether located within or outside city limits. In this report an effort has been made to account for expenditures and income of hospitals within the city.

2. Although the City's Expense Budget lists budgeted expenditures hospital by hospital, it does not show actual payments hospital by hospital. The total amounts paid, furnished to the Hospital Council by the Bureau, pertain not only to hospitals inside and outside the city but also to proprietary and state hospitals and to independent dispensaries.

3. Payments by the Bureau of Charitable Institutions are classified by type of program (general, medical, tuberculosis, psychiatry, and so forth) but not by type of hospital (general, allied special, tuberculosis, psychiatric, and so forth). It would be erroneous to attribute all payments for tuberculosis patients to tuberculosis hospitals.

4. The published hospital-by-hospital budgeted figures combine payments for the care of certain inpatients and for custodians. They exclude, however, budgeted expenditures under the physically handicapped program, including premature infants, which are shown only as a total. Moreover, the hospital-by-hospital figures reflect anticipated gross expenditures by government before account is taken of contributory payments by patients.

5. The budget of the Bureau of Charitable Institutions does not embrace all of the programs involving City payments to voluntary hospitals. Among the omissions are payments for participating in the emergency ambulance sevice (which appear under the budget of the Department of Hospitals) and payments to mental hygiene clinics of hospitals (which appear under the budget of the Community Mental Health Board). The latter are, in turn, lumped under contracts with all voluntary mental hygiene clinics.

6. Payments by the City do not follow the same timing as income earned by voluntary hospitals, which is presumably reported on an accrual basis. Differences in timing between the date of accrual and date of cash receipts vary hospital by hospital and probably also program by program.

Because of these difficulties it was decided to derive the figures on government payments to voluntary hospitals from other sources. Chief among them is the report *Statistical and Financial Information*, published annually by the United Hospital Fund.[2] This report shows the number of public-charge patient days in all voluntary hospitals in New York City, not only in member hospitals, by type of care. A companion report entitled *Sundry Financial and Statistical Information*[3] presents for the member hospitals figures on the average City payment per patient day and the average daily contribution of public-

charge patients. These two publications furnished the bases for estimating City payments for the care of inpatient public charges.

Additional sources were employed to calculate income from tax
funds, as follows:

1. *Payments for emergency ambulance service.* This item is taken
from the annual Cost Statement of the Department of Hospitals,[4]
where it appears as a deduction from the Department's budget.

2. *Payments for custodians.* This item is taken from unpublished
data furnished by the United Hospital Fund, supplemented by information from the Bureau of Charitable Institutions for non-member
hospitals.

3. *Payments for mental hygiene clinics.* This item is taken from a
special report prepared by the Community Mental Health Board.
Matching contributions by the institutions were deducted.

4. *Payments under Medicare.* A total amount was furnished by
Associated Hospital Service of New York for 1957 and by the Blue
Cross Association for 1958. Each total was distributed between the hospitals in New York City and the other member hospitals of the Associated Hospital Service and by hospital ownership in the same proportions as all Associated Hospital Service inpatient payments.

REIMBURSEMENT FROM NEW YORK STATE AND UNITED STATES

In municipal hospitals the amount of reimbursement received by
the City of New York from the state and federal governments can be
obtained from the income statement of the Department of Hospitals,
as adjusted for the Hospital Council. In the case of the voluntary hospitals there is no such single statement of reimbursement by type of
program. A number of sources were employed, as follows:

1. *Payments under Department of Welfare program.* The amount
of reimbursement from the state and federal governments was taken
from the annual income statement of the Department of Hospitals, as
adjusted. The adjustment consists of separating reimbursement received
by the City in behalf of patients in voluntary hospitals from reimbursement received in behalf of patients in municipal hospitals. Furthermore, it was estimated that reimbursement to general-care hospitals came to 93 percent of total reimbursement, on the basis of a
special tabulation of claims made by the New York City Department
of Welfare for one month. The distribution of the amount reimbursed
under this program between state and federal sources follows the
percentage distribution of another special tabulation of claims, also
prepared by the Department of Welfare.

2. *Patients under Department of Health programs.* For physically
handicapped children, including premature infants, the data were ob-

tained from the New York City Department of Health. Reimbursement for the care of tuberculosis patients was computed by multiplying the number of patient days, as reported to the Hospital Council
in its annual inventory, by the appropriate daily rate of State reimbursement.

3. *Patients under Community Mental Health Board programs.* For
inpatients the amount of reimbursement was calculated as follows:
after government payments to the hospitals were computed by multiplying the daily rate of payment by the number of psychiatric patient
days approved under the program, the product was multiplied by the
proportion that the State contribution to the Board's budget constitutes of total tax funds spent by the Board. For outpatients the same
ratio of State participation is applied to expenditures from tax funds,
as derived above.

14 FINANCIAL POSITION OF VOLUNTARY HOSPITALS

In New York City voluntary hospitals have traditionally incurred a certain amount of deficit on their operations, and they meet this with income from philanthropy. It is now proposed to trace the trend in the size of operating deficits, with special emphasis on recent years; to identify the sources of deficits; and to ascertain the frequency with which individual hospitals incur deficits and how effectively they cope with them. To complete the presentation of data begun earlier, all voluntary general-care hospitals are dealt with at the outset. For reasons of practical necessity in processing voluminous data, the analysis is then confined to the member general hospitals of the United Hospital Fund. It is conducted in two stages: (1) member hospitals viewed in the aggregate and (2) the same hospitals taken one at a time.

Size of Operating Deficit

TRENDS IN GENERAL-CARE HOSPITALS, 1934–57

Between 1934 and 1957 the annual operating deficit of voluntary general-care hospitals in New York City increased two and one half times, whereas expenditures increased almost six times. As a result, the proportion of operating deficit to expenditures declined more than one half, from 28 to 12 percent. Almost all of this decline took place between 1934 and 1948, corresponding with the decline in the relative importance of philanthropy.

Table 14.1 shows the amount of operating deficit in relation to expenditures for three selected years. Expenditures are defined here to include the sum of operating and nonoperating expenditures, exclusive of expenditures for research and undergraduate medical education.

Table 14.1. RELATIONSHIP OF OPERATING DEFICIT TO EXPENDI-
TURES FOR VOLUNTARY GENERAL-CARE HOSPITALS,
NEW YORK CITY, 1934, 1948, AND 1957
(IN THOUSANDS OF DOLLARS)

Year	Operating Deficit	Expenditures	Percent of Operating Deficit to Expenditures
1934	9,912	35,257	28.1
1948	13,752	110,261	12.5
1957	24,243	201,449	12.0

SOURCE: Hospital Council of Greater New York.

Comparison with the data in Table 13.3 shows that in 1948 and in 1957 income from philanthropy was adequate not only to erase the aggregate operating deficit but sufficient to create a surplus. In this context a surplus means that the sum of the net surpluses of all hospitals with a surplus exceeded the sum of the net deficits of all hospitals with a deficit. A surplus at one hospital is, of course, not transferable to another with a deficit.

MEMBER GENERAL HOSPITALS OF UNITED HOSPITAL FUND, *1956–58*

In view of the persistent rise in hospital cost in recent years and the uncertainties of response on the income side, it is important to study in detail the income and expenditure position of voluntary hospitals for a recent period. A three-year period seems appropriate, although reference is made to comparable data for earlier years, where indicated. The remainder of this chapter deals with the financial position of the member general hospitals of the United Hospital Fund in the years 1956, 1957, and 1958.

Table 14.2. RELATIONSHIP OF OPERATING DEFICIT TO EXPENDI-
TURES FOR PATIENT CARE FOR UNITED HOSPITAL
FUND MEMBER GENERAL HOSPITALS, NEW YORK CITY,
1956, 1957, AND 1958 (IN THOUSANDS OF DOLLARS)

Year	Operating Deficit	Patient-Care Expenditures	Percent Operating Deficit to Patient-Care Expenditures
1956	13,647	143,475	9.5
1957	18,771	160,137	11.7
1958	21,210	174,076	12.2

SOURCE: United Hospital Fund of New York, unpublished data.

Although the data in Table 14.2 are similar to those in Table 14.1, there are sufficient conceptual differences between them to account for the discrepancies between the two sets of figures for the year 1957. Table 14.1 has the higher figures because it reflects a broader concept of expenditures and, more important, includes a larger number of hospitals.

The operating position of the member general hospitals of the United Hospital Fund as a group has deteriorated. The amount of operating deficit increased by $5.1 million between 1956 and 1957 and by an additional $2.4 million between 1957 and 1958. The proportion of deficit to expenditures has also continued to rise.

Factors in Operating Deficit

THREE MAJOR SOURCES

One question that persistently arose during this study was how to account for the size of operating deficit in voluntary hospitals. In 1957, for example, average inpatient day cost in member general hospitals, as published by the United Hospital Fund, was $25.77; average inpatient day income was $24.94; and average patient day loss was therefore $0.83.[1] Since the member general hospitals of the Fund rendered 5,270,594 days of care that year, their loss on inpatient care must have amounted to $4,607,000. Any difference between the deficit of $18,771,000 shown in Table 14.2 and the figure of $4,607,000 can only be attributed to factors other than inpatient care.

Further investigation showed the additional factors to be (1) the cost of caring for newborn infants and (2) losses on services for ambulatory patients. (Losses on the emergency ambulance service are included in the latter.) The operating deficit (in thousands of dollars) from the care of patients was distributed as follows in 1957:

Source	Distribution of Deficit	
	Amount	Percent
All sources	18,771	100.0
Inpatients	4,607	24.5
Newborn	4,707	25.1
Ambulatory patients	9,457	50.4

The percentage distribution of losses from the care of patients fluctuates from year to year. In 1958 the inpatient figure was four percentage points higher than in 1957, and the newborn and ambulatory patient figures were correspondingly lower. There are, however, certain long-term trends that can be discerned from a comparison of the distribution of losses by source in 1948 and in 1957.

1. The proportion of losses attributable to inpatients declined from almost one half of the total to one fourth.

2. The proportion of losses attributable to newborn care rose from less than one fifth to one fourth.

3. The proportion of losses attributable to the care of ambulatory patients rose from one third to one half. Among the component services to ambulatory patients there were both upward and downward shifts, as follows: (a) losses attributable to the emergency department rose from 3 to 7 percent of total losses; (b) losses in the outpatient department rose from 33 to 46 percent; (c) losses on the emergency ambulance service declined from 2 to 0.5 percent; and (d) surplus on services to private ambulatory patients declined from 5 to 3 percent.

It may be that by virtue of its separation from patient day cost, the cost of newborn care tends to be unduly neglected in calculating a hospital's revenue requirements. Users of United Hospital Fund statistics do not always realize, despite explicit explanations in the column headings of the published tables, that the cost of care of newborn is shown separately from the cost of care of other patients and is without a counterpart on the income side. One result is that steps designed to obtain more income for voluntary hospitals are often incomplete.

With the care of ambulatory patients assuming increased importance as a source of hospital deficit, questions arise regarding the magnitude of outpatient costs and outpatient losses. In the course of interviews conducted during this study, numerous points of view on this matter were encountered. These can be summarized under three major positions.

One position is that outpatient department costs are calculated in accordance with standard cost-accounting formulas. However arbitrary the elements entering into such formulas may be, they are objective and do not yield capricious results for any individual hospital service.

A second position is that the formula is valid in general but is not properly applied in this instance. The claim is that too large a fraction of the hospital's work load and expenditures is allocated to the outpatient department, which is, at most, a forty-hour-a-week operation. The result is to overstate the cost of the outpatient department.

The third position is that average unit costs should not be used as a basis for determining charges or assessing the adequacy of charges. Here the argument is both theoretical and practical.

Among the three positions outlined, the second one, suggesting a possibly faulty application of the formula, would require a special study. This was not done. As for the first and third positions, it is evident that the cost allocation formula is objective but may still not be an appropriate basis for establishing charges or assessing their adequacy. One knows from both economic theory and business practice that a firm with two or more products or services to sell takes into consideration the demand for each item as well as the differential (marginal) cost of producing it. Where more than a single product is produced, average cost has no bearing on selling price, because it cannot be calculated without ambiguity. It would be a grave error for a firm to try to match average income against average cost for each unit of service sold.[2]

In the specific case of the outpatient department, experience to date suggests that its revenue potential is lower than that of most other hospital services. It seems desirable to encourage the tendency to give weight to the revenue potential of hospital services, which became manifest in the recently concluded rate negotiations between local hospitals and Associated Hospital Service. To allow for the cost of outpatient care by deducting the income of the outpatient department from total expenditures is one step to a solution of this difficult problem in hospital financing.

Cost data have, of course, other uses, particularly as tools of internal management. Nothing said here is meant to touch on this aspect of cost accounting in which the United Hospital Fund has long pioneered.

In its annual appeals to the City of New York for increases in appropriations for the care of public-charge patients in voluntary hospitals, the United Hospital Fund presents data on the trend in losses on public-charge inpatients and on outpatient department services. For recent years the losses reported by United Hospital Fund member general hospitals are as follows (in thousands of dollars):

Year	Total	Public-Charge Inpatients	Outpatient Department
1956	17,211	9,575	7,636
1957	19,639	10,982	8,657
1958	21,844	12,752	9,092

These figures exceed operating losses on the care of patients in the same years shown in Table 14.2. The reverse was true in the 1940s, before the City adopted the current certification policy that has resulted in a sizable increase in the number of public-charge patient days in voluntary hospitals.

The impact of the new policy is conveyed by the drastic shift in figures that occurred between 1949 and 1950. The losses (in thousands of dollars) are as follows:

Year	Patient Care	Public-Charge Inpatients and Outpatient Department
1949	12,093	9,939
1950	11,488	11,888
Change	− 605	+ 1,949

In one year computed losses on public-charge inpatients plus losses on outpatients rose by almost $2 million, whereas total losses on the care of patients declined. It is evident that, to some extent, the increase in the computed loss on City-charge inpatients is the arithmetic result of the City's liberal certification policy. The more patient days there are certified, the larger is the hospital's computed loss on care rendered to City patients, as long as the City's daily payment is less than the hospital's average cost. This method fails to show the losses facing hospitals because certain patients are not certified as public charges and fails to take into account the losses that are no longer incurred because public charge patients have replaced free patients.

Change in Formula. The amount shown as the computed loss on City-charge inpatients is also affected by changes in cost accounting. For the year 1958 the figure would have been substantially above the $12.75 million previously shown, had the formula prevailing until 1953 remained in use. As a result of certain technical modifications proposed by a United Hospital Fund ad hoc committee, whereby educational activities were to be treated as if they were general overhead type of expenses, the relationship between average daily cost in the semiprivate service and in the ward was reversed. In 1953 cost in the ward was approximately the same as for the entire hospital, whereas cost in the semiprivate service was 95 percent of the over-all figure. By 1958, semiprivate cost was 100 percent of the over-all figure, whereas ward cost was 95 percent.

This change in the allocation of cost by type of accommodation was worth $1.38 per patient day in 1958. With 1,181,000 public-charge patient days reported, the sum involved was $1,630,-000.

Rate Policy and Certification Policy. For a given sum that a city or county pays voluntary hospitals for the care of patients, it can be credited with discharging its obligations in full or be charged with evading its obligations, depending on its certification policy and on its rate policy. If government pursues a tight (or tough) certification policy but pays hospitals at a daily rate closely geared to cost, it presumably "owes" the hospitals nothing. Conversely, if government pursues a liberal certification policy but pays hospitals at a daily rate well below cost, it "owes" the hospitals an amount of money that can be calculated with precision. Yet, it is a moot question whether voluntary hospitals fare better financially under the first policy than the second.

New York City has several hospitals located on its periphery that care for patients from both the city and an adjacent county. Only one of these hospitals cares for a significant number of ward patients from both. This hospital reports that it fares better under the policies pursued by the City of New York. That is to say, for a given group of ward patients the combined effect of the City's certification and rate policies yields a larger income to the hospital than the combined effect of the neighboring county's certification and rate policies. The county government pays the hospital in relation to cost, as calculated by the New York State Department of Social Welfare [3] but certifies only emergency admissions and refuses to pay anything in behalf of patients who carry health insurance, however inconsequential the benefits of such insurance may be.

Notwithstanding, it appears upon further reflection that the computation of losses on City-charge inpatients has a validity that transcends mere arithmetic. The fact is that the City's daily rate to voluntary hospitals is both the minimum and maximum amount that a hospital can earn for the care of this group of patients. If the daily rate for public-charge patients is below the hospital's average cost, its daily income from other patients must be above average cost or it must have access to income from philanthropy.

It may be possible to justify subsidization of ward patients by hospitals on a number of grounds, including their availability for teaching. Not to be overlooked is the tradition in New York City of joint effort by philanthropy and government in providing the free care needed by the community. In the short run one could also justify caring for public-charge inpatients at a rate lower than average cost on the ground that the beds might otherwise go to waste. The ultimate point is the same: to afford any or all of these objectives, a hospital must be able to draw on other sources of income.

INCOME FROM WARD PATIENTS OTHER THAN PUBLIC CHARGES

Since losses on the outpatient department are involved both in the data presented in the United Hospital Fund's appeal to the City and in total operating losses from the care of patients, they can be eliminated from both in order to facilitate analysis. The following data show 1958 losses or earnings (in thousands of dollars) in the United Hospital Fund member general hospitals in each type of accommodation:

Accommodation and Pay Status	Amount of Loss (-) or Earnings (+)
Public charge inpatients	- 12,752
All inpatients	- 11,190
Ward	- 17,734
Semiprivate	+ 2,302
Private	+ 4,242

Losses on the care of public-charge inpatients alone exceed losses on the care of all inpatients, because a surplus is earned on the care of private and semiprivate inpatients. Losses on the care of public-charge inpatients fall short of losses on the care of all ward patients, because daily income from ward patients who are not public charges also falls below average daily cost. However, computed average loss per patient day was four and one half times greater for public charge patients than for other ward patients—$11.34 compared with $2.52.

This was not always the case. In 1948 the average daily loss on public-charge patients was $8.30 and for other ward patients $4.95, a ratio of less than 2 to 1. Since then the loss on public-charge patients has increased by $3 a day, and the loss on other ward patients has declined by almost $2.50.

The shift in the ratio of losses between public-charge and other ward patients is associated, in part, with shifts in the composition of ward patients in member general hospitals. As public-charge patient days rose from 34 percent of ward days in 1948 to 53 percent in 1958, they came to include many of the patient days that formerly were classified as free. The latter category of patients, which accounted for 245,000 patient days in 1948, has almost disappeared. At the same time, ward patients other than public charges have come to include an increasing number of patients with Blue Cross membership, for whom hospitals have been paid a rate approximately $2 lower than for semiprivate patients. In 1958 Associated Hospital Service subscribers received 18 percent of all ward patient days, or nearly two fifths of the patient days received by ward patients other than public charges. Hospitals have also raised charges to self-paying patients in the ward and have evidently succeeded in raising collections as well.

It is noteworthy that between 1948 and 1958 per diem income

on ward patients who are not public charges showed a larger percentage increase than for any other group of patients and next to private patients, the largest increase in dollar amount.

Table 14.3. AVERAGE PATIENT DAY INCOME (IN DOLLARS) BY
          TYPE OF ACCOMMODATION AND PAY STATUS
          WITHIN THE WARD FOR UNITED HOSPITAL
          FUND MEMBER GENERAL HOSPITALS,
          NEW YORK CITY, 1948 AND 1958

Accommodation and Pay Status	1948	1958	Increase Amount	Increase Percent
Private	23.19	40.62	17.43	75
Semiprivate	15.66	29.60	13.94	89
Ward	8.18	19.03	10.85	133
Public charge	5.95	14.88	8.93	150
Other	9.30	23.70	14.40	155

SOURCE: United Hospital Fund of New York, *Financial and Statistical Information Relating to Member Hospitals and Hospital Statistics for Greater New York, 1948 and 1958* (New York, 1949 and 1959); and United Hospital Fund, *Sundry Financial and Statistical Information Relating to Hospitals in New York City, December 31, 1948 and December 31, 1958* (New York, 1949 and 1959).

It may seem surprising that each of the two components of ward patients had a higher percentage increase in patient day income than did all ward patients. The explanation lies in the pronounced shift in the composition of ward patients toward the lower paying public charges.

Net Deficits of General Hospitals

Operating deficits from the care of patients are shown in Table 14.2 for United Hospital Fund member general hospitals. To compute the net balance at the end of each year, income from philanthropy for general operating purposes is also shown in Table 14.4.

For the entire group the net financial position has deteriorated from a surplus of $4,150 million in 1956 to a deficit of $680 million in 1958.

What holds true for the group as a whole is likely to apply to a majority of its members but need not apply to each member. It is, moreover, conceivable that large hospitals exert such a disproportionate weight on the total income and expenditures of the

Table 14.4. INCOME FROM PHILANTHROPY FOR GENERAL PUR-
POSES AND SIZE OF OPERATING DEFICIT FOR UNITED
HOSPITAL FUND MEMBER GENERAL HOSPITALS,
NEW YORK CITY, 1956, 1957, AND 1958
(IN THOUSANDS OF DOLLARS)

Year	Income from Philanthropy	Operating Deficit	Surplus (+) or Deficit (-)
1956	17,795	13,647	+ 4,148
1957	20,113	18,771	+ 1,342
1958	20,534	21,210	− 676

SOURCE: United Hospital Fund of New York, unpublished data. Also see Appendix
18.A.

group as to obscure the experience of smaller institutions. Accordingly, an analysis was undertaken of the financial position of
individual hospitals in three recent years.

FINANCIAL POSITION OF INDIVIDUAL HOSPITALS

The analysis proceeds in three stages, showing at each the
number of hospitals with a surplus or small deficit and the number of hospitals with a larger deficit.

1. At the first stage the difference shown is between operating
income and operating expenditures. This is operating surplus or
operating deficit.

2. At the next stage the difference is between total income
and total expenditures (including nonoperating income on the
one hand, and nonoperating expenditures on the other). This
difference is here designated as net balance.

3. At the final stage account is taken of bequests that may be
used for current purposes by adding them to income. The resulting difference is called final balance, and this is either the same as
net balance in the absence of such a bequest or a more favorable
figure.

At no stage has a charge for depreciation been taken into
account.

At the operating deficit or surplus stage, a small deficit has
been defined as under $100,000 or less than 10 percent of operat-
ing expenditures, whichever is smaller. At the net balance and
final balance stages, a small deficit has been defined as under

$50,000 or less than 2.5 percent of expenditures, whichever is smaller.

If the classification of hospitals that obtained in 1958 is applied to each of the three years, there were 53 member general hospitals of the United Hospital Fund. The number of hospitals with an operating surplus or small deficit declined between 1956 and 1958, whereas the number with large deficits increased. (The number of hospitals with some operating deficit, large or small, equals the number of hospitals with a large deficit plus 10.)

Year	Number of Hospitals with Operating Surplus or Small Deficit	Number of Hospitals with Large Operating Deficit
1956	25	28
1957	19	34
1958	18	35

The ratio of the number of hospitals with an operating surplus or small deficit to the number with a large operating deficit has changed from approximately 1 to 1 to 1 to 2. Almost all of the deterioration in operating position took place between 1956 and 1957.

At the second stage, after application of income from philanthropy, all other nonoperating income, and nonoperating expenditures, the financial position of the hospitals appears to have deteriorated to the same degree.

Year	Number of Hospitals with Net Surplus or Small Deficit	Number of Hospitals with Large Net Deficit
1956	43	10
1957	38	15
1958	35	18

The ratio of the number of hospitals with a net surplus or small deficit to the number with a large net deficit has declined from almost 4.5 to 1 to 2 to 1. Although more hospitals shifted into the larger net deficit group between 1956 and 1957 than between 1957 and 1958, the adverse trend has continued.

Hospitals are sometimes able to improve their net balance position through the receipt of bequests that may be used for current purposes. If these sums are taken into account, the distribution of hospitals was as follows:

Year	Number of Hospitals with Final Surplus or Small Deficit	Number of Hospitals with Large Final Deficit
1956	47	6
1957	41	12
1958	37	16

With the passage of the years bequests that may be used for current purposes have become less effective in overcoming a net deficit. The main reason is that the total amount of such bequests happened to decline from $6.5 million in 1956 to less than $3.0 million in 1957 and to $2.5 million in 1958.

It is reasonable to conclude that the financial position of voluntary hospitals (as represented by the United Hospital Fund member general hospitals) deteriorated considerably between 1956 and 1957 and continued to do so, but more slowly, between 1957 and 1958. Since incomplete data for 1955 indicate scarcely any change between 1955 and 1956, the adverse trend appears to be a recent one.

CHARACTERISTICS OF HOSPITALS WITH NET DEFICIT AND WITH OPERATING SURPLUS

Altogether a net deficit exceeding $50,000 a year or 2.5 percent of expenditures occurred 43 times in the three years, 1956, 1957, and 1958. Twenty-four of the 53 United Hospital Fund member general hospitals had deficits of this size, 14 of them more than once. The distribution of hospitals by the number of deficit years follows:

Number of Deficit Years	Number of Hospitals
1	10
2	9
3	5

All nine of the hospitals with two deficits reported them in consecutive years. Apparently, if there is a tendency toward self-correction, it takes longer than one calendar year to manifest itself. Each of the 14 hospitals with large deficits in two or three years had a cumulative deficit for the three-year period. Among the 10 hospitals that had a large deficit in one year, 4 had a cumulative surplus for the period, and 6 had a cumulative deficit.

Included among the latter group is 1 hospital that had small deficits in the other two years and 4 hospitals that had a small deficit in one other year.

Altogether, 20 hospitals had a cumulative deficit for the three-year period—5 with a large deficit in each of three years, 9 with a large deficit in two of three years, and 6 with a large deficit in one year. What characteristics do these 20 hospitals hold in common, and what characteristics distinguish them from hospitals with a surplus? The latter comprise a group of 13 hospitals with an operating surplus in every year (7) or in two of the three years (6).

The two groups of hospitals were analyzed for five characteristics that might have a significant bearing on a hospital's deficit or surplus. The characteristics are: proportion of public-charge patient days to total; level of patient day cost; availability of income from philanthropy; role of outpatient department losses in its finances; and rate of occupancy.

Percentage of Public-Charge Patient Days. The City's daily payment is below average cost for voluntary general hospitals as a group. Such payment constitutes the maximum daily income that a hospital can earn for the care of a public-charge inpatient. It follows that a hospital with a large proportion of public-charge to total patient days is likely to incur a deficit, unless its daily in-patient cost is below average or it has access to supplementary sources of income.

The distributions of the two hospital groups by the proportion of public-charge to total inpatient days proved to be similar.

Percent of Public-Charge Inpatient Days to Total	Number of Hospitals with Net Deficit	Number of Hospitals with Operating Surplus
0– 9	4	4
10–19	5	3
20–29	7	4
30 and over	4	2
	20	13

There are three hospitals in which public charges receive more than 50 percent of all patient days, two with a net deficit and one with an operating surplus.

Daily Inpatient Cost. The hypothesis is that a hospital operating at low cost is less likely to have a deficit than one operating at high cost. This proposition can also be stated conversely: a hospital without access to supplementary sources of income and dependent almost exclusively on income from patients cannot afford to operate at high cost. For this analysis the criterion of high or low cost is the extent to which a hospital's own cost deviates from the average daily cost of all member general hospitals of the United Hospital Fund.

The distribution of the two groups of hospitals by the size of deviation in daily cost between a hospital and the average follows for the year 1958:

Deviation from Average Daily Cost of All Voluntary Hospitals	Number of Hospitals with Net Deficit	Number of Hospitals with Operating Surplus
Greater by $1 or more	10	1
Within $1	4	0
Less by $1 or more	6	12
	20	13

The hypothesis regarding the relationship between patient day cost and a hospital's deficit or surplus seems to be borne out. Hospitals with a surplus are almost exclusively lower cost hospitals, whereas those with a deficit tend to have higher cost.

Percentage of Income from Philanthropy to Operating Expenditures. A hospital with access to significant amounts of supplementary income is in a better position than a hospital without such access to support a deficit when it occurs. Is it, therefore, likely to incur one with greater frequency?

The two groups differ in access to income from philanthropy.

Percent of Income from Philanthropy to Expenditures	Number of Hospitals with Net Deficit	Number of Hospitals with Operating Surplus
0–2	0	3
3–6	4	7
7–9	6	1
10 and over	10	2
	20	13

The data support an affirmative answer to the above question.

Percentage of Outpatient Department Loss to Operating Expenditures. Here the attempt is to take cognizance of the outpatient department's contribution to the hospital's operating deficit. Since one group of hospitals has an operating surplus, an indirect approach is indicated, namely, through the percentage of outpatient department loss to operating expenditures.

In the latter respect the distributions of the two groups of hospitals in 1958 are not greatly dissimilar. Nevertheless, the difference between them appears to be real.

Percent of Outpatient Department Loss to Operating Expenditures	*Number of Hospitals with Net Deficit*	*Number of Hospitals with Operating Surplus*
0–2	4	6
3–4	8	4
5–6	3	3
7–8	5	0
	20	13

For the 20 hospitals with a net deficit the size of loss in the outpatient department was related to total operating deficit.

Proportion (Percent) of Outpatient Department Loss to Operating Loss	*Number of Hospitals*
0–19	7
20–39	7
40–59	3
60 and over	3
	20

The hospitals are widely scattered in this distribution, and no conclusions can be drawn.

Rate of Occupancy. At a low rate of occupancy a large proportion of a hospital's expenditures continue, whereas income from patients declines. Conversely, at a high occupancy rate the increase in income exceeds that in expenditures. It may be assumed that, all other factors being equal, a high rate of occupancy is more likely to be associated with a surplus than with a deficit, and conversely.

The distributions of the two groups of hospitals by rate of occupancy in 1958 follow:

Rate (Percent) of Occupancy	Number of Hospitals with Net Deficit	Number of Hospitals with Operating Surplus
Under 70	3	1
70–79	3	6
80–89	11	4
90 and over	3	2
	20	13

Surprisingly, perhaps, the hospitals with a surplus had the lower rates of occupancy.

Distribution by Borough. The geographic distributions of the two contrasting groups of hospitals differ markedly with respect to two of the boroughs, Manhattan and Richmond (Staten Island).

Borough	Number of Hospitals with Net Deficit	Number of Hospitals with Operating Surplus
Bronx	3	1
Brooklyn	5	5
Manhattan	11	3
Queens	1	1
Richmond	0	3
All boroughs	20	13

The three voluntary hospitals on Staten Island had an operating surplus in each of the three years.

Conclusions. From the above analyses it is concluded that hospitals with a net deficit tend to have higher costs than hospitals with an operating surplus, tend to receive a greater measure of philanthropic support, and probably incur a relatively larger loss in the outpatient department. They also tend to have a slightly higher, not lower, rate of occupancy. There is no difference between the two groups of hospitals in their proportion of public-charge inpatients.

These last two are striking findings and suggest that the process of incurring and sustaining deficits is a complex one. Some of the factors involved are specific to the individual situation and probably elude concrete measurement and statistical analysis.

HOSPITALS' ABILITY TO SUPPORT NET DEFICITS

In the final analysis the important question is whether hospitals with net deficits can sustain them. In order to answer it, a number of factors were taken into account, namely, the trend in a hospital's deficits, its access to other resources (such as working capital and permanent investment funds), the hospital's ability to attract unrestricted bequests (as demonstrated by experience in recent years), its membership in a central agency or federation, and the potential of that agency for bringing financial support to the hospital. The final result is leavened with elements of subjective judgment.

It was not possible to characterize the financial capabilities of 1 of the 20 hospitals with a cumulative net deficit over the three-year period, for lack of adequate data. For the remaining 19, the following classification was made:

Ability to Sustain Deficit	Number of Hospitals
Deficits took place in first year or two	2
Can afford deficits of size experienced	4
Doubtful, at prevailing size	3
Would be doubtful without backing of central agency	2
Cannot afford prevailing size of deficit, but backing of central agency may make a difference	2
Cannot afford prevailing size of deficit	6

If the last two groups are taken together, 8 hospitals of 53 are classified as unable to afford net deficits of the amount they have experienced. Five of them are located in Manhattan, 1 is in the Bronx, and 2 are in Brooklyn. Two of the 8, 1 in the Bronx and 1 in Manhattan, have experienced problems of adjustment following relocation. There is good reason to believe that the size of their net deficits will soon decline, if not disappear.

With respect to the factors previously explored, the eight hospitals are distributed uniformly among the several class intervals in rate of occupancy, proportion of public-charge to total patient days, and level of patient day cost. They fall outside the lowest class in the proportion of philanthropic income to expenditures but are otherwise distributed evenly among the other class intervals. In the relationship of outpatient department loss to operating expenditures, they tend to be concentrated in the lower class intervals.

HOSPITALS WITH DEFICITS TODAY AND TEN YEARS AGO

Unpublished data from the New York State Hospital Study permit a comparison to be made between hospitals with deficits today and hospitals with deficits in 1947 and 1948. At that time a hospital was classified as having a net deficit if expenditures exceeded income by $10,000 or more.

Of the 20 hospitals with a net deficit in the period 1956 to 1958 one did not exist a decade ago. The distribution of the other 19 by net financial position at the end of 1947 and 1948 follows:

Deficit or Surplus Status	Number of Hospitals
Net deficit in 1947 and 1948	7
Net surplus (or small deficit) in both years	8
Net deficit one year and net surplus one year	4

One half of the 19 hospitals with a net deficit during the period 1956–58 had a net deficit a decade ago and the other half had a surplus.

Of the 7 hospitals with a deficit in both periods, 1 could not be classified with respect to its ability to bear a deficit. The remaining 6 were classified as follows for the recent period:

Ability to Sustain Deficit, 1956–58	Number of Hospitals
Can afford deficits of size experienced	3
Doubtful, at prevailing size	1
Would be doubtful without backing of central agency	1
Cannot afford prevailing size of deficit	1

It is no surprise that only one of the hospitals with a net deficit in both periods is classified as unable to afford a deficit.

The comparison over time shows that the financial position of a given hospital can change a great deal within a span of ten years. There were 6 hospitals with a net deficit in 1947 and 1948 that did not have a deficit in recent years. Indeed, 2 of them had an operating surplus in each of the years 1956, 1957, and 1958.

Summary

The net position of voluntary hospitals in New York City is analyzed for the group and for individual institutions. Most of the data pertain to the member general hospitals of the United Hospital Fund.

VOLUNTARY HOSPITALS AS A GROUP

1. In recent years, particularly between 1956 and 1957, the operating position of voluntary general hospitals in New York City deteriorated.

2. Three sources account for the operating deficit of hospitals: losses on the care of inpatients; losses on the care of outpatients; and expenditures on newborn infants. In 1957 these sources contributed, respectively, one quarter, one half, and one quarter of total operating loss. During the past decade the proportion of loss attributable to inpatients has declined, whereas that due to outpatients has increased.

3. The size of the loss attributable to the care of outpatients raises questions regarding allocations of hospital cost and the bases for hospital charges.

4. The increase in the amount lost on the care of public-charge inpatients is to some extent the arithmetic result of the liberal certification policy adopted by the City of New York in the late 1940s. A hospital located on the periphery of the city and dealing with both the City of New York and a suburban county reports that it fares better financially under the combination of certification and payment policies followed by the City.

5. The City's daily rate to a voluntary hospital is both the minimum and maximum income that the hospital can earn from the care of a public-charge patient. It must, therefore, be able to absorb the difference between the City's payment and its own revenue requirements through access to supplementary sources of income.

INDIVIDUAL HOSPITALS

6. The financial position of individual voluntary hospitals was examined. The number of hospitals with a large deficit increased between 1956 and 1957 and increased further, at a slower rate, between 1957 and 1958.

7. Altogether, 24 of 53 hospitals had one or more large deficits in the years 1956 to 1958, and 20 had a cumulative net deficit over the three-year period. When compared with 13 hospitals with operating surplus in three or at least two of the three years, the

20 hospitals with a net deficit tend to have a higher patient day cost, receive a higher degree of philanthropic support, and probably incur a relatively larger loss on the outpatient department. The deficit hospitals also tend to have a slightly higher rate of occupancy. There is no difference between the two groups of hospitals in the proportion of public-charge inpatients. These findings suggest that the process of incurring and supporting deficits is complex, not always susceptible of statistical analysis, and most likely to be understood when studied hospital by hospital.

8. Nineteen of the 20 hospitals with cumulative net deficits for the three-year period were classified according to their ability to support a net deficit. It was concluded that 6 cannot afford their prevailing deficits and that another 2 cannot afford them either, but that the backing of a central agency may make a difference.

9. The financial position of a voluntary hospital can change a great deal within ten years. Two of the hospitals with a net deficit in 1947 and in 1948 had an operating surplus in each of the years 1956, 1957, and 1958.

10. The conclusion that recent years have witnessed a deterioration in the financial position of voluntary hospitals in New York City is reinforced by the finding that, once a large deficit appears, it tends to persist for more than one calendar year.

15   INCOME OF MUNICIPAL HOSPITALS

By definition income and expenditures are equal in the municipal hospital system. Expenditures are budgeted in advance and closely controlled. They can be changed materially by an across-the board salary increase during the fiscal year or by authorization of new outlays occasioned by a drastic change in program. Income from sources other than the City of New York varies in accordance with the composition of the patient load in terms of pay status and eligibility for State reimbursement. Income from the City is a residual item.

Trend in All Municipal Hospitals

Table 15.1 shows trends in total income of municipal hospitals and in the distribution of income by source.

Table 15.1. DISTRIBUTION OF INCOME BY SOURCE FOR ALL MUNICIPAL HOSPITALS, NEW YORK CITY, 1934, 1948, AND 1957 (IN THOUSANDS OF DOLLARS)

Source	1934		1948		1957	
	Amount	Percent	Amount	Percent	Amount	Percent
All sources	19,548	100.0	65,883	100.0	155,499	100.0
Private payments	336	1.7	2,577	3.9	9,994	6.4
Tax Funds	19,031	97.4	63,224	96.0	145,358	93.5
Philanthropy	181	0.9	82	0.1	147	0.1

SOURCE: Hospital Council of Greater New York. See Appendixes 15.A and 12.A.

Between 1934 and 1957 total income of municipal hospitals increased eight times. Income from philanthropy is negligible; fluctuations in its amount reflect differences in the report forms employed and in data processing. Income from tax funds increased seven and one half times, and private payments thirty times.

In the period 1948–57 tax funds increased less than two and one half times, whereas private payments increased fourfold. The latter reflects the combined influence of a number of factors: inclusion of income from employees' meals and board, which increased as cash salaries were substituted for maintenance; continued operation of private and semiprivate services at Sydenham Hospital, acquired by the City in 1949; admission of significant numbers of Blue Cross subscribers, with expansion of Blue Cross enrollment to cover one half of the city's population; setting charges to patients at or near daily cost, subject to a discount geared to ability to pay; and, as reported by the Department of Hospitals, a more intensive collection effort.

Despite the thirty-fold increase in the amount of private payments, they constitute only 6 percent of total income. Tax funds still account for more than 93 percent of the total.

There is no basis in the data compiled by the Department of Hospitals for dividing private payments between general-care hospitals and long-term hospitals. Accordingly, the estimates developed for the year 1957 reflect the simplifying assumption that private payments occur only in the former. Miscellaneous receipts from employees for meals and lodging were divided between the two types of hospital on an arbitrary basis.

There are, however, ample data for classifying expenditures by type of hospital. These are provided by the Department of Hospitals in its annual cost statement,[1] which solves for the outsider many of the riddles posed by a line-by-line expense budget that is subject to accruals and savings (see Chapter 9). The cost statement goes beyond the Department's Expense Budget by transferring from the expense budgets of other City departments certain cash expenditures that are clearly chargeable to the operation of municipal hospitals and by deleting those items that are not related to the operation of municipal hospitals. The estimates in this report go beyond the cost statement in allowing for interest on debt (see Appendix 15.A).

Availability of data does not, however, resolve the conceptual problems of classifying hospital facilities. For present purposes it was decided to classify psychiatric, tuberculosis, and long-term units of municipal hospital centers as long-term facilities in the year 1957. For the years 1934 and 1948 the figures are used as compiled at the time and presumably reflect the classification of facilities then current. Since the concept of the municipal hospital center in New York City is only a decade old, part of the increase in expenditures in long-term hospitals may be more apparent than real: what was formerly a psychiatric unit of a general hospital, whose expenditures are not segregated, is now a psychiatric hospital of a hospital center, reporting separate expenditure figures.

Income of municipal long-term hospitals increased more than ten times between 1934 and 1957.

Table 15.2. DISTRIBUTION OF INCOME BY SOURCE FOR MUNICI-
PAL LONG-TERM HOSPITALS, NEW YORK CITY,
1934, 1948, AND 1957 (IN THOUSANDS OF DOLLARS)

	1934		1948		1957	
Source	Amount	Percent	Amount	Percent	Amount	Percent
All sources	4,473	100.0	13,367	100.0	46,538	100.0
Private payments	26	0.6	0	0	363	0.8
Tax funds	4,442	99.3	13,362	100.0	46,153	99.2
Philanthropy	5	0.1	5	*	22	*

* Amount negligible.

SOURCE: See Table 15.1.

In municipal long-term hospitals income from sources other than tax funds is negligible. The proportion of tax funds is, as expected, smaller in general-care hospitals.

Table 15.3. DISTRIBUTION OF INCOME BY SOURCE FOR MUNICI-
PAL GENERAL-CARE HOSPITALS, NEW YORK CITY,
1934, 1948, AND 1957 (IN THOUSANDS OF DOLLARS)

	1934		1948		1957	
Source	Amount	Percent	Amount	Percent	Amount	Percent
All sources	15,075	100.0	52,516	100.0	108,961	100.0
Private payments	310	2.0	2,577	4.9	9,631	8.8
Tax funds	14,589	96.8	49,862	94.9	99,205	91.1
Philanthropy	176	1.2	77	0.2	125	0.1

SOURCE: See Table 15.1.

Between 1934 and 1957 the total income of municipal general-care hospitals increased seven times. Substantial increases may be expected in the future (see Chapter 19).

Whereas private payments increased thirty times between 1934 and 1957, tax funds increased almost seven times. Private payments constituted only 9 percent of total income in 1957.

Detailed Sources of Income for General-Care Hospitals, 1957

PRIVATE PAYMENTS

A detailed listing of the sources of private payments has been prepared for the year 1957. For each component the amount is shown, as well as the proportion of private payments and of total income.

Table 15.4. DISTRIBUTION OF PRIVATE PAYMENTS BY SOURCE FOR MUNICIPAL GENERAL-CARE HOSPITALS, NEW YORK CITY, 1957 (IN THOUSANDS OF DOLLARS)

Source	Amount	Percent of Private Payments	Percent of Total Income
Total income: 108,961			
All sources	9,631	100.0	8.8
Associated Hospital Service	3,260	33.9	2.9
Workmen's Compensation	500	5.2	0.5
Patients	5,038	52.3	4.6
Other private income	833	8.6	0.8

SOURCE: New York City Department of Hospitals, Statement Showing Sources and Amounts of Revenue (Claimed or Collected) for Hospital Services Rendered during 1957 and 1958, prepared for Hospital Council of Greater New York, September 30, 1959 (typewritten); for adjustment see Appendix 15.A.

Included in private payments are $430,000 collected from private and semiprivate patients at Sydenham Hospital. All other income from patients represents collections from ward patients who were able to pay the Department's stated charges, in full or in part, or carried health insurance.

Municipal hospitals have three sets of daily rates for patients and a fourth set for reimbursement by the State of New York. There are rates for Workmen's Compensation patients, promulgated by the State Workmen's Compensation Board, which apply to such patients admitted in an emergency to the municipal hospital wards or to emergency departments. The same rates apply to liability cases. The second daily rate is paid by Associated Hospital Service for its subscribers. Since 1950 this has been iden-

tical with the daily medical and surgical rate paid by the City of
New York to voluntary hospitals for the care of public charges.
The third set of rates applies to self-paying patients. In recent
years these have been set at the average daily cost of each type of
hospital care, as computed in the Department's annual cost statement. Rates charged to patients are subject to downward adjustment, in accordance with the patient's ability to pay.

It is difficult to justify tying the Associated Hospital Service
daily payment to municipal hospitals to the City's daily payment
to voluntary hospitals. Rather, it seems appropriate that the formula by which Associated Hospital Service pays hospitals apply to
all, without discrimination as to hospital ownership. Equality of
treatment is not meant to, and would not, preclude classification
of hospitals for payment in accordance with objective standards of
quality of care, as agreed upon, or in relation to the scope of services rendered. It may be necessary to take cognizance of patients'
prolonged stay in the hospital.

The City of New York does not charge for outpatient care in
municipal hospitals. In recent years the question of establishing
such a charge, either in the outpatient department or the emergency department or both, has received considerable attention.
When asked for its advice in the summer of 1956, the Hospital
Council of Greater New York endorsed the imposition of a charge
of $1 a visit as a matter of principle, with an adjustment downward
for those who cannot afford to pay the stated fee. The Hospital
Council observed: "This is merely to extend the principle of
charging according to ability to pay that is already established in
the inpatient service." [2] (see Chapter 2).

It is realized that this step alone will not solve some of the
difficulties under which the outpatient departments of municipal
hospitals (and of many voluntary hospitals) operate. Improved
care for ambulatory patients is one of the major areas of unmet
and inadequately met need in the field of medical care through
organized facilities for the sick.

Income from philanthropy in municipal hospitals includes a
small sum received from a foundation in payment for patient care.
Four fifths of the $125,000 represents contributions by the United
Hospital Fund and the Greater New York Fund to the women's

committees of municipal hospitals. (Income from the hospitals' own trust funds was omitted, because in the past expenditures of these monies were negligible.)

In municipal general-care hospitals in 1957 income from tax funds amounted to $99.2 million. Included were $11.2 million from other levels of government—the State of New York and the federal government. The remaining $88 million came from the City of New York.

Income from tax funds means something different to municipal hospitals and to voluntary hospitals. To the latter income from government is essentially payments made by the City. Although voluntary hospitals are not unaware of the presence or absence of State aid for a given group of public-charge patients, they do not deal with New York State as a vehicle of payment. (The vocational rehabilitation program is an exception to this statement, but the amount of money involved is small—$100,000 for the entire state.) To City officials, however, the distinction between State money and City money is very real. With the amount of expenditures given, a dollar received from the State is seen as a local dollar saved.

The amounts respectively contributed by the federal, state, and city governments to financing hospital care in New York City are discussed in the next chapter. Suffice it to note here that the City is reimbursed by the State for care rendered in municipal hospitals under the same programs as in voluntary hospitals. (Again there is one exception, involving little money. Municipal hospitals do not receive payment from vocational rehabilitation).

The rate at which the State reimburses the City for care in municipal hospitals is negotiated. It is somewhat lower (about 7 percent) than the rate charged to the general public, because the State insists that certain items of expenditure be excluded from the computation.

Income to the City

Income to the City from operating the municipal hospital system is estimated in this report at $33.6 million, almost the same as the collections of $33,584,000 reported by the Department of Hospitals.[3] The closeness of the two totals in 1957 is fortuitous, since the component elements differ considerably (see Appendix 15.A). The major differences are these: this report has taken into account income from the State under the budget of the Community Mental Health Board ($4.5 million) and miscellaneous receipts, mostly from employee's meals and lodgings ($1 million), and has deducted payments under Department of Welfare programs for patients in voluntary hospitals ($2.5 million) and at Farm Colony ($1 million) and tuberculosis payments for an extra calendar quarter ($2 million).

Since the Social Security Act became law in 1935 the amount of reimbursement the City receives for the care of patients has increased. It is reasonable to project a continuing increase in the State's share on two bases: (1) recent establishment of reimbursement for outpatient care rendered to recipients of public assistance and (2) an increase in the number of hospital patients with public-assistance status, as more patients acquire such status in nursing homes and in public-home infirmaries (see Chapter 16). The federal share has increased, as a result of the enactment of legislation on medical care for the aged.

An increase may also be expected in the number of patients paid for by Associated Hospital Service, whose proportion has increased from 3.5 percent of all admissions in 1950 to 9 percent in 1957 (see Chapter 3). Collections have not, however, kept pace with the trend in patients. Two factors are primarily involved: the low daily rate of payment by Associated Hospital Service to the City, previously mentioned, and the high proportion of discount days to total Blue Cross patient days (see Chapter 17). Lags in billing contribute to large fluctuations in payments from year to year.

Summary

1. The income of municipal hospitals in New York City rose from $19.5 million in 1934 to $155.5 million in 1957.

2. Throughout this period income from philanthropy remained negligible. Private payments increased in both amount

and relative importance. Nevertheless, tax funds remained the major source of financial support, constituting more than 93 percent of the total.

3. Private payments increased from $300,000 in 1934 to $10 million in 1957. Sydenham Hospital, which alone among municipal hospitals maintains private and semiprivate services, accounts for less than 5 percent of all private payments.

4. Payments to municipal general-care hospitals by Associated Hospital Service constitute 3 percent of total income. The last may be compared with the figure of 9 percent—the proportion of all municipal hospital patients who are potentially reimbursable by Blue Cross. The difference between the two figures is attributable to (1) the large proportion of Blue Cross patient days paid for at the discount rate of 50 percent and (2) a daily rate of payment well below cost.

5. Municipal hospitals do not charge for care in the outpatient department. Establishment of such a charge has been under consideration for several years.

Appendix 15.A

INCOME AND EXPENDITURES OF MUNICIPAL HOSPITALS, 1957

EXPENDITURES

The figures on expenditures in municipal hospitals are not taken from the Expense Budget of the Department of Hospitals. For purposes of this report the Department's budget has several shortcomings:

1. It includes certain items of expenditure by the City of New York, such as payments to voluntary hospitals for emergency ambulance service, that are not costs to municipal hospitals.

2. It fails to reflect certain cash expenditures in behalf of municipal hospitals incurred by other departments and agencies of the City. Most prominent among the missing items are fringe benefits for the City's employees and a charge for electricity and gas.[4]

3. It is prepared for a fiscal year ending June 30. In a year when a major facility opens or closes the usual device of converting fiscal year data to calendar year data by means of a two-year moving average does not yield satisfactory results.

4. A budgetary appropriation is, of course, not synonymous with an expenditure. By the end of the year a supplementary appropriation may have been required or an unspent balance may remain.

The Hospital Council was fortunate in obtaining from the Bureau of Administration, Department of Hospitals, a series of mimeographed cost statements that compensate for the above lacks. The annual cost statement, which has been prepared according to the present concepts since 1951, has the additional advantage of showing hospital by hospital the allocation of total expenditure among inpatient services, outpatient department, and home care. The inpatient figures further segregate in each hospital expenditures in large units for the care of patients with tuberculosis or mental illness. Expenditures in public-home infirmary units are also segregated.

The data developed in the cost statement were adjusted by the addition of interest on long term debt. This was calculated as the product of the amount of funded debt incurred in behalf of the Department of Hospitals by the average rate of interest on all debt, as reported by the Comptroller of the City of New York.[5] Allocations between general-care and long-term hospitals were related to respective appropriations for capital purposes in the past decade.

No adjustment was made for services furnished to municipal hospitals by other departments of the City. The kind of data needed to do this had not been developed.

INCOME

Total income of municipal hospitals is equal to expenditures. Income from the City of New York is a balancing figure, after income from all other sources is taken into account.

For this study the Department's statement for the year 1957 was adjusted and supplemented in several respects.

1. For collections from or in behalf of patients the Bureau of Administration made available a more detailed list of items. This permitted a finer regrouping of the figures according to the ultimate source of payment, that is, consumers, government, and philanthropy.

2. For income from Blue Cross payments reported by Associated Hospital Service were substituted. This was done for two reasons: (1) to incorporate payments made to Sydenham Hospital; and (2) to obtain full comparability among Associated Hospital Service payments to all hospital ownership groups (see Chapter 17).

3. Under income derived from claims processed by the Department of Welfare, the Department of Hospitals separated income earned in behalf of patients in voluntary hospitals and income earned in behalf of patients in municipal hospitals. The former figure was then deducted.

4. Under the Department of Welfare programs 83 percent of the income of municipal hospitals was attributed to general-care hospitals and 17 percent to long-term hospitals. These are based on a special one-month tabulation of claims performed for the Hospital Council by the Department of Welfare of the City of New York.

5. Certain miscellaneous receipts accruing to the City in behalf of municipal hospitals that are not processed by the Division of Collections of the Department of Hospitals were recognized as similar to "other operating income" received by voluntary hospitals. These consist mostly of payments by hospital employees for meals and lodging. The data were furnished by the Bureau of Administration, Department of Hospitals.

6. Under the Community Mental Health program expenditures in municipal hospitals for psychiatric services, as shown in the cost statement of the Department of Hospitals, were taken as the basis for estimating reimbursement by the State. The ratio of State reimbursement to expenditures in municipal hospitals was assumed to be the same as the ratio of State funds to total tax funds in the Expense Budget of the Community Mental Health Board.

7. Income for patients with tuberculosis was reduced, because in 1957 five calendar quarters' worth of reimbursement had been received from the State Department of Health.

8. Distributions by the United Hospital Fund and the Greater New York Fund to the women's auxiliaries of municipal hospitals were added to income and, simultaneously, also to expenditures.

16 ROLE OF GOVERNMENT

New York City traditionally cares for the sick poor in both voluntary and municipal hospitals. This policy is reflected, to varying degrees, in government's participation in the financing of both groups of hospitals. The authority and responsibility of government in this area are long established and well recognized. They are also delimited by law and by custom.

Background

In the municipal hospital system tax funds constituted more than 93 percent of total income in 1957. This compares with 97 percent in 1934, before enactment of the Social Security Act, when income from tax funds referred exclusively to City funds. Federal and state moneys first became available for hospital care in 1938. They amounted to very little that first year—$150,000—and did not attain $1 million annually until the middle of World War II.

Government assistance to voluntary hospitals in New York City can be traced back to colonial times, when the Legislature of the Colony appropriated money to assist in the building of New York Hospital. Later on the Legislature of the State voted annual sums toward the operating expenditures of this hospital.[1] Lump sum payments to voluntary hospitals ceased in 1872, and were prohibited by amendment to the State Constitution two years later.[2]

It is possible to trace back to 1831 lump-sum payments by the City of New York to voluntary dispensaries. Grants to voluntary hospitals at stated daily rates began with payments for the care of children and lying-in mothers in the 1860s. By 1900 the Budget of the City listed a daily rate of 60 cents for medical cases and

80 cents for surgical cases treated in voluntary general hospitals. This marks the approximate beginning of the modern era of financial relations between the City and voluntary hospitals. Four years earlier the voluntary hospitals' real estate tax exemption had been formally voted by the State, and some five years later came payment by the City for special policemen or custodians.

Relations with Voluntary Hospitals

In the modern era most of the income from tax funds accruing to voluntary hospitals is for the care of public-charge inpatients. Of 80 general-care hospitals in New York City under voluntary control, 66 receive funds under the Charitable Institutions Budget of the City. Four small hospitals are each listed for less than $10,000 a year.

HISTORY OF DAILY RATE

During most of the last sixty years changes in the City rate of payment to voluntary hospitals were few and far between. Just prior to World War I the daily rate was $1.25—the surgical and medical rates were merged in 1915—and immediately after the end of the War it was $1.75, after two changes of 25 cents each. When the depression came the daily rate was $3, and, when the depression ended, the daily rate was still $3. Immediately after the end of World War II, the daily rate was $3.25. Thereafter, increases were granted with considerable frequency, so that between July, 1946, and July, 1959, ten changes took place (see Table 16.4). The main reason for the more frequent and larger increases in rates in the recent past is that at higher levels of hospital cost the supplementary sources of funds available to voluntary hospitals to help defray the cost of free care are no longer adequate.

In 1959 an understanding was reached between voluntary hospitals and the City calling for an increase in the daily medical and surgical rate from $20 to $22 on July 1, 1960, to $23 on July 1, 1961, and to $24 on July 1, 1962. This was the first time that rates had been projected ahead. In the summer of 1960, however, the rate of $24 was instituted, without mention of future changes. (The rate was raised to $26 in the summer of 1961.)

Although the medical and surgical rate reflects the trend in the

City's rate policy, the elements of the rate structure for the several categories of care are not always consistent with one another. For example, the rate for maternity care, which is paid on a per case basis, was $100 in the spring of 1960. This is five times the daily rate of $20 then prevailing for medical and surgical patients. Since the City does not pay voluntary hospitals for the care of newborn (unlike the State, which reimburses the City for newborn care in municipal hospitals), the sum of $100 was disproportionately low.

CHANGES IN CERTIFICATION POLICY

The City's policy in certifying patients in voluntary hospitals as public charges cannot be described with numerical precision. With the overcrowding of municipal hospitals in the depression and also in recognition of the shrinking of income from philanthropy at that time, the City adopted a liberal attitude toward paying voluntary hospitals for care rendered to patients unable to pay for it. During World War II and thereafter the number of public charges in voluntary hospitals declined markedly. By 1948 the City was approving for payment only patients who were emergencies at the time of admission. Meanwhile, overcrowding had returned to municipal hospitals. Since voluntary hospitals had considerably lower rates of occupancy in their wards, the City once again changed policies.

As stated in an annual report of the Department of Hospitals: "The Departmental rules and requirements for admission to the voluntary hospitals were . . . interpreted liberally to permit an increase [sic] number of admissions to the wards of the voluntary hospitals." [3] For a patient in a voluntary hospital to be approved for payment by the City, he still had to meet the City's criteria of financial eligibility but no longer needed to be an emergency admission.

The Department of Hospitals states that today these criteria are applied uniformly in both hospital systems. As shown later in this chapter, the criteria employed under the programs administered by the New York City Department of Health are different from those employed under the Department of Hospitals' own programs or those it administers in behalf of the New York

City Department of Welfare. In addition, any patient with tuberculosis, regardless of his financal status, is declared a public charge by law, if he so elects.

The income schedules promulgated by the City are intended to serve as flexible guides for its financial investigators. Other factors bearing on a patient's ability to pay for hospital care, including ownership of assets, fixed financial obligations, and probable length of illness, are also taken into account.

RETROACTIVE POLICY ON CITY PAYMENTS

The number of public-charge patient days in voluntary hospitals increased by more than one half between 1948 and 1958. The increase would have been even larger had it not been for one of the rules governing City payment to voluntary hospitals under which a patient who is certified as a public charge for any part of his hospital stay is, for purposes of City payment, so treated for his entire stay. The City's daily rate is both the minimum and maximum that a voluntary hospital can receive in behalf of a patient certified as a public charge (see Chapter 14). This limit applies not only to the time interval for which the patient is certified as a public charge but applies retroactively to his entire hospital stay.

The City's obligation to a voluntary hospital is calculated by subtracting the patient's accumulated payments from the amount computed by multiplying the City's daily rate by the patient's total length of stay. Payments made by the patient or in his behalf at the beginning of his stay, which exceed the amount the City would have paid at its stated daily rate, are applied to the latter part of the stay when the patient is no longer able to pay. As a result, there are many instances in which it is not worth while for a hospital to seek a patient's certification as a public charge because City payment cannot begin until the patient has been in the hospital a very long time.

The situation can best be conveyed by the example of a patient with membership in Blue Cross who goes on half benefits after 21 days. In 1957 the City rate for medical and surgical patients was $16. At that time a hospital could not begin to receive payment from the City until the beginning of the patient's third month in the hospital if its Blue Cross rate was $24 and not until the middle of the patient's eighth month if its Blue Cross rate was $32. The odds against a Blue Cross patient's staying in a hospital longer than two months are 170 to 1, and for seven and one half months they are 10,000 to 1.

The following table shows the day of a patient's hospital stay on which City payment could begin for a patient with Blue Cross membership who began with 21 full service benefit days. The day on which City payment begins varies with the hospital's daily Blue Cross rate and with the City's daily rate. In this example the City rates for medical and surgical care prevalent in 1957 ($16) and in 1960 ($20) are employed.

Associated Hospital Service Rate (in Dollars)	Day of Patient's Hospital Stay When City Payment Could Begin	
	City Rate, $16	City Rate, $20
20	36	22
24	64	33
28	148	50
32	223	85
36	229	140

Two points should be noted. (1) The higher a hospital's Blue Cross rate, the longer the hospital must wait before it can expect to claim payment from the City. (2) The higher the City rate, the shorter is the hospital's wait. The reasonableness of a policy that rewards hospitals by paying them for more patient days as the City's rate of payment increases and penalizes them for a higher, and presumably more adequate, Blue Cross rate, is open to question. This is not to deny that adequate safeguards should surround City payments under a policy that treats a patient as a public charge only from the date of his certification.

Distribution of Income from Tax Funds

In Chapter 12 tax funds in New York City hospitals, short term plus long term, were shown to have increased from $24 million in 1934 to $71 million in 1948 and to $170 million in 1957. They declined from two fifths of total hospital income in 1934 to one third in 1948 and rose to two fifths in 1957.

Table 16.1 shows that tax funds devoted to hospital care have increased faster than the City's Expense Budget.

Table 16.1. PROPORTION OF EXPENSE BUDGET OF CITY OF NEW YORK DEVOTED TO HOSPITAL CARE, 1948 AND 1957 (IN MILLIONS OF DOLLARS)

			Increase	
Item	*1948*	*1957*	*Amount*	*Percent*
Tax funds for hospital care	71.3	169.6	98.3	138
Total expense budget	1,096.3	1,925.4	829.1	76
Percent hospital care to total expense budget	6.5	8.8	2.3	35

SOURCE: Table 12.1; *Expense Budget of City of New York,* Fiscal Years 1948, 1949, 1957, and 1958 (New York, 1947, 1948, 1956, and 1957).

The major share of hospital income from tax funds accrues to the municipal system. A recent study traces the expenditures of municipal hospitals back to 1914. At that time the combined operating expenditures of the institutions under the jurisdiction of the three predecessor agencies of the Department of Hospitals—the Department of Health, the Department of Welfare, and Trustees of Bellevue and Allied Institutions—came to $5.5 million. By 1924 annual expenditures had doubled. In 1929, the year the Department of Hospitals was organized, the expenditures of its institutions amounted to $16.8 million.[4] For 1934, 1948, and 1957 the data presented in this report show expenditures of $20 million, $66 million, and $155 million, respectively.

The proportion of income from tax funds accruing to municipal hospitals first rose and then declined, as follows:

Year	Proportion (Percent) of Tax Funds Accruing to Municipal Hospitals	Proportion (Percent) of Tax Funds Accruing to Voluntary Hospitals
1934	80.5	19.5
1948	88.7	11.3
1957	86.0	14.0

At 86 percent of the total, the share of municipal hospitals in income from tax funds is significantly higher today than in 1934. For general-care hospitals the proportion of tax fund income accruing to each of the ownership groups has varied within two percentage points of the above, so that in 1957 the municipal group received 84 percent of the total.

State Reimbursement

Reimbursement by the State to the City, whether for patients in voluntary hospitals or in municipal hospitals, is on a program by program basis. Although essentially the same programs are reimbursed in both groups of hospitals, rates of reimbursement differ, reflecting differences in the City's own expenditures per patient day in each system.

STATE AID PROGRAMS

Broadly speaking, State reimbursement for care rendered in a hospital falls under three major sets of programs—those supervised by the City's Department of Welfare, Department of Health, and Community Mental Health Board.

Under the programs supervised by the Department of Welfare, the State pays the City the following.

1. Fifty percent of the City's expenditures for inpatient care for all recipients of public assistance who fall under one of the four federal categories (Old Age Assistance, Aid to Dependent Children, Aid to the Blind, and Aid to the Permanently and Totally Disabled), after allowance for the federal share, which is treated by the State as if it accrued directly to the City.

2. Fifty percent of the City's expenditures for inpatient care for all recipients of home relief (including veterans' relief) who were on the assistance rolls thirty days or more prior to admission to the hospital. According to the New York City Department of Welfare the thirty-day rule does not impose a hardship on the City.

3. One hundred percent of the City's expenditures for all nonresidents who are adjudged to be medically indigent.

4. Two and one half dollars toward each outpatient department visit by a recipient of public assistance, as defined under the regulations.

Under the programs supervised by the Department of Health, the State pays the City:

1. Fifty percent of the City's expenditures for physically handicapped children. Premature infants are included under this program.

2. Fifty percent of the City's expenditures for patients with tuberculosis, up to a maximum of $5 per patient day.

3. The entire payment of $0.50 or $1.00 per plate under the program of promoting the routine taking of chest x-rays of patients admitted to general hospitals.

Beginning in 1955 the State matches the City's expenditures, net of receipts, under the Community Mental Health Board program, up to a total grant of $1 dollar per resident of New York City. Under this program inpatient care is reimbursed by the State only if provided in psychiatric units of general hospitals. Since the City's expenditures that are eligible for reimbursement exceed the total amount of the State grant, the State's share fell below 50 percent of total expenditures from tax funds—to 47 percent in 1957 and 43 percent in 1958. (The State per capita grant was raised to $1.20 in fiscal year 1961.)

This description of State reimbursement suggests that its role in financing hospital care in New York City is limited. The State's fiscal relations with the City of New York are, however, varied and complex, and hospital care is only one of many programs involved. From the standpoint of the City what counts is the total amount of State aid, rather than the headings under which the dollars accrue. Nevertheless, as pointed out below, the presence or absence of reimbursement may in itself influence a program's development.

FEDERAL, STATE, AND CITY SHARES

The estimates in Table 16.2 show that only a small amount of federal money comes into the city for hospital care. Any estimate of the extent of federal participation in financing hospital care in New York City is subject to question, since it reflects the assumptions made by local welfare authorities in allocating the federal government's contribution among expenditures for food, shelter, clothing, medical care, and so forth. The estimates presented in this report are based on data furnished the Hospital

Council by the City's Department of Welfare; their general order of magnitude is believed to reflect accurately the situation in 1957.

Table 16.2. DISTRIBUTION OF INCOME FROM TAX FUNDS
BY LEVEL OF GOVERNMENT ACCORDING TO
TYPE OF HOSPITAL, NEW YORK CITY, 1957
(IN THOUSANDS OF DOLLARS)

Level of Government	All Hospitals		General-Care Hospitals		Long-Term Hospitals	
	Amount	Percent	Amount	Percent	Amount	Percent
All levels	169,630	100.0	118,312	100.0	51,318	100.0
Federal government	1,452	0.9	932	0.8	520	1.0
New York State	27,652	16.3	14,834	12.5	12,818	25.0
City of New York	140,526	82.8	102,546	86.7	37,980	74.0

SOURCE: Hospital Council of Greater New York. See Appendixes 13.B and 15.A.

Eighty-three percent of all income from tax funds is from the City of New York, 16 percent from New York State, and 1 percent from the federal government. The State's share is twice as high in long-term hospitals as in general-care hospitals—one quarter compared with one eighth of total tax funds. The federal government's share is negligible in both instances.

In 1948 reimbursement by the State amounted to $8 million, according to unpublished estimates developed by the New York State Hospital Study. Although the State's payments have increased three and one half times—from $8 million to $28 million —its proportion of total tax funds has risen by only one half—from 11 to 16 percent.

The amount of State reimbursement is likely to increase as the relative importance of long-term facilities increases. It is also reasonable to anticipate a continuing increase in the number of hospital patients with public-assistance status who are eligible for State reimbursement. This will come about not because the public-assistance caseload is increasing but because patients with a prior or intermittent stay in a public-home infirmary or nursing home are eligible to acquire public-assistance status. This they cannot do while in the hospital.

Another source of increased State reimbursement is the program of paying for outpatient department care rendered to persons on public assistance. Instituted in September, 1958, this program has not realized expectations as a source of State funds. In voluntary hospitals 12.5 percent of all visits are being reimbursed and in municipal hospitals 8 percent. When visits not eligible for reimbursement under the existing program are eliminated from the base, the adjusted proportions of reimbursed to total visits are 13.5 and 9.5 percent, respectively, compared with an initial planning figure of 20 percent for each hospital system.

The reasons underlying the unexpectedly low proportions of reimbursed to total visits are not evident. During this study a number of explanations were encountered, foremost being the difficulty in proving that a patient has actually seen a physician, as manifested by the signature of a licensed physician. In the municipal hospital system there is the additional factor that persons administering the clinics are not accustomed to recording information for financial purposes.

The City receives $2.50 from the State for each reimbursable visit in voluntary and municipal hospitals and pays $5 for each eligible visit in voluntary hospitals. With the number of outpatient department visits in the two hospital systems approaching equality, the higher proportion of reimbursable visits in voluntary hospitals results in a net cost to the City treasury. Under prevailing conditions each percentage point of difference between the two systems in the proportion of reimbursable to total visits represents a net loss of $125,000 a year.

SELECTIVE INFLUENCE OF REIMBURSEMENT

The relatively small proportion of funds accruing from reimbursement may perhaps obscure its potential influence on the development of medical care programs. It will be recalled that reimbursement occurs program by program, so that its influence is selective and concentrated. In the past decade alone amendments to the Social Security Act have contributed first to the City's embarking on an extensive program of referring patients to proprietary nursing homes and later to the establishment of public-home infirmary units in its own hospitals. Availability of reimbursement led directly to the institution of City payment for outpatient department care rendered to public assistance recipients in voluntary hospitals. Availability of reimbursement is probably a factor in the growth of psychiatric units in general hospitals.

The City departments supervising the several reimbursement —and payment—programs differ in their approach to this mechanism. The Department of Health employs it as a means for improving care while minimizing the financial impact of sickness on the patient's family. The criteria of financial eligibility employed by the Department of Health are more liberal than those employed by other departments, on the ground that the physically handicapped children's program deals mostly with patients with long-term illnesses; that these illnesses are typically extra expensive, requiring skilled care by many individuals; and, finally, that public health officials must be aware of the continuing financial needs of families. At the same time the Department tries to enlist some financial participation by the family.

Under the inpatient programs supervised by the Community Mental Health Board, it is reported, the period of payment is limited to ninety days, with the result that a public-charge patient's stay in the psychiatric unit of a general hospital tends to be limited to ninety days.

To recognize the potential influence of reimbursement—and payment—mechanisms on selected programs does not mean that their importance should be overestimated. These mechanisms also have their limitations. For example when the public-home infirmary care program was established in municipal hospitals, it was expected to accommodate 3,000 persons by the end of 1958.[5] For a number of reasons, including lack of support from the medical staffs in several large institutions and a lack of suitable patients, this number has not been attained. Starting out with 1,000 patients, the program had 1,500 at the end of 1957 and 1,800 at the end of 1959. It is unlikely that the peak census will reach 3,000 in the foreseeable future, in the absence of major federal legislation.

Reimbursement for outpatient department visits by public assistance recipients was instituted with the aim of achieving improvements in the quality of care. It is increasingly obvious that, although such improvements are highly desirable, they can be accomplished only with great difficulty and perhaps only if drastic changes are made in staffing and organization.

Applications of Techniques to Dual Rate Policies

The techniques employed in this report to estimate amounts of reimbursement proved useful for dividing payments in behalf of the indigent from those made in behalf of the medically indigent. (An indigent person, it will be recalled, is a recipient of public assistance, and a medically indigent person is one who can normally pay his way but cannot afford the cost of hospital care at the time of illness.)

For the purpose of this set of computations certain payments from tax funds were excluded, on the ground that they pertain neither to indigent nor to medically indigent patients. Among them are expenditures on the emergency ambulance services of voluntary and municipal hospitals, contributions by the City to voluntary hospitals toward the support of custodians, and federal expenditures for dependents of the military. Also excluded for present purposes are expenditures for patients with tuberculosis (who are automatically designated as public charges) and interest on debt in municipal hospitals (which is not a reimbursable item of cost).

In 1957 exclusions of $10,040,000 served to reduce the amount of tax funds in question in general-care hospitals from $118,312,000 (Table 16.2) to $108,272,000. Table 16.3 shows the division of the total between medically indigent and indigent patients in each hospital system.

Table 16.3. EXPENDITURES FROM TAX FUNDS IN GENERAL-CARE HOSPITALS BY CATEGORY OF RECIPIENT AND HOSPITAL OWNERSHIP, NEW YORK CITY, 1957 (IN THOUSANDS OF DOLLARS)

Category of Recipient	All Hospitals	Voluntary	Municipal
All categories	108,272	16,453	91,819
Medically indigent	88,492	12,363	76,129
Indigent	19,780	4,090	15,690
Ratio of medically indigent to indigent	4.5 to 1	3 to 1	5 to 1

SOURCE: Hospital Council of Greater New York. See Appendixes 13.B, 15.A, and 3.A.

Over-all the ratio of tax funds spent for medically indigent patients to tax funds spent for indigent patients was 4.5 to 1, in municipal hospitals 5 to 1, and in voluntary hospitals 3 to 1. These ratios are helpful in analyzing the results of alternative rate policies.

The ratio in voluntary hospitals is lower not because their patients on public assistance constitute a higher proportion of total ward patients than in municipal hospitals but because voluntary hospitals have access to funds other than taxes to help pay for care to the poor. If all patients in the wards of voluntary hospitals, not only public charges, are assumed to be indigent or medically indigent, the ratio of medically indigent to indigent patient days is of the order of 7 to 1. Thus, for every indigent patient in the wards of voluntary hospitals, there are 3 medically indigent patients supported by tax funds and 4 more medically indigent patients who are supported by other funds. Among the latter are subscribers to Blue Cross and probably members of other insurance plans. For the two systems combined the adjusted ratio of medically indigent to indigent patient days is 6 to 1.

The ratio of 3 to 1 shown in Table 16.3 for voluntary hospitals has direct implications for the City's rate policy. From time to time the question is raised whether government might not pay voluntary hospitals a higher rate for indigent patients than for medically indigent patients. Under the prevailing distribution of patient days in New York City, a differential in daily rates of any significant size could readily result in a financial loss for the voluntary hospitals. If it were assumed that the hospitals receive 70 percent of cost at the current rate of payment, they would do just as well at 75 percent under a single rate policy as by receiving 90 percent in payment for indigent patients and the current 70 percent in payment for medically indigent patients. If the City insisted on a wider differential between the two rates, the hospitals would stand to lose. When the weight of medically indigent patient days is predominant, there is practically no room for the application of rate differentials.

A similar (adverse) conclusion was reached on the question of a dual rate policy for aged public charges (65 years and over). They constitute 26 percent of all public-charge patient days in voluntary general hospitals (see Chapter 3), giving a ratio of 1 aged public-charge patient day to 3 non-aged days. The reasoning is similar to the above. The answer might be different, however, if the question at issue were a dual policy of reimbursement that distinguishes between groups now covered and groups not now covered.

Broader Policy Implications

It is important to recall that it is the City's criteria of financial eligibility and their application that determine the total number of public-charge patients. Their division between municipal and voluntary hospitals depends, however, on a number of factors, the most important of which is the City's policy toward certifying patients in voluntary hospitals.

When the City decided to accept as public charges patients in voluntary hospitals who were not emergencies at the time of admission its own hospitals were seriously overcrowded. This certification policy has continued into a period when, by most standards, occupancy in the municipal hospital system as a whole is normal and on the low side in several of its members. The time will come when the City of New York must balance paying considerably more money to voluntary hospitals through continuing rate increases against the need to realize the maximum return on its expenditures in municipal hospitals by filling available beds. Once the beds are in existence and staffed for optimum operation, the second alternative is the cheaper one.

In municipal hospitals the proportion of tax funds to total income is likely to remain high in the long run, and the proportion of private payments correspondingly low. There is no reason to expect a drastic change in the relative importance of the several sources of income as long as the City remains the residual source of financial support.

Thus, if expenditures of tax funds on hospital care are to be kept within bounds, major reliance on voluntary hospitals is more likely to be effective than major reliance on municipal hospitals. For the City and voluntary hospitals to work together, a number of things are necessary. Chief among them are an equitable sharing of the patient load between the two hospital groups and a feeling on the part of both the City and voluntary hospitals that each is making a fair contribution to the provision of free care in this community and not taking advantage of the other. What is called for is explicit recognition of the size of the problem and a high degree of mutual trust and cooperation.

Voluntary hospitals differ widely in the proportion of public-charge to total patient days (see Chapter 14). With the City playing a significant role in the income of a large number of such hospitals, a uniform rate of payment is not likely to prove effective. Such a rate is almost bound to be a low rate, to forestall allegations of waste, on the one hand, and of profiteering, on the other. In light of experience there appears to be no reason why the City's rates of payment cannot be adapted to meet the revenue requirements of individual hospitals (see Chapter 21).

Summary

1. Government first contributed tax funds to the support of voluntary hospitals in New York City in colonial times. The modern era of financial relations between government and voluntary hospitals, in which government buys services at a stated rate in behalf of persons certified as public charges, began about 1900.

2. Between 1948 and 1957 tax funds devoted to hospital care increased as a proportion of the City's Expense Budget by one third.

3. In municipal hospitals tax funds are by far the predominant source of income. The primary responsibility rests on the City of New York, which meets all expenditures and keeps all collections.

4. The City's daily rate of payment to voluntary hospitals has increased much more rapidly during the postwar period than ever before. Concurrently its criteria of eligibility for certifying patients as public charges have been the same in voluntary hospitals as in municipal hospitals.

5. In New York City hospital income from tax funds is largely income from the City of New York. In 1934, prior to the passage of the Social Security Act, there was no reimbursement by the state or federal government. Reimbursement reached $1 million during World War II and $8 million in 1948. By 1957

State and federal funds amounted to $29 million. The proportion of reimbursement income to total tax funds increased from 0 percent in 1934 to 11 percent in 1948 and 16 percent in 1957.

6. In the fall of 1958 a new program was initiated, under which outpatient department visits by recipients of public assistance became eligible for reimbursement by New York State. It was originally estimated that 20 percent of total visits in municipal hospitals and in voluntary hospitals would qualify for reimbursement. In fact the proportion of total visits reimbursed comes to 8 percent in municipal hospitals and to 12.5 percent in voluntary hospitals.

7. One way in which the amount of reimbursement is likely to increase in the future is through patients' acquiring public-assistance status in public-home infirmaries and nursing homes, a status they cannot attain while in the hospital. Since long-term patients are in the hospital intermittently, some are now eligible for reimbursement who might not have been in the past.

8. The reimbursement mechanism exerts selective influence on the development of programs of care. Examples are given of the successful wielding of such influence and also of failure to achieve stated goals.

9. Expenditures of tax funds are divided between medically indigent and indigent patients in the ratio of 4.5 to 1. The ratio in municipal hospitals alone is 5 to 1 and in voluntary hospitals 3 to 1.

10. In voluntary hospitals there are, in addition, ward patients not paid for by tax funds. For every patient day in the ward reported for an indigent person, there are three medically indigent patient days paid for by tax funds and four medically indigent days paid for by net income on private patients and philanthropy. Altogether, the ratio of medically indigent to indigent patient days in both hospital systems is 6 to 1.

11. A dual rate policy, under which the City would pay voluntary hospitals a lower rate for the care of medically indigent patients than of indigent patients, is not practicable.

12. Major reliance on voluntary hospitals is more likely to be effective than major reliance on municipal hospitals in keeping within bounds the expenditure of tax funds on hospital care.

Table 16.4. DAILY RATE OF PAYMENT BY CITY TO VOLUNTARY
GENERAL HOSPITALS FOR MEDICAL AND SURGI-
CAL TREATMENT OF PUBLIC CHARGES,
NEW YORK CITY, 1900–61

Year	Rate (in Dollars)	Year	Rate (in Dollars)
1900	.80 [a]	1946–47 [b]	4.50
1907	.90 [a]	1947–48 [b]	6.00
1908	1.10 [a]	1948–49 [b]	7.50
1914	1.25 [a]	1949–51 [b]	8.00
1915	1.25	1951 [c]	10.00
1918	1.50	1951–52 [d]	11.00
1919	1.75	1952–54 [b]	12.00
1919–21 [b]	2.00	1954–55 [e]	14.00
1921–28 [b]	2.50	1956–59 [f]	16.00
1928–43 [b]	3.00	1959–60 [b]	20.00
1943–46 [b]	3.25	1960–61 [b]	24.00

[a] Surgical rate. Medical rate was lower: *1900*, $.60; *1907*, $.70; *1908*, $1.00; *1914*, $1.10.
[b] Period beginning on July 1 and ending June 30.
[c] July 1–August 31.
[d] September 1–June 30.
[e] July 1, 1954 to December 31, 1955.
[f] January 1, 1956 to June 30, 1959.
SOURCE: New York City Comptroller, Bureau of Charitable Institutions.

17 ROLE OF BLUE CROSS

The growth of voluntary health insurance is the single major change in the method of paying for hospital care accomplished in this country in the past generation. The Social Security Administration estimates that in 1958 hospital care insurance benefits in the United States represented 54 percent of private expenditures.[1]

Proportion of Patients and of Payments

It is not feasible to make a comparable estimate of the role of voluntary health insurance in New York City, because pertinent data are lacking for commercial health insurance. The carriers are unable to delimit their benefit payments to a small area, such as New York City. The routine records of hospitals regarding enrollment of patients under commercial insurance are incomplete, because commercial carriers pay most of their benefits to subscribers as cash indemnities.

It is known from other sources, however, that commercial insurance is considerably less important in this area than in the nation. With somewhat more than 70 percent of the population insured for hospital care in both the city and nation, the ratio of Blue Cross to commercial insurance enrollees in the city is 10 to 4 [2] and in the nation 3 to 4.[3]

In studying the role of voluntary health insurance in financing hospital care in New York City, it is, therefore, appropriate to focus the discussion on Associated Hospital Service of New York (AHS), the local Blue Cross plan. Even if comparable data of equal reliability were available for the commercial insurance plans, Blue Cross would still command the major emphasis.

Under the founding statute enacted in 1934, AHS serves a seventeen-county area in New York State, including the five counties comprising New York City. Until recently almost all data issued from AHS covered the entire service area, and the experience of New York City hospitals could not be separated. A single exception was the information on AHS claims paid to member hospitals of the United Hospital Fund, which the Fund has published in its quarterly reports on hospital occupancy for the past five years. The Hospital Council is pleased to present here for the first time data on the relative importance of AHS—its patients and its payments—in New York City hospitals.

AHS payments to long-term hospitals in New York City are small, amounting in 1957 to less than $100,000. This report deals, therefore, with the role of AHS in general-care hospitals.

AHS pays hospitals for care rendered to inpatients and also to outpatients for emergency treatment or minor surgical procedures not requiring hospitalization. Payments for outpatients are a very small fraction of the total, amounting in 1957 to $227,-000, or 0.3 percent of all AHS payments to hospitals in New York City.

TRENDS IN AHS PATIENTS, PATIENT DAYS, AND PAYMENTS

Early Years. Complete data regarding the role of AHS in general-care hospitals in New York City are available beginning in 1950. That year less than one third of all patients and one fourth of all patient days were accounted for by AHS subscribers. Prior to 1950 the data are more fragmentary. In municipal hospitals there were 800 AHS patients in 1939 with 11,000 patient days,[4] compared with 13,000 and 144,000, respectively, in 1950.

For voluntary hospitals a time series is available on the proportion of AHS patients and patient days in 30 United Hospital Fund member general hospitals.[5]

The figures follow for selected years:

Year	Percent AHS to Total Patients	Percent AHS to Total Patient Days
1941	14	12
1942	14	13
1944	15	14
1945	19	18
1946	23	21
1948	32	29
1950	40	35

The above percentages for 1950 are very close to those calculated for all voluntary general-care hospitals in New York City. Between 1945 and 1950 the relative importance of AHS doubled. The rate of increase in the 1950s was much slower (see Table 17.4).

1950–58. Table 17.1 presents annual data on AHS patients, patient days, and payments in all general-care hospitals in New York City. Tables 17.8, 17.9, and 17.10 present these data separately for voluntary, municipal, and proprietary hospitals.

Table 17.1. AHS PATIENTS, PATIENT DAYS, AND PAYMENTS
FOR ALL GENERAL-CARE HOSPITALS,
NEW YORK CITY, 1950–58

Year	Patients (in Thousands)	Patient Days (in Thousands)	Payments (in Thousands of Dollars)
1950	294	2,613	35,000
1951	312	2,790	40,826
1952	335	2,942	46,733
1953	344	3,027	50,678
1954	355	3,175	55,476
1955	371	3,403	63,097
1956	398	3,576	70,200
1957	435	3,902	82,010
1958	455	4,081	93,005

SOURCE: Tables 17.8, 17.9, and 17.10.

Between 1950 and 1958 the number of AHS patients and patient days in hospitals in New York City increased more than one half, and payments increased one and two thirds times. Payments used to increase by $5, $6, or $7 million a year; but between 1956 and 1957 they increased by $12 million and between 1957 and 1958 by $11 million.

DISTRIBUTION AMONG THREE HOSPITAL SYSTEMS

A big majority of AHS subscribers use private or semiprivate accommodations. Because proprietary hospitals care only for private and semiprivate patients, their share of AHS patients is greater than of total patients. The converse holds true of municipal hospitals, all but 2,000 of whose patients receive care in the ward.

With 18 percent of total patients and 30 percent of all private and semiprivate patients, proprietary hospitals had 25 percent of

Table 17.2. DISTRIBUTION OF TOTAL PATIENTS, PRIVATE AND
SEMIPRIVATE PATIENTS, AND AHS PATIENTS
(IN THOUSANDS) BY HOSPITAL OWNERSHIP
FOR GENERAL-CARE HOSPITALS,
NEW YORK CITY, 1957

Ownership	Total Patients		Private and Semiprivate Patients		AHS Patients	
	Number	Percent	Number	Percent	Number	Percent
All hospitals	988	100.0	576	100.0	435	100.0
Voluntary	597	60.5	400	69.5	305	70.1
Municipal	217	21.9	2	0.3	19	4.4
Proprietary	174	17.6	174	30.2	111	25.5

SOURCE: Hospital Council of Greater New York, annual inventory; Tables 17.8, 17.9, and 17.10.

AHS patients. Municipal hospitals had 22 percent of total patients but only 4 percent of AHS patients, because they had a
negligible fraction of private and semiprivate patients. Voluntary
hospitals had 60 percent of total patients but 70 percent each of
private and semiprivate patients and of AHS patients.

Because of differences in average length of patient stay, the
distribution of patient days among the three ownership groups
departs from that of patients. As expected, the distribution of
AHS payments approaches that of patient days more closely than
that of patients.

Table 17.3. DISTRIBUTION OF AHS PATIENT DAYS AND PAYMENTS
FOR INPATIENTS BY HOSPITAL OWNERSHIP
FOR GENERAL-CARE HOSPITALS,
NEW YORK CITY, 1957

Ownership	Patient Days		Payments	
	Number (in Thousands)	Percent	Amount (in Thousands of Dollars)	Percent
All hospitals	3,902	100.0	82,010	100.0
Voluntary	2,850	73.0	60,458	73.7
Municipal	254	6.5	3,260	4.0
Proprietary	798	20.5	18,292	22.3

SOURCE: Tables 17.8, 17.9, and 17.10.

Only voluntary hospitals account for the same proportion of
AHS payments as of patient days. In municipal hospitals the proportion of payments is the lower figure, whereas in proprietary

hospitals the proportion of patient days is the lower figure. The chief explanatory factor is the difference among the ownership groups in the proportion of discount days to total AHS patient days. (It will be recalled that for a discount day a hospital receives 50 percent of the full daily rate from AHS and makes up the difference by charging the patient one half of its stated charges.) In 1957 the proportion of discount days in proprietary, voluntary, and municipal hospitals was, respectively, 8, 18, and 42 percent. In municipal hospitals the daily rate of payment is also a factor; pegged at the City's rate of payment to voluntary hospitals, it was in 1957 approximately two thirds of the average AHS rate for semiprivate nonmaternity patients in voluntary and proprietary hospitals.

REFERRAL OF AHS SUBSCRIBERS FROM MUNICIPAL HOSPITALS

Over the last six years efforts have been made to reduce the number of AHS patients in the municipal system. The Commissioner of Hospitals has directed his hospitals to refer to a voluntary hospital any person seeking admission who has AHS insurance and is not an emergency at the time of admission. Since 1958 the Greater New York Hospital Association has sponsored a pilot project at a municipal hospital in Manhattan, aimed at facilitating the finding of such patients and their referral to a neighboring voluntary hospital. At the same time the cooperation of voluntary hospitals was enlisted.

On the evidence to date it appears that no large number of potential inpatients are being discovered and transferred to voluntary hospitals. The proportion of all AHS patients who receive care in municipal hospitals has remained stable; this means that with the expansion of AHS enrollment in New York City, the proportion of all municipal hospital patients who have Blue Cross has increased. Some of the factors at play are discussed elsewhere, in connection with the use of ward accommodations by patients with insurance (see Chapter 4).

IMPORTANCE OF AHS PATIENTS IN EACH HOSPITAL SYSTEM

From Table 17.2 it is evident that AHS patients must constitute a small proportion of patients in municipal general-care hospitals and substantial proportions of patients in voluntary and proprietary hospitals. Just how large these figures are is shown in Table 17.4, which also shows the corresponding figures for patient days.

Table 17.4. PROPORTION OF AHS PATIENTS AND PATIENT DAYS
TO TOTAL PATIENTS AND PATIENT DAYS IN EACH
OWNERSHIP GROUP FOR GENERAL-CARE HOSPITALS,
NEW YORK CITY, 1957

Ownership	*Percent AHS Patients to Total*	*Percent AHS Patient Days to Total*
All hospitals	44.1	37.2
Voluntary	51.0	47.3
Municipal	9.0	8.0
Proprietary	63.7	62.2

SOURCE: See Table 17.2.

In municipal general-care hospitals 9 percent of the patients have AHS membership; in voluntary hospitals 51 percent, approximately equal to the proportion of the city's population with AHS membership; and in proprietary hospitals 64 percent.

The proportions of AHS patient days follow the same pattern but are consistently lower. This means that in every hospital ownership group AHS patients have a shorter stay than other patients. (This is true despite the fact that AHS reports more patient days on a payment basis—approximately 1 percent—than it would if it followed the statistical concept of a patient day employed by hospitals.)

The percentages for all hospitals combined are revealing. AHS, which insures one half of the population in New York City, is responsible for 44 percent of the patients in the city's hospitals and for 37 percent of the patient days. In other words, not only do AHS patients spend a shorter time in the hospital than the rest of the population, but they are admitted to hospitals less frequently. The shorter stay of AHS patients is consistent with the findings of other studies; patients with insurance tend to have shorter hospital stays than patients without insurance.[6] The lower admission rate is, however, surprising, running counter to the findings of other studies on this score.[7] (Indeed, the admission rate of New York City residents with AHS coverage is overstated in the above data, since nonresidents are included. Among nonresidents hospitalized in New York City the proportion with AHS membership is higher than among residents.)

IMPORTANCE OF AHS IN HOSPITAL FINANCES

How large is the role of AHS in financing hospital care in New York City? The answer to this question requires a two stage analysis: (1) AHS payments to hospitals and (2) supplementary charges to AHS subscribers.

AHS Payments. Table 17.5 shows the proportion of AHS payments to hospital income in each ownership group and for all hospitals. The total income of proprietary hospitals is a rough estimate, based on data submitted to the American Hospital Association (see Appendix 12.A). Percentages are computed on two bases: (1) total income and (2) operating income, that is, total income minus income from philanthropy and receipts for research and undergraduate medical education. Only voluntary hospitals are affected by the alternative computations.

Table 17.5. PROPORTION OF AHS PAYMENTS TO TOTAL INCOME AND TO OPERATING INCOME IN EACH OWNER-SHIP GROUP FOR GENERAL-CARE HOSPITALS, NEW YORK CITY, 1957

Ownership	Percent AHS Payments to Total Income	Percent AHS Payments to Operating Income
All hospitals	23.0	26.8
Voluntary	28.2	34.1
Municipal	2.9	2.9
Proprietary	51.5	51.5

SOURCE: Tables 17.8, 17.9, and 17.10, and Hospital Council of Greater New York.

Table 17.5 shows:

1. AHS payments constitute a small proportion of the income of municipal hospitals, much smaller than the AHS proportion of patient days. The responsible factors have been noted: (a) a high proportion of discount days and (b) a low daily rate of payment. Even at Sydenham Hospital AHS payments for private and semi-private patients constitute only 11 percent of total income.

2. In proprietary hospitals, it is estimated, AHS payments constitute more than one half of total income.

3. In voluntary hospitals AHS payments constitute 28 percent of total income and one third of operating income.

4. In all general-care hospitals in New York City, AHS payments constitute approximately one quarter of income, plus or minus two percentage points, depending on whether operating income or total income is the base.

To summarize the analysis up to this point, in the field of general-care hospitalization the relative importance of AHS is as follows:

Item	Proportion (Percent) of AHS to Total
Population	50
Patients	44
Patient days	37
Income	25 ± 2

Supplementary Charges to AHS Patients. What happens when supplementary payments by AHS subscribers are taken into account?

In broad terms, the standard AHS contract provides for service benefits to nonmaternity patients in semiprivate or ward accommodations for a period of 21 days. (More than 8 percent of AHS subscribers, all or part of whose premiums are paid by their employers, have a full benefit period of 70 or 120 days.[8] For items of care covered as a service benefit there is no charge to the patient; the hospital has agreed to accept the AHS remittance as payment in full.

As of the summer of 1960 three categories of AHS patients were billed for sizable sums:

1. *Maternity patients.* A maternity patient receives a lump sum of $80 from AHS. The patient is expected to pay the difference between the amount billed by the hospital and $80, whatever it may be. Specified complications of pregnancy are, however, covered as service benefits.

2. *Private patients.* A patient in a private accommodation is covered in full for ancillary services but receives a daily allowance of $10 toward the hospital's room and board charge. The patient is expected to pay the difference. (In the fall of 1960 the AHS benefit for private patients was changed to equal that for semiprivate patients. The patient is now responsible for the difference

between the hospital's charges to a private patient and the AHS payment for a semiprivate patient.)

3. *Discount patients.* For 180 days, after the first 21 days, AHS pays the hospital at one half of the full daily AHS rate. The patient is billed at one half of the hospital's posted charges, and he is expected to pay this out of pocket.

The AHS patient is also charged for certain miscellaneous services, such as blood and x-ray therapy, and personal items, such as telephone and newspapers.

The amount that AHS patients pay to hospitals is not known. The AHS does, however, keep a record of the hospitals' supplementary charges to its subscribers, not all of which are necessarily collected. These charges were analyzed for the member general hospitals of the United Hospital Fund. These resemble all voluntary general-care hospitals in New York City in the relative role of AHS and its patients, as shown by the following:

	Percent AHS to Total	
Item	United Hospital Fund Member General Hospitals	All Voluntary General-Care Hospitals
Patients	49.6	51.0
Patient days	46.1	47.3
Operating income	33.9	34.1

When supplementary charges to patients in member hospitals of the United Hospital Fund are taken at face value, the proportion of operating income earned for the care of AHS patients rises to 45 percent, close to the proportion of AHS patient days, 46 percent. The proportion of AHS income becomes even more favorable if the base for computing the proportion is reduced to income from and in behalf of inpatients, by eliminating payments by ambulatory patients and auxiliary earnings. On the new basis the proportion of income earned for the care of AHS patients rises to 52 percent.

Perhaps too much has been proved. An allowance should certainly be made for failure to collect some of the charges to patients. Still, the difference between 52 and 46 percent is not likely to be eliminated by a high loss ratio on collections. Do AHS patients contribute more than their proportionate share of hospital income?

To answer this question it is necessary to turn to separate data for the three types of hospital accommodation. It may be that the predominant use by AHS patients of private and semiprivate accommodations, which are higher priced than the ward, leads to a difference between the proportion of AHS patient days and of income earned for the care of AHS patients, even though there is no difference within each type of accommodation.

Data for the year 1957 follow for the member general hospitals of the United Hospital Fund.

Table 17.6. PROPORTION OF AHS PATIENT DAYS AND OF INCOME FROM AHS PATIENTS IN EACH TYPE OF ACCOMMO-DATION FOR UNITED HOSPITAL FUND MEMBER GENERAL HOSPITALS, NEW YORK CITY, 1957

Type of Accommodation	Percent AHS Patient Days to Total	AHS Payments Plus Charges to Patients as Percent of Inpatient Income
All accommodations	46.1	51.5
Private	48.6	50.5
Semiprivate	66.0	63.7
Ward	23.1	31.0

SOURCE: United Hospital Fund of New York.

It will be recalled that all figures that include charges to patients are subject to the reservation that charges probably exceed collections. The size of the difference is not known.

Subject to this qualification, certain conclusions may be drawn from a comparison of the two columns in Table 17.6:

1. *Private service.* A larger average daily income is collected from AHS patients than from other patients.

2. *Semiprivate service.* Daily income from AHS patients is apparently lower than from other patients. The size of the difference is of approximately the same order as for private patients, but in the opposite direction.

The semiprivate service is the only part of the hospital in which the relative importance of AHS and its patients approaches 65 percent. This figure has frequently been cited as the proportion of voluntary hospital income derived from AHS.

3. *Ward patients.* Daily income from AHS patients is appreciably higher than from other patients. An important reason is that a majority of other ward patients are public charges, for whom the daily payment to the hospital is well below that of AHS. The AHS daily payment for a ward patient is approximately $2 less than that for a semiprivate patient.

4. *Over-all.* The difference between the AHS proportion of patient days and the AHS proportion of inpatient income (including charges to AHS subscribers) is accounted for in large part —almost three quarters—by the greater use of private and semiprivate accommodations by AHS patients. If most charges to AHS patients materialize as collections, AHS patients in United Hospital Fund member general hospitals may be said to have paid their way in 1957.

Summary. It is now possible to complete the analysis of the relative importance of AHS and its patients in financing hospital care in New York City. If it is assumed that supplementary payments by AHS patients are negligible in municipal hospitals and of the same order of magnitude in proprietary hospitals as in the semiprivate service of voluntary hospitals, then income from and in behalf of AHS patients was three tenths of the total income of all general-care hospitals in New York City and one third of their operating income. The corresponding AHS proportions in voluntary hospitals were 37 and 44 percent, respectively.

Selected Issues in Relations among Hospitals, Blue Cross, and Subscribers

The material presented in this chapter should be amplified for certain purposes and qualified for others.

1. The fact that AHS patients in voluntary hospitals as a group appear to pay their way does not mean that they pay their way in every hospital. This has created problems for the AHS payment mechanism calling for fundamental changes in approach.

2. The volume of supplementary charges to AHS patients suggests that voluntary hospitals may have a larger measure of control over their charges to patients than is generally realized. The degree of control can be measured.

3. It is possible to estimate the distribution of supplementary

charges among the several categories of patients not covered in full by service benefits. These estimates are useful for calculating the cost of specified changes in benefits.

FORMULA FOR CALCULATING THE DAILY RATE OF PAYMENT

When the present method of setting AHS rates was established on September 1, 1948, hospitals with high charges to semiprivate patients relative to cost in the first part of 1948 enjoyed a financial advantage, whereas those with relatively low charges were at a disadvantage. Despite numerous adjustments since 1948 in the daily rate paid to individual hospitals, inequities have persisted and sometimes even increased. This is demonstrated, on the one hand, by the large number of AHS member hospitals that did not file for an increase in the daily rate in the fall of 1959, when a justification in terms of cost was required. On the other hand, a number of hospitals that have not had a change in program sufficient to justify a new daily rate on the basis of audited cost claim sizable losses from the care of AHS patients, of the order of $2, $3, or $4 a day.

To understand the present situation it would help to go back to 1948, when the formula now used was being developed. In the years immediately after World War II hospital cost was rising rapidly. This was an unusual experience for hospitals and a novel one for AHS, since it had been established in the depth of the depression. It became necessary to raise the rate of payment, which at that time was still uniform for all member hospitals. (Since 1943 the rate was no longer a flat daily sum but a sliding scale, varying inversely with a patient's length of stay.) Negotiations between representatives of the hospitals and AHS to raise the rate were frequently protracted. The process of receiving necessary approval of a revised rate from the State Superintendent of Insurance as to reasonableness and the State Department of Social Welfare as to adequacy [9] occasioned further delay. The longer it took to change a rate, the more costly it proved to the hospitals, because there was no provision for the retroactive application of a new rate.

Moreover, since AHS patients, patient days, and payments were assuming increasing importance in the hospital economy, a uniform rate of payment was no longer satisfactory. Some hospitals were losing substantial amounts on the care of AHS patients, whereas others profited. For a couple of years partial afforts to mitigate the losses were made by means of additional special payments to individual hospitals out of a limited pool of money. In 1945 and 1946 the special payments were distributed among hospitals in proportion to their computed losses on the care of AHS patients relative to regular charges.[10] Such payments were clearly a stopgap until a fundamental revision in the payment formula could be effected.

It seemed essential to develop mechanisms of payment that would incorporate three features: (1) different rates of payment to individual hospitals, in order to reflect differences in cost experience and, therefore, in revenue needs; (2) an automatic response to increases in hospital cost, to eliminate the need for periodic negotiation; and (3) uniform percentage increases for all hospitals, as a continued assurance of equitable treatment. A fourth feature was thought desirable, namely, that the amounts of future increases should be outside the influence of individual hospitals.

All four features were incorporated in a formula that defined a base payment for each hospital and then adjusted the rate every quarter in accordance with the movement of general economic indicators. In this case the economic indicators were to be wage rates in selected industries in the United States and the retail cost of food in New York City, with the two factors given weights of 80 and 20 percent, respectively. (In 1957 the respective weights were changed to 90 and 10 percent.)

Originally it was thought that the base payment would be related to each hospital's cost. That proved to be impracticable. Instead, field audits were conducted in 22 voluntary hospitals, in which costs could be compared with charges.[11] After these and other studies were completed, the new payment formula for semiprivate nonmaternity patients established for each hospital a base equal to 95 percent of its average per diem charges to AHS during the period January–May, 1948.

The idea of a formula that adjusts the rate of payment automatically and applies uniformly to all hospitals has considerable appeal. Notwithstanding, it is clear by now that the 1948 formula is not equal to the task of providing adequate reimbursement and fair treatment to all. This is true, despite the use of devices to lend flexibility to the mechanism, including provision for an audit of costs when a hospital's program changes significantly and for across-the-board increases in the daily rate when increases in hospital cost outstrip the rise in the economic indicators. The latter step has been authorized by the State Superintendent of Insurance four times, three times without any restrictions and most recently with the proviso that the increase would require justification by each hospital in terms of its own cost.

The reasons for the failure of the 1948 formula, it is believed, are twofold. (1) Substitution of charges for cost meant that from the outset some hospitals were favored over others. The rise in the economic indicators over the years has aggravated the initial differences among hospitals. (2) The idea behind a base payment that will rise along with an index of wages and salaries is that increases in hospital cost reflect changes in wages and salaries in the economy and are not likely to go beyond that. The fact is that the rate of increase in hospital cost has exceeded that of wages and salaries in the economy at large. The number of employees in hospitals has increased, in part because hospitals, as personal service industries, have not been able to offset the reduction in working hours with increased employee productivity. In addition, the 1948 formula was not geared to reflect increases in cost associated with medical advances in general or with a gradual and steady improvement of program in an individual hospital. Nor does the formula reflect increases in cost arising from the transformation of students' services from contributions to the hospital to net outlays, as exemplified by the services of student nurses (see Chapter 19).

The recent discussions between hospitals and AHS regarding a new method of calculating the daily rate of payment were, therefore, welcome. The bases for these discussions were certain proposals advanced simultaneously by the School of Public Health and Administrative Medicine of Columbia University and by a special committee of the Greater New York Hospital Association. These aimed to relate the AHS rate of each hospital to its own expenditures and revenue needs and to take cognizance of the different capacities of the three types of hospital accommodation to yield income.[12]

One aspect of a payment formula warrants additional attention, namely, how to reward good quality of care, on the one hand, and how not to encourage and pay for inefficient operation of hospitals, on the other hand. Consideration should be given to setting up appropriate classes of hospitals, with a separate ceiling and floor for the daily rate established for each class of hospitals. Classification by size of hospital, or by range of services, or by scope of teaching program is employed by other Blue Cross plans in New York State.

Throughout the country Blue Cross plans have developed a great many refinements in their methods of paying hospitals. It is important to avoid complicated methods of payment that cannot be understood by hospitals and may discourage their participation in Blue Cross.

HOSPITALS' CONTROL OVER CHARGES

To what extent are voluntary hospitals now restricted by contract or by public policy in setting charges for the care of patients? In the case of an inpatient certified as a public charge the hospital has no control over daily income. The hospital also has no control over the room rate or the individual charges on an itemized bill rendered to a patient covered by Workmen's Compensation. The hospital does, however, retain various degrees of control over charges for certain classes of patients with AHS membership; these can be quantified.

From the special sample of voluntary general hospitals in New York City developed for this study by the United Hospital Fund, a percentage distribution of patient days by pay status was obtained for the year 1958, as follows: [13]

Pay Status	Percent of Patient Days
Workmen's Compensation	2.8
Public charges	19.7
Associated Hospital Service	49.2
All other	28.3
	100.0

At first glance it would seem that voluntary hospitals can control charges over no more than 28 percent of their patient days. Closer examination of the matter suggests, however, that it is an overstatement to treat all days of care received by AHS subscribers as if they were full service benefit days. The hospital retains full control over charges to AHS patients receiving maternity care without complications; a significant degree of control over charges to nonmaternity patients who occupy private accommodations; and a moderate degree of control over charges to nonmaternity patients in receipt of discount benefits.

On the basis of data furnished by AHS, the above figure of 49 percent for AHS subscribers can be divided into four components according to the degree of control over charges retained by the hospital:

Degree of Hospital Control	Percent of Patient Days
None	32.0
Some	17.2
Full	4.7
Significant	5.2
Moderate	7.3

When Workmen's Compensation and public charge patients are taken into account, voluntary general hospitals as a group are found to have some degree of control over charges for 46 percent of their patient days and full or a significant measure of control for 38 percent. These are lower degrees of control than voluntary hospitals exercised in the past but higher than might be inferred at first glance. The degree of control retained by an individual hospital may, however, depart widely from the average.

As AHS benefits are expanded, hospitals tend to lose control over charges for a larger proportion of patient days. This loss is offset by the automatic character of the rate adjustment when the AHS rate is related to changing cost.

COST OF SELECTED CHANGES IN BENEFITS

For the year 1958 it was possible to estimate the distribution of charges to AHS patients in United Hospital Fund member general hospitals according to the type of patient involved. As previously noted, there are three major groups of AHS patients who receive hospital bills of significant size: maternity, patients in the discount period, and private patients. For maternity patients separate charge figures were available; for the other two groups, as well as for miscellaneous billings, estimates were developed by distributing a given total.

Since the three major groups overlap, precise definition of each group, as here employed, is necessary.

1. *Maternity*—patients admitted for delivery, in all three types of accommodation.

2. *Patients in discount period*—nonmaternity patients in the hospital after 21 days and prior to 201 days, in all three types of accommodation.

3. *Private patients*—nonmaternity patients in private accommodations during the first 21 days in the hospital.

Distribution of Supplementary Charges among AHS Patients. Table 17.7 shows the estimated distribution of supplementary charges to patients in United Hospital Fund member general hospitals by the category of charge.

Table 17.7. ESTIMATED DISTRIBUTION OF SUPPLEMENTARY CHARGES TO AHS PATIENTS BY CATEGORY OF CHARGE FOR UNITED HOSPITAL FUND MEMBER GENERAL HOSPITALS, NEW YORK CITY, 1958

Category	Amount (in Thousands of Dollars)	Percent
Maternity	4,837	27.6
Discount period	6,490	37.0
Private accommodation	4,741	27.0
Miscellaneous	1,475	8.4
Total	17,543	100.0

SOURCE: Hospital Council of Greater New York.

Charges for the discount period are the largest single item, constituting 37 percent of the total. If the full benefit period were extended from 21 to 120 days, as has been proposed, supplementary charges to patients for the discount period would decline by seven eighths, or approximately $5.7 million. AHS payments to hospitals would perhaps increase by a smaller amount.

In maternity care, charges to patients exceed AHS payments. In 1958, when charges to patients were $4.8 million, AHS payments for maternity patients were $3.4 million.

Supplementary charges to private nonmaternity patients during the period of full benefits are approximately equal to charges to all maternity patients. Total charges to private nonmaternity patients, including charges of approximately $700,000 during the discount period, are almost equal to AHS payments for this group. Sometimes these charges are incurred by patients who cannot afford them, persons of modest means for whom semiprivate beds were not available at the time of admission.

Charges for miscellaneous items amount altogether to 8 percent of the total. The most important single item here is the purchase of blood. For semiprivate nonmaternity patients, according to a survey performed several years ago, blood and blood plasma accounted for more than 60 percent of the miscellaneous supplementary charges; other hospital services for 15 percent; and personal items for the remainder.[14]

Expansion in Benefits, with Provision for Deductible. The use of hospitals by AHS subscribers is well below the average for all Blue Cross plans in the country. Yet utilization of hospitals by Blue Cross subscribers is increasing here as elsewhere while hospital cost is rising. Moreover, an insistent demand is being expressed for expanding the benefits of the standard contract, including provision of a longer period of full benefits and coverage of psychiatric services for inpatients and of certain services for ambulatory patients. Some or all of these provisions are available to members of other Blue Cross plans and are rapidly coming to be considered an integral part of a comprehensive Blue Cross program. There is no reason why New York City should lag.

As one possible means of restraining a rise in AHS premiums, consideration might be given to introducing a deductible feature, such as requiring the patient to pay for the first day or two of his hospital stay. Such a deductible provision is not aimed at reducing hospital use by deterring the admission of patients but should be considered solely for its value in lowering insurance premiums. The patient would be expected to pay a predictable sum toward his hospital bill at the time of illness on top of the premium he and his employer paid when he was well.

It is estimated that a one-day deductible clause would be worth approximately 11 percent of all AHS payments for nonmaternity care, if the other elements of the benefit structure remained the same. A deductible clause of two days would be worth approximately 20 percent of all such AHS payments, and a deductible clause of three days, almost 30 percent.

Consideration might be given to offering the deductible provision as an optional feature. It may be desirable to limit the deductible provision to the room and board component of hospital care, leaving coverage of ancillary services undisturbed. In any event care should be taken to limit the potential liability of the patient and to avoid his undertaking an open-end commitment.

Reactions to deductible features vary. One half of the Blue Cross plans in the United States have had some experience with them.[15]

Summary

1. In New York City, unlike the rest of the country, Blue Cross is the predominant voluntary insurance plan for hospital care. With 70 percent of the population insured, 50 percent is enrolled with Blue Cross.

2. Almost all payments by Associated Hospital Service, the local Blue Cross plan, are for inpatient services rendered in general-care hospitals. AHS payments to long-term hospitals and to general-care hospitals for the care of ambulatory patients are small.

3. Between 1950 and 1958 AHS patients and patient days in general-care hospitals in New York City increased by more than one half. AHS payments increased one and two third times.

4. Relative to the total patient load, AHS plays the largest role in proprietary hospitals, next largest in voluntary hospitals, and the smallest by far in municipal hospitals. This order is understandable, since most AHS patients use private and semiprivate accommodations.

5. AHS subscribers have a lower admission rate than the population as a whole. This finding goes counter to most other studies, which have found that persons with insurance have a higher admission rate than patients without insurance.

6. AHS subscribers have a shorter hospital stay than other patients. This is consistent with the findings of other studies.

7. AHS payments to hospitals are accompanied by a substantial amount of payments by subscribers. The amount of such payments is not known, but AHS keeps a record of supplementary charges to patients. If such charges are taken at face value, income from the care of AHS patients (the sum of AHS payments and supplementary charges to patients) equals approximately three tenths of total income and one third of the operating income of all general-care hospitals in New York City. These figures compare with the following figures on the role of Blue Cross in New York City and in its general-care hospitals:

Proportion (percent) of population with Blue Cross insurance   50
Proportion (percent) of all patients   44
Proportion (percent) of all patient days   37

8. In voluntary hospitals AHS payments plus charges to subscribers approach 65 percent of total income only in the semiprivate service.

9. The formula for paying hospitals adopted by AHS in 1948 was an attempt to cope in an objective and automatic fashion with differences in cost among hospitals and with increases in cost. This attempt failed because (1) at the outset it was necessary to substitute charges for cost and (2) the index numbers incorporated in the formula failed to reflect adequately subsequent increases in hospital cost.

10. Voluntary hospitals have some degree of control over charges for 46 percent of their patient days and full, or a significant measure of, control for 38 percent. These are lower degrees of control than voluntary hospitals exercised in the past, but higher than is generally believed.

11. The chapter concludes with a discussion of expansion of Blue Cross benefits, including a longer period of full benefits and coverage of psychiatric services for inpatients and of certain services for ambulatory patients. The possible introduction of a deductible feature is raised; this is meant not to deter hospital admissions but to restrain the rise in insurance premiums. If a deductible were adopted, it should represent a limited cash commitment on the patient's part at the time of illness.

Appendix 17.A

TABLES ON AHS PATIENTS, PATIENT DAYS,
AND PAYMENTS

The timing of data in Tables 17.8, 17.9, and 17.10 is as of the year of payment rather than that of services rendered. Where billing is irregular, the data may display fluctuations that did not occur in fact.

For the years 1950–53 the number of patient days accounted for by maternity patients in voluntary and proprietary hospitals was estimated from the number of claims, on the basis of data on length of stay published by the United Hospital Fund.[16]

In municipal hospitals the number of patient days during the same period was estimated from data on payments. The daily rate of payment was known, and the proportion of discount days was extrapolated backward.

Payments to municipal hospitals include those for the private and semiprivate services at Sydenham Hospital, which ranged from $150,-000 in 1950 to $236,000 in 1957 and $260,000 in 1958.

Table 17.8. AHS PATIENTS, PATIENT DAYS, AND PAYMENTS FOR
VOLUNTARY GENERAL-CARE HOSPITALS,
NEW YORK CITY, 1950–58

Year	Patients (in Thousands)	Patient Days (in Thousands)	Payments (in Thousands of Dollars)
1950	206	1,962	25,813
1951	219	2,079	30,225
1952	231	2,155	34,158
1953	239	2,234	37,434
1954	249	2,346	41,141
1955	262	2,518	47,010
1956	280	2,640	52,147
1957	305	2,850	60,458
1958	327	3,071	70,833

SOURCE: Computed by Hospital Council of Greater New York from data furnished by Associated Hospital Service of New York.

Table 17.9. AHS PATIENTS, PATIENT DAYS, AND PAYMENTS FOR
MUNICIPAL GENERAL-CARE HOSPITALS,*
NEW YORK CITY, 1950–58

Year	Patients (in Thousands)	Patient Days (in Thousands)	Payments (in Thousands of Dollars)
1950	13	144	1,401
1951	13	166	1,490
1952	15	184	1,942
1953	15	178	1,803
1954	15	210	2,062
1955	16	225	2,413
1956	18	229	2,783
1957	20	254	3,260
1958	19	237	3,138

* Private and semiprivate services at Sydenham Hospital are included.
SOURCE: Associated Hospital Service of New York.

Table 17.10. AHS PATIENTS, PATIENT DAYS, AND PAYMENTS FOR
PROPRIETARY GENERAL-CARE HOSPITALS,
NEW YORK CITY, 1950–58

Year	Patients (in Thousands)	Patient Days (in Thousands)	Payments (in Thousands of Dollars)
1950	75	494	7,691
1951	80	532	9,111
1952	89	586	10,733
1953	90	599	11,440
1954	90	619	12,274
1955	93	660	13,674
1956	100	708	15,270
1957	111	798	18,292
1958	109	772	19,035

SOURCE: Associated Hospital Service of New York.

18   ROLE OF PHILANTHROPY

In New York City almost all income from philanthropy accrues to voluntary hospitals. Municipal hospitals receive some small sums through their women's auxiliaries, which participate in the distribution of funds by the United Hospital Fund of New York and the Greater New York Fund. Proprietary hospitals are organized for profit and do not receive any contributions.

About a century ago when voluntary hospitals were being founded in New York City by religious and nationality groups, philanthropy paid for a good part of the free care rendered to the sick poor. Subsequently voluntary hospitals extended care to paying patients as well, and net earnings on private patients became available to defray part of the cost of free care. In the past generation hospital expenditures in New York City have increased markedly, and income from philanthropy has failed to retain its relative position in financing hospital care.

In this report income from philanthropy is defined as comprising contributions and grants from private sources—individuals, churches, foundations, and business—and earnings on investments. An exception is made in the case of bequests and legacies available for current purposes; they are excluded because of their erratic occurrence. As a practical matter, most contributions for designated purposes are excluded because they cannot be identified as deriving from philanthropic sources by the central data collecting agency, the United Hospital Fund. Income from investments for designated purposes is, however, estimated and included in this report. Grants from government, whatever their purpose, are excluded from philanthropy.

There are voluntary hospitals in New York City that have no ward service or outpatient department and do not require any philanthropic support. A hospital can retain voluntary status here by virtue of being a nonprofit corporation, in the sense that no person or group connected with it derives a profit from its operation. It need not render charitable service.[1]

It is estimated that in 1958 one third of the 69 voluntary general hospitals in New York City received less than 5 percent of their income from philanthropy, including 8 hospitals with practically no such income; one third received between 5 and 10 percent; and one third, more than 10 percent, including 7 hospitals with 20 percent or more. One research hospital that relies almost totally on philanthropic income is excluded from this distribution.

Introduction

The concept of income from philanthropy, as above defined, is the same for both 1948 and 1957. In application there are differences between the two years because the sources of the basic data differ. There are, however, certain differences in concept between these two years and 1934. Imbedded in the 1934 data are bequests and legacies available for current use and also certain appropriations of principal, both of which are excluded in later years. The net effect of these departures from uniformity is apparently to overstate philanthropic income in 1934 and to understate it in 1948. In other words, the increase in philanthropy between 1934 and 1948 was greater than reported and that between 1948 and 1957 was smaller than reported.

On the basis of the statistics reported in Chapters 12 and 13, income from philanthropy in hospitals in New York City increased from approximately $9 million in 1934 to $19 million in 1948 and to $29 million in 1957. The proportion of philanthropy to total income declined from 15 to 9 to 7 percent, respectively, for all hospitals and from 25 to 15 to 13 percent, respectively, in voluntary hospitals. The decline was much steeper during the period 1934–48 than during 1948–57.

The same trends obtain in general-care hospitals. Here the amount of income from philanthropy rose from approximately $9 million in 1934 to $15.5 million in 1948 to $27 million in 1957. As a proportion of total income philanthropy declined from 16 to 9 and to 8 percent, respectively, for all general-care hospitals and from 25 to 14 and to 13 percent, respectively, in voluntary general-care hospitals.

The primary division of income from philanthropy is between contributions and earnings on investments. Between 1934 and 1957 each of these components tripled in amount. There is, however, an interesting difference in timing.

Table 18.1. DISTRIBUTION BY COMPONENT OF INCOME FROM PHILANTHROPY FOR VOLUNTARY GENERAL-CARE HOSPITALS, NEW YORK CITY, 1934, 1948, AND 1957 (IN THOUSANDS OF DOLLARS)

Component	1934		1948		1957	
	Amount	Percent	Amount	Percent	Amount	Percent
All components	8,627	100.0	15,480	100.0	27,060	100.0
Contributions	5,001	58.0	11,844	76.5	15,887	58.7
Centrally raised	1,489	17.2	6,435	41.6	7,950	29.4
Donated services of Sisters	486	5.6	638	4.1	1,306	4.8
Other	3,026	35.2	4,771	30.8	6,631	24.5
Income from investments	3,626	42.0	3,636	23.5	11,173	41.3

SOURCE: Hospital Council of Greater New York; Appendix 18.A.

The proportion of contributions to total income from philanthropy was the same in 1957 as in 1934, having first increased and then declined. The proportion of income from investments in 1957 was also the same as in 1934, having first declined and then increased.

The proportion of centrally raised contributions in 1957 fell midway between that in 1934 and 1948. In 1948 these contributions could be seen as rising four times as fast as total income from philanthropy. By 1957 the rate of increase in centrally raised funds was still far ahead of any other item of income from philanthropy for the period 1934–57, but the difference in rate of increase between this item and the others had narrowed. The reason is that between 1948 and 1957 the amount of centrally raised funds increased by one fourth, whereas total income from philanthropy increased by three fourths.

By contrast, income from investments tripled between 1948 and 1957, although it had scarcely changed between 1934 and 1948. There is some reason to believe that this component of income was understated in 1948 by approximately $1 million. The fact remains that the change between 1934 and 1948 was small, whereas the increase between 1948 and 1957 was sizable.

Table 18.2. PERCENTAGE INCREASES IN COMPONENTS OF IN-
COME FROM PHILANTHROPY FOR VOLUNTARY
GENERAL-CARE HOSPITALS, NEW YORK CITY,
1934–48, 1948–57, AND 1934–57

Component	1934–48	1948–57	1934–57
All components	78	75	212
Contributions	137	34	218
Centrally raised	332	24	434
Donated services of Sisters	31	105	168
Other	58	39	119
Income from investments	0	208	208

SOURCE: Table 18.1.

In the value of donated services of Sisters four fifths of the increase for the period 1934–57 took place between the years 1948
and 1957.

Only "other contributions" showed equal rates of increase in
the two time periods.

In sum, conclusions regarding the several components of philanthropy in financing hospital care would be quite different from
the vantage point of 1957 than from the vantage point of 1948.

What lies ahead? The more numerous the points in a time
series and the more accurate the data, the sounder the projection
that can be made. For the member hospitals of the United Hospital Fund it was possible to obtain data reflecting uniform concepts for selected years, beginning in 1940. In the remainder of
this chapter data are presented for the Fund member general-care
hospitals for 1940, 1948, and for one or two recent years, including 1957.

Centrally Raised Funds

For voluntary hospitals in New York City centrally raised
money consists largely of contributions from the United Hospital
Fund, the Greater New York Fund, and the Federation of Jewish Philanthropies. In 1957 the three agencies accounted for 92
percent of all centrally raised funds accruing to member general-
care hospitals of the United Hospital Fund. Numerous agencies
accounted for the remaining 8 percent, including Catholic Charities, Federation of Protestant Welfare Agencies, and miscellaneous foundations.

In 1934 the Greater New York Fund was not yet in existence.

The United Hospital Fund's grants to member general-care hospitals amounted to $391,000, approximately one fourth of all centrally raised funds received by voluntary general-care hospitals in New York City. The Federation of Jewish Philanthropies contributed $1,075,000.[2]

For 1940, the last prewar year, figures are available for all three major agencies. Table 18.3 presents data for 1940, 1948, and 1957.

Table 18.3. DISTRIBUTION BY SOURCE OF CENTRALLY RAISED FUNDS RECEIVED BY UNITED HOSPITAL FUND MEMBER GENERAL HOSPITALS, NEW YORK CITY, 1940, 1948, AND 1957 (IN THOUSANDS OF DOLLARS)

	1940		1948		1957	
Source	Amount	Percent	Amount	Percent	Amount	Percent
All sources	2,802	100.0	5,832	100.0	7,948	100.0
United Hospital Fund	1,085	38.7	1,778	30.5	1,901	23.9
Greater New York Fund	496	17.7	859	14.7	1,488	18.7
Federation of Jewish Philanthropies	1,221	43.6	2,983	51.2	3,909	49.2
Other agencies	n.a.	n.a.	212	3.6	650	8.2

SOURCE: United Hospital Fund of New York.

Centrally raised contributions almost tripled in amount between 1940 and 1957. The Greater New York Fund, a relatively new organization in 1940, and the Federation of Jewish Philanthropies kept pace with the over-all rate of increase, whereas the United Hospital Fund's contribution increased only by three fourths. As a result, the latter's share of centrally raised funds declined from almost two fifths in 1940 to less than one quarter in 1957. Both in 1948 and in 1957 the Federation's contribution represented one half of all centrally raised moneys received by the general-care member hospitals of the United Hospital Fund.

UNITED HOSPITAL FUND

The United Hospital Fund is the oldest of the three major central fund-raising organizations in New York City, having been organized in 1879 as the Hospital Saturday and Sunday Association of New York City. The current name was adopted in 1916, and in 1920 membership in the Fund was opened to hospitals in the boroughs of Brooklyn, Queens, and Richmond.

Collections. For many years fund raising was slow. By the turn of the century annual collections amounted to $70,000. Campaign contributions and other income available for distribution reached $103,000 in 1906 and then declined. By 1910 they were $115,000. Funds available for distribution exceeded $200,000 for the first time in 1918 and rose strikingly to $939,000 in 1919. Then they declined once again, reaching $537,000 in 1924. They rose to $769,000 in 1929 and declined again, reaching a low of $439,000 in 1933, in the depth of the depression.

After a major reorganization of the Fund, campaign collections and other income available for distribution reached $1,744,000 in 1935. They continued to increase in the following two years and declined in 1938, when the Greater New York Fund was established and took over solicitation of publicly owned corporations. In 1940 United Hospital Fund moneys available for distribution amounted to $1,566,000. During World War II a slow increase began, and this accelerated during the early postwar period.

In 1952 funds available for distribution reached $2,676,000, of which $2,214,000 came from the current campaign and $463,000 from other sources.[8] By 1954 income from other sources available for distribution was down to $127,000, whereas campaign contributions remained steady. In 1955 campaign contributions rose to $2,720,000. Since then they have fluctuated around $2.6–$2.7 million.[4]

Criteria for Distributing Funds. At first the United Hospital Fund distributed money to its member institutions according to the number of free days of care rendered. As statistical data were accumulated, it became evident that differences among hospitals in patient day cost tend to persist. Accordingly, in the years immediately prior to World War I it was decided to take cost into account in computing the number of free days of care rendered by a hospital.[5] This was done essentially by dividing a hospital's total income from ward patients by its own patient day cost (subject to a ceiling). When the result is subtracted from the number of ward patient days, the difference is the computed number of free days.

In 1924 the services of the outpatient department were recognized in the distribution formula,[6] with the number of free visits computed in a manner similar to the number of free ward days.

These two figures are converted into free-care units by equating a computed free day with a specified number of computed free visits.

In the 1935 distribution the "women's committees" received their first grants in support of their social service and other auxiliary activities. The Fund's report for 1934 also shows grants to meet the special emergency needs of hospitals that arose from the depression.[7] The special grants were not determined by formula but were awarded by a committee after review of the financial needs of individual hospitals.

In 1948, when direct benefit payments were instituted at the recommendation of a special committee, the method of distribution became substantially the one used today. Direct benefit payments are incentive payments to hospitals to participate actively in the United Hospital Fund campaign. Payment is made when a hospital's fund raising committee exceeds its assigned quota.

The distribution mechanism, and especially the part pertaining to free care, depends for its fairness in application on the maintenance of uniform records by the member hospitals and on the submission of uniform reports. Owing to its long and unique experience, the United Hospital Fund of New York has become one of the nation's leading repositories of statistical and financial information on the economy of the voluntary hospital. The Fund has taken the lead in publicizing such information and in applying it to improve the management of hospitals and to promote more adequate financing of hospital care.

Amount and Pattern of Distribution. The United Hospital Fund distributes its own moneys and also acts as agent for the Greater New York Fund in relation to hospitals. In the financial statistics reported by the United Hospital Fund the moneys contributed by the two sources are kept separate.

The general-care member hospitals of the United Hospital Fund received the following sums in selected years:

Year	Amount (in Thousands of Dollars)
1940	1,085
1948	1,778
1956	1,823
1957	1,901
1958	1,933
1959	1,736

Table 18.4. ALLOCATION OF UNITED HOSPITAL FUND MONEYS TO MEMBER GENERAL-CARE HOSPITALS ACCORDING TO BASIS OF DISTRIBUTION, NEW YORK CITY, 1940, 1948, 1957, AND 1959 (IN THOUSANDS OF DOLLARS)

Basis of Distribution	1940		1948		1957		1959	
	Amount	*Percent*	*Amount*	*Percent*	*Amount*	*Percent*	*Amount*	*Percent*
All bases	1,085	100.0	1,778	100.0	1,901	100.0	1,736	100.0
To hospital	717	66.1	1,333	75.0	1,527	80.3	1,879	79.4
Free care	714	65.8	1,063	59.8	1,150	60.5	1,018	58.6
Ward	542	50.0	842	47.4	743	39.1	707	40.7
Outpatient department	172	15.8	221	12.4	407	21.4	311	17.9
Direct benefit payments	0	0	251	14.2	374	19.6	356	20.5
Discretionary grants	3	0.3	19	1.0	3	0.2	5	0.3
To women's committees	368	33.9	445	25.0	374	19.7	357	20.6

SOURCE: United Hospital Fund of New York, *Statistical and Financial Information Relating to Member Hospitals and Hospital Statistics for Greater New York, Year 1939, 1947, 1956, and 1958* (New York, 1940, 1948, 1957, and 1959).

In recent years the basis for distributing United Hospital Fund moneys has remained substantially unchanged. Significant changes have, however, taken place since 1940 and 1948.

Discretionary grants have been small, almost negligible, during the entire period shown in Table 18.4. They reached a peak of $238,000 in 1937, to meet the emergency needs of hospitals. Direct benefit or incentive payments to hospitals for campaign effectiveness have increased to the point where they equal the amounts distributed to women's committees. Grants to women's committees were approximately the same in 1957 and 1959 as in 1940. As a proportion of total United Hospital Fund grants, they have, however, declined from one third in 1940 to one fourth in 1948 and to one fifth in recent years. The distribution to women's committees includes some direct benefit payments and some discretionary allocations for special projects.

As a result of all these changes, the proportion distributed on the basis of free care has declined from the entire amount in 1934 to two thirds in 1940 and to three fifths in 1948 and in recent years. The proportion of the total distributed for free ward care was approximately one half in 1940 and 1948 and two fifths in recent years. The proportion allocated for free care in the outpatient department has tended to fluctuate between one eighth and one fifth, with an upward trend for the entire period.

From the standpoint of the individual institution the procedure for distributing the United Hospital Fund's moneys is arithmetic and not discretionary. Over-all, judgment is involved in deciding how much of the total to distribute under the free-care formula and how much to the women's committees, after direct benefit payments are deducted.

As long ago as the mid-1930s the Hospital Survey for New York expressed the view that in the future a larger proportion of the United Hospital Fund moneys should be distributed to hospitals in need, provided that the institutions so assisted are rendering an indispensable service to the community.[8] To adopt this suggestion would be to depart from the automatic application of arithmetic formulas. It is recognized that the exercise of judgment in distributing philanthropic funds entails the risk of inequitable treatment and, perhaps as serious, of allegations of inequitable treatment. To avoid this risk, however, may be to fail to help essential voluntary hospitals with special financial needs (see Chapter 14).

THE GREATER NEW YORK FUND

The Greater New York Fund was organized in May, 1938, to solicit contributions for welfare and health activities from publicly owned corporations and employee groups. The United Hospital Fund was designated to serve as its agent for distributing funds to hospitals. At times certain hospitals were members of the Greater New York Fund but not of the United Hospital Fund; today the hospital memberships of the two Funds are identical.

In distributing its moneys the Greater New York Fund treats hospitals as if they were one institution, allocating to them their proportionate share of the total deficit of the members of the Greater New York Fund. For this purpose deficit is defined as operating deficit minus income from investments. The sum allocated to hospitals on the basis of deficit is then distributed to individual hospitals, with a few exceptions, according to the criteria of allocation employed by the United Hospital Fund, with direct benefit payments excepted.[9]

Amount Distributed. Between 1940 and 1957 the amount of Greater New York Fund moneys received by United Hospital Fund member general-care hospitals tripled. Since then there has been a further increase.

Year	Amount (in Thousands of Dollars)
1940	496
1948	859
1956	1,250
1957	1,488
1958	1,455
1959	1,709

Two fifths of the increase between 1956 and 1957 is not real but due to the reclassification of a large hospital from long-term to general care.

Two factors underlie the increase in the Greater New York Fund's contributions to hospitals. (1) Its campaign collections have been rising; and the Greater New York Fund distributes almost everything it raises, maintaining no reserves. (2) Its hospital members have accounted for a steadily rising proportion of the philanthropic deficit calculated for all member agencies.

Table 18.5. ALLOCATION OF GREATER NEW YORK FUND MONEYS TO UNITED HOSPITAL FUND MEMBER GENERAL-CARE HOSPITALS ACCORDING TO BASIS OF DISTRIBUTION, NEW YORK CITY, 1940, 1948, 1957, AND 1959 (IN THOUSANDS OF DOLLARS)

Basis of Distribution	1940		1948		1957		1959	
	Amount	Percent	Amount	Percent	Amount	Percent	Amount	Percent
All bases	496	100.0	859	100.0	1,488	100.0	1,709	100.0
To hospital	434	87.6	645	75.1	1,145	77.0	1,344	78.6
Free care	n.a.	n.a.	634	73.9	1,127	75.8	1,326	77.5
Renewal claims	n.a.	n.a.	11	1.2	18	1.2	18	1.1
Discretionary grants	n.a.	n.a.	n.a.	n.a.	•	•	•	•
To women's committees	62	12.4	214	24.9	343	23.0	365	21.4

• $500 or less.

SOURCE: United Hospital Fund of New York, Statistical and Financial Information Relating to Member Hospitals and Hospital Statistics for Greater New York, Year 1939, 1947, 1956, and 1958 (New York, 1940, 1948, 1957, and 1959).

In 1940 the ratio of United Hospital Fund moneys to the Greater New York Fund moneys received by general-care member hospitals of the United Hospital Fund was 2 to 1. The same ratio held in 1948, but by 1957 it was only 5 to 4, and by 1959 1 to 1.

Pattern of Distribution. The bases of distribution have been less variable for the contributions of the Greater New York Fund than for those of the United Hospital Fund (Table 18.5).

Renewal claims are obligations to certain member institutions assumed by the Greater New York Fund at its inception. They were intended to replace the income that these institutions formerly received through their own solicitations of corporations and employee groups. For hospitals the amount to be replaced was small.

The amounts involved in discretionary grants are negligible. Today they almost invariably represent payments of a minimum sum to member hospitals ($500) when application of the free-care formula yields a lower figure.

More than three fourths of the money distributed is for free care, and this is allocated among individual hospitals in exactly the same proportion as the free-care moneys distributed by the United Hospital Fund. If a division were desired between payments for care in the ward and in the outpatient department, it would be identical with that shown in Table 18.4.

In recent years the amount distributed by the Greater New York Fund for free care has been rising. In 1959 it exceeded for the first time the amount distributed for this purpose by the United Hospital Fund. A comparison of the free-care moneys received by the general-care member hospitals of the United Hospital Fund from the two sources follows:

Year	Moneys Distributed for Free Care (in Thousands of Dollars)		Difference between United Hospital Fund and Greater New York Fund (in Thousands of Dollars)
	By United Hospital Fund	By Greater New York Fund	
1940	714	424	+ 290
1948	1,063	634	+ 429
1956	1,088	935	+ 153
1957	1,150	1,127	+ 23
1958	1,132	1,127	+ 5
1959	1,018	1,326	− 308

• Estimated from Table 18.5.

The remainder of the Greater New York Fund's distribution accrues to women's committees. They have received increasing amounts but a declining proportion of the Fund's total distribution. Again, for the first time in 1959 the sum distributed to women's committees by the Greater New York Fund exceeded that distributed by the United Hospital Fund.

FEDERATION OF JEWISH PHILANTHROPIES

The Federation of Jewish Philanthropies was organized in 1917 to serve as a central fund-raising agency for the welfare and health activities sponsored by Jewish groups in Manhattan and the Bronx. In 1942 a merger was effected between the New York and Brooklyn federations.

The Federation network comprises 9 general hospitals in the four major boroughs and 1 psychiatric hospital, in addition to several institutions for the care of long-term patients and other quasi-medical agencies. Not every hospital under Jewish ownership belongs to the Federation.[10]

The Federation distributes money to its affiliated hospitals on the basis of an annual budgetary review. Included in the grant to each hospital are funds for general operating purposes and for specific purposes, such as support of full-time chiefs of clinical service. This program was adopted to broaden and improve teaching and to create an environment conducive to research.

Annual distributions by the Federation to its general-care hospitals follow:

Year	Amount (in Thousands of Dollars)
1938	1,139
1940	1,221
1948	2,983
1956	2,700
1957	3,909
1958	3,775

Since more than two thirds of the increase of $1.2 million between 1956 and 1957 reflects a change in classification of one large hospital, only one third is real. If this hospital were assigned the same classification in 1948 that it had in 1958, the amount distributed by the Federation of Jewish Philanthropies would be approximately the same in both years, which were a decade apart.

Federation hospitals receive few direct contributions and have small earnings from investments for general purposes.

CONCLUSIONS ON CENTRAL FUND RAISING

Table 18.3 shows contributions from other agencies, as well as from the United Hospital Fund, the Greater New York Fund, and the Federation of Jewish Philanthropies. Other agencies are not discussed because too many are involved.

The amount distributed by the United Hospital Fund has been fairly constant during the past decade, fluctuating between $1,700,00 and $1, 950,000 a year. The proportion allocated to free care has also remained constant, at approximately three fifths. Direct benefit payments have increased and payments to women's committees have decreased commensurately. Discretionary grants for special projects are negligible.

The amount distributed by the Greater New York Fund doubled between 1948 and 1959. The 1959 sum almost equalled that distributed by the United Hospital Fund; and the Greater New York Fund's allocation for free care exceeded that of the United Hospital Fund for the first time.

If changes in the classification of hospitals are disregarded, the Federation grants to hospitals were as high in 1948 as in 1958. The tendency has been toward a substantially constant total, however variable the amounts received by individual institutions. Over the past decade an increasing amount has been allocated to the support of full-time chiefs of clinical service (see Chapter 9).

Donated Services of Sisters

In New York City today this component of income from philanthropy represents almost exclusively the value of donated services in Catholic hospitals. In 1938 10 percent of the total was reported by Protestant institutions.[11]

Donated services of Sisters are noteworthy for two reasons. They are of special importance for one group of hospitals. They behave, moreover, in markedly different fashion from the other components of income from philanthropy. When a hospital receives a cash donation, its financial position is almost invariably improved. A conceivable exception is when restrictions on the use of a gift can render its receipt unduly burdensome. However,

when a hospital is allowed to raise the imputed value of the donated services of Sisters, nothing happens to its financial position
immediately. True, the hospital's income has been increased on
the books; but so have its expenditures, by exactly the same
amount. Increasing the value of the donated services of Sisters can
be a first step in improving a hospital's financial position, provided
that the higher costs can be readily translated into higher charges
and larger cash collections. There is nothing automatic about this
step.

The value of donated services of Sisters, as reported on the income side of the member hospitals' accounts, has increased as follows:

Year	Amount (in Thousands of Dollars)
1940	511
1948	542
1956	1,111
1957	1,306
1958	1,604

Between 1940 and 1948 the increase was small. The value of
donated services of Sisters doubled between 1948 and 1956 and has
increased even more rapidly since then.

Several factors help to explain these increases, including (1)
more current and, therefore, higher valuations placed on the positions occupied by Sisters, in line with the general rise in hospital
salaries; (2) upgrading in the positions held by Sisters; and, more
recently, (3) recognition of overtime work beyond a forty-hour
week, if duly recorded. The number of Sisters in Catholic hospitals in New York City has actually declined since 1948.[12]

It may be that in the course of time fewer charges (withdrawals) are being made against this account. If so, the amount
shown in the income account, "value of donated services of Sisters," is increasingly close to the amount initially recorded on the
expense side. The above figures may, therefore, overstate the rate
of increase in the value of Sisters' services.

Other Cash Contributions

Available data for 1940 on cash contributions by individuals
and churches to the general-care member hospitals of the United

Hospital Fund are not comparable with those for 1948 and later years. Accordingly, the 1940 figures are not shown.

	Amount
Year	*(in Thousands of Dollars)*
1948	3,793
1957	5,085
1958	5,414

The increase of one third between 1948 and 1957 is on a par with the rate of increase in the amount of centrally raised funds. It is, however, only one half as great as the increase in investment income for general purposes (see below).

Cash contributions are reported by every voluntary hospital. Even so, there is a tendency for a large proportion of the total to be concentrated among a small number of hospitals. In 1958, for example, 9 hospitals of 62 received one half of the total; and 18 received two thirds. The degree of concentration shown by cash contributions is less than that shown by contributions from the Greater New York Fund (9 hospitals received one half of the total and 16 two thirds) or the United Hospital Fund (7 hospitals received one half and 13 two thirds) and much less than that shown by income from investments.

Income from Investments

Since the United Hospital Fund does not keep a record of investment income on funds for designated purposes, its figures on investment income are limited to income for general purposes. Such income includes earnings from the investment of permanent fund assets (including endowments safeguarded by law) and of general fund assets (working capital).

INVESTMENT INCOME FOR GENERAL PURPOSES

For the United Hospital Fund general-care member hospitals investment income for general purposes has increased as follows:

	Amount
Year	*(in Thousands of Dollars)*
1935	2,591
1940	3,268
1948	4,296
1956	6,786
1957	7,324
1958	7,510

There is no figure available for the year 1934. Beginning in 1935 investment income rose every year until it stabilized during World War II. Steady increases took place after the war. These were usually small, but occasionally the increase was as much as $0.5 million a year.

Investment income for general purposes almost tripled between 1935 and 1958. For the shorter period 1940–57, the increase was one and one quarter times, compared with an almost threefold increase for centrally raised funds. In the period 1948–57, however, investment income increased by two thirds, twice as fast as centrally raised funds.

ESTIMATED INVESTMENT INCOME FOR DESIGNATED PURPOSES

Income on invested funds for designated purposes must have increased faster than investment income for general purposes. The reason is that during the period 1948–57 funds for general purposes held by the general hospital members of the United Hospital Fund increased by one half, whereas funds for designated purposes increased one and one third times. (Incidentally, the difference between the increase in investment income for general purposes of two thirds and in investment funds for general purposes of one half is explained by a rise in bond and stock yields.)

Table 18.6. VALUE OF PERMANENT AND TEMPORARY FUNDS HELD BY UNITED HOSPITAL FUND MEMBER GENERAL HOSPITALS, BY PURPOSE, NEW YORK CITY, 1948 AND 1957 (IN THOUSANDS OF DOLLARS)

Type of Fund and Purpose	1948	1957	Increase 1948–57	
			Amount	Percent
General purposes	88,958	132,672	43,714	48.2
Permanent funds, principal	74,049	115,759	41,710	56.4
General funds invested	14,909	16,913	2,004	13.4
Designated purposes	32,027	75,575	43,548	135.7
Permanent funds, principal	27,667	50,974	23,307	84.2
Temporary funds, reserve	4,360	24,601	20,241	464.0

SOURCE: United Hospital Fund of New York, *Analysis of Financial Statement Submitted by General Hospital Members for the Years 1946–48 and 1955–57* (New York, 1949 and 1958).

If it is assumed that one half of the amount in temporary funds for designated purposes is available for investment, as well as most of the principal of permanent funds, investments for general purposes were more than twice as large in 1957 as those for designated purposes. In 1948 the corresponding ratio was more than 3 to 1.

These relationships underlie the 1957 estimate of $3.6 million as investment income for designated purposes received by the general-care member hospitals of the United Hospital Fund in 1957. This amount compares with the reported figure of $7,324,-000 as investment income for general purposes.

In 1948, when investment income for general purposes was $4,296,000, investment income for designated purposes, it is estimated, was of the order of $1 to $1.3 million.

DEGREE OF CONCENTRATION OF INVESTMENT INCOME

A small number of hospitals receive most of investment income; this may be defined as a high degree of concentration. Because investment income for general purposes includes some earnings from the investment of working capital, its distribution is slightly less concentrated than that of the principal of permanent funds for general purposes. For example, 2 of 62 hospitals received one half of all such income, 5 received two thirds, and 8 received three quarters; for permanent fund holdings, the corresponding numbers of hospitals were 2, 4, and 6, respectively.

Permanent fund principal for designated purposes (exclusive of building funds) is even more highly concentrated. In 1957, 2 of 62 hospitals held two thirds of the assets, 4 hospitals held four fifths, and 5 hospitals, nine tenths.

Earnings from Private Patients

Voluntary hospitals have traditionally regarded net earnings from private patients as available to help defray the cost of free care. For the general-care member hospitals of the United Hospital Fund such earnings increased as follows:

Year	Amount (in Thousands of Dollars)
1940	2,491
1948	3,575
1956	4,196
1957	4,280
1958	4,614

Between 1940 and 1957 net earnings from private patients increased by less than three quarters, and between 1948 and 1957 they increased by only one fifth. In view of the higher rate of increase in most other sources of philanthropic income and the still higher increase in the cost of hospital care, net earnings from private patients constitute a relatively diminishing source of hospital income.

Summary and Comments

SUMMARY OF FINDINGS

In all voluntary general-care hospitals in New York City the relative role of income from philanthropy declined by one half between 1934 and 1948 but very little between 1948 and 1957. In the latter period the increase in the amount of such income from $15.5 to $27.1 million was almost enough, on a relative basis, to match the increase in total income.

Trends in the components of philanthropic income are summarized for the general-care member hospitals of the United Hospital Fund as background for discussing their implications.

1. Between 1948 and 1957 centrally raised funds increased by one third, in contrast to the period 1940–48 when they more than doubled. During the past decade the amount distributed by the United Hospital Fund has been nearly stable, and distributions by the Federation of Jewish Philanthropies seem to have leveled off. Although distributions by the Greater New York Fund have been rising, they constituted in 1958 less than one fifth of all centrally raised funds.

2. The value of donated services of Sisters increased one and one half times between 1948 and 1957, having remained constant during the period 1940–48. This component of income from philanthropy is widely distributed among Catholic hospitals.

3. Direct cash contributions from individuals and churches increased by one third between 1948 and 1957, the same rate as centrally raised funds. From year to year this component of income from philanthropy fluctuates erratically.

4. Between 1948 and 1957 investment income for general purposes increased by two thirds, more than double the rate of increase between 1940 and 1948.

5. Investment income for designated purposes, it is estimated,

increased approximately three times as fast as investment income for general purposes between 1948 and 1957.

6. Net earnings from private patients increased by one fifth between 1948 and 1957, compared with more than two fifths in the period 1940–48.

7. Of all components of income from philanthropy, direct cash contributions show the least tendency toward concentration. Next in degree of concentration are contributions by the Greater New York Fund and by the United Hospital Fund. Contributions by the Federation of Jewish Philanthropies and the value of donated services of Sisters do not lend themselves to this type of comparison, since by definition each is limited to a segment of the voluntary hospital system. Investment income for general purposes tends to be highly concentrated among a few hospitals, although not so highly as permanent fund principal for designated purposes (and, presumably, investment income for designated purposes).

DISCUSSION

The contribution of income from philanthropy to hospital finances is still sizable in New York City, where it is considerably greater than in the country as a whole or in other large cities (see Chapter 20). Moneys for general purposes and moneys for designated purposes are both increasing in amount, with the latter increasing more rapidly. What do these developments signify?

Funds for General Purposes. The traditional pattern in New York City has been for income from philanthropy to share with tax funds in paying for free care. Philanthropy is interpreted broadly in this connection, to include net earnings from private patients.

Some students of hospital finances insist that paying for hospital care received by the indigent and medically indigent is the responsibility of government. When the City of New York sets a daily rate below cost, they point out, it is failing to meet this responsibility.[13]

On the other hand, there are those who would like to perpetuate the pattern of joint effort between philanthropy and government.[14] In New York City centrally raised philanthropic funds pay for free care, either explicitly through a free-care allocation or through grants related to hospitals' deficits. The same purpose is being served by the value of donated services of Sisters. At least in part, direct cash contributions and investment income for general purposes are similarly employed.

Funds for Designated Purposes. To some the movement toward earmarking of funds is a step in the right direction. They see as the primary role of philanthropic contributions to hospitals the provision of venture capital for the promotion of high quality care through better teaching and more research. Although research is increasingly being financed by the federal government, it can be furthered by philanthropy through initial financing of the cost of personnel and facilities required to attract government grants.

The same developments can be interpreted, at least in part, as possibly leading to undesirable emphases in hospital programs. Frequently, when earmarked money is available for a designated purpose, it may lead to distortion in the order in which programs are undertaken. The hospital does not necessarily do what is urgently needed from the standpoint of the institution's total mission, but it does what it can most readily pay for.

There is sufficient experience in financing medical education to suggest that a prospective recipient should approach an offer of earmarked money with some caution. In the early stages of a program's development, earmarking may be not only desirable but essential to progress; at later stages, it may become a hindrance. It seems advisable to follow as flexible a policy as possible, whereby earmarked funds are coupled with contributions for general purposes.

Conclusion. At present there is still leeway in New York City to decide on the future uses of income from philanthropy. One can choose to follow the traditional pattern of providing ward care and outpatient care in both voluntary and municipal hospitals and of financing them jointly from tax funds and income from philanthropy. Alternatively, one can redirect the use of income from philanthropy away from free care to developmental and pilot projects, which would serve to raise the standards of patient care and advance medical education and medical research. The two courses are not mutually exclusive.

Appendix 18.A

ESTIMATE OF INCOME FROM PHILANTHROPY, 1957

Almost all income from philanthropy accrues to voluntary hospitals.

In municipal hospitals income from philanthropy, as reported here, consists of (1) annual distributions to women's auxiliaries by the United Hospital Fund and the Greater New York Fund and (2) payments by nonprofit foundations for patient care.

Among voluntary hospitals it is necessary to distinguish between member hospitals of the United Hospital Fund and all others.

For nonmember hospitals financial data were obtained directly from the hospitals. In most instances the response to a request for information was the submission of a financial statement. In others approximate figures were furnished over the telephone. In no instance did the Hospital Council have access to reports filed by individual hospitals with official agencies.

For the United Hospital Fund member hospitals a number of sources and devices were employed. Essentially, the several components of supplementary income tabulated by the Fund were broken down and regrouped, as follows:

1. *Contributions by the United Hospital Fund and the Greater New York Fund.* Data were taken from *Statistical and Financial Information*, published annually by the United Hospital Fund. The figures shown in the Fund's report for 1957 are received by the hospitals in 1958.

2. *Federation of Jewish Philanthropies.* Data were taken from worksheets developed by the United Hospital Fund for the purpose of analyzing the deficit position of member hospitals.

3. *Contributions by other central agencies.* Data were taken from worksheets maintained by the Department of Distribution, United Hospital Fund.

4. *Value of donated services of Sisters.* Data were furnished by the United Hospital Fund upon request.

5. *Other cash contributions.* Data were taken from the Department of Distribution's source book, as above. It was necessary to adjust for the difference between the amount of income received by the women's committees reported in the source book and that reported in *Financial and Statistical Information*.

6. *Income on investment for general purposes.* Data were taken from the source book.

7. *Income on investment for designated purposes.* A rate of return was calculated on general fund and permanent fund investments for general purposes. This rate of return was applied to investments for designated purposes, both permanent and temporary, to obtain in-

vestment income. The data on invested assets were furnished by the United Hospital Fund, upon request.

The United Hospital Fund has three other accounts under Supplementary Income: Transfers of Appropriations for Special Purposes, Income for Research and [Undergraduate] Medical Education, and Miscellaneous. In the present report, the sum of these three accounts is treated as "other" income, after deduction of two sets of items. One deduction is investment income for designated purposes, as above. The other deduction is for the purpose of avoiding double counting of certain transactions. An example of the latter is deletion of receipts from the City of New York for the services rendered by one voluntary hospital to its affiliated municipal hospital, since expenditures of the latter are included in the cost statement of the Department of Hospitals.

There are certain differences between the data on income from philanthropy in 1934, 1948, and 1957 that should be noted:

1. Unlike the figures for 1948 and 1957, those for 1934 include bequests for current purposes.

2. The figures for 1934 include appropriations for designated purposes, whereas those for 1948 do not. The figures for 1957 include investment income for designated purposes but not appropriations for special purposes made from other sources of income. The latter are shown under "other income" (see Chapter 13).

19   COST OF HOSPITAL CARE

Between 1934 and 1957 expenditures in general-care hospitals in New York City rose from $55 million to $360 million, or 550 percent. Most of the increase in expenditures is attributable to an increase in unit cost.

Increase in Cost

The derivation of this finding is outlined in Appendix 19.A. Suffice it to note here that certain simplifying assumptions were made: (1) the analysis is limited to expenditures for inpatients in general hospitals, in order to avoid the problems posed by the changing composition of the basket of services produced by hospitals; (2) the figures on patient day cost, as calculated and reported by hospitals, are accepted as valid; and (3) the intensity of care embodied in a hospital patient day has remained unchanged or, alternatively, has changed in a fashion that can be measured.

If the quality of the unit of service (patient day) has not changed, the increase in patient day cost during the period 1934–57 contributed 94 percent of the increase in expenditures and the increase in patient days, only 6 percent. In the early period, 1934–48, the corresponding figures were 88 and 12 percent, respectively, and in the later period, 1948–57, they were 97 and 3 percent, respectively (see Table 19.4).

These findings would be more meaningful if they were not based on the assumption that the hospital patient day has been of constant intensity—an assumption that is so obviously contradicted by experience.[1] A measure of the change in activity in hospitals can be devised by recognizing that the volume of services rendered by the laboratory or radiology department may be more closely associated with the number of admissions than with the number of patient days. Perhaps more obvious is the fact that the long term reduction in the average stay of obstetrical patients from 10 to 5 days has not resulted in a decline of one half in the use of the delivery suite per admission. In the calculations set forth in Appendix 19.A it is assumed that the services which are concentrated over a patient's shorter stay are the so-called ancillary services, and these constituted nearly 30 percent of patient day cost in 1957. When the increased activity in hospitals is taken into account, the relative contribution of unit cost to the increase in hospital expenditures is reduced. The reduction is small—from 94 to 91 percent for the period 1934–57 (see Appendix 19.A, p. 485).

It would have been desirable to take account of other changes in the quality of hospital care, such as menu, personal service, degree of privacy. That was not feasible. It is unlikely, however, that improved methodology would reverse the above findings. In discussing the financing of hospital care in New York City in the future, primary emphasis must be asssigned to unit cost.

SIZE OF INCREASE

Between 1934 and 1957 patient day cost in general hospitals in New York City rose from $5.26 to $26.40, or 400 percent. The dollar amounts represent weighted averages for the three ownership groups, which were calculated from patient day cost reported by, or estimated for, each group, without adjustment for lack of uniformity in the elements of cost. (Patient day cost in proprietary hospitals was so high in 1934, because the rate of occupancy was under 50 percent.)

Table 19.1. CHANGES IN PATIENT DAY COST OF GENERAL HOSPITALS BY OWNERSHIP, NEW YORK CITY, 1934, 1948, AND 1957

Hospital Ownership	Amount (in Dollars)			Percent Increase		
	1934	1948	1957	1934–48	1948–57	1934–57
All hospitals	5.26	13.18	26.40	150	100	402
Voluntary	6.04	14.62	25.77	143	76	327
Municipal	3.38	10.38	27.51	207	165	714
Proprietary	12.24	17.65	26.18	44	48	114

SOURCE: Table 19.4.

The average (geometric mean) rate of increase in patient day cost in hospitals in New York City was higher between 1948 and 1957—8 percent per year—than between 1934 and 1948—6.75 percent.

The increase in cost in municipal hospitals has been much greater than in voluntary hospitals. Separation for accounting purposes of the psychiatric and tuberculosis units of municipal hospital centers has served to magnify the increase in cost in municipal general hospitals in the second period. Nevertheless, much of the difference in trend between the two hospital systems is real. Owing in part to the marked decline in rate of occupancy and in part to the more complete enumeration of the elements of cost, patient day cost of municipal hospitals rose more than twice as fast as in voluntary hospitals in the period 1948–57. By the year 1955 the two cost curves had crossed, and for the first time average cost was reported to be higher in municipal general hospitals than in voluntary hospitals. Between 1957 and 1958 the reported difference in cost between the two hospital systems declined from $1.74 to $0.44 ($28.04 in municipal general hospitals and $27.60 in voluntary). In 1959, however, when the Department of Hospitals separated expenditures for emergency departments and allowed for the cost of caring for newborn, voluntary general hospitals once again had the higher cost ($29.58 compared with $28.72).

Students of hospital finance agree that hospital cost will continue to rise. The size of the probable increase can best be projected and the steps that might be taken to mitigate the increase can best be considered on the basis of an understanding of the forces that influence hospital cost. Such understanding is, moreover, useful for other purposes, such as examination of hospital staffing policies and development of effective payment mechanisms by large purchasers of hospital care (see Chapter 17).

DISTRIBUTION OF INCREASE BY MAJOR DEPARTMENT

It has been shown that certain components of hospital cost, such as the ancillary services, have increased much faster than other components, the so-called "hotel" services.[3] The same data may be employed to determine the relative contribution of each group of hospital departments to the total increase in hospital cost.

It is important to distinguish between data that reflect direct departmental expenses and those that show departmental costs after the allocation of indirect costs. In effect, the latter data charge to various patient services the expenses incurred by the general departments of the hospital in their behalf. Three principal methods of cost analysis are in use.[4] These may yield different values for the same hospital service at a given time, and a shift from one method to another is almost bound to distort comparisons of cost over time. Moreover, as noted in Chapter 14, the allocation of overhead is always a matter of judgment. However objective the process may be, it rests on an arbitrary base. Comparisons of direct departmental expenses are immune to these vagaries but are affected by the transfer of functions from one department to another.

Direct Expenses. Comparisons of direct departmental expenses are available for New York City hospitals from two sources, the United Hospital Fund of New York and the Blue Cross study conducted by Columbia University. Since some of the results derived from the two sets of data are similar, the former are shown in the text and the latter, in Table 19.8. The classification of expenses by major departmental grouping follows that employed by the Columbia University study.[5]

The total figure in Table 19.2 is higher than patient day cost in Table 19.1, because certain costs chargeable to outpatient and emergency departments have not yet been allocated.

The highest rates of increase are shown by special professional services and by administration and general expenses. The former comprise the laboratory and radiology, and the operating and delivery suites—the hospital's diagnostic and treatment facilities par excellence. The latter include fringe benefits of employees, in addition to administration, purchasing, and insurance.

The amount of increase in special professional services is the same as in nursing. Each contributed less than one fourth of the increase of $13.15 in patient day cost. Other general professional

Table 19.2. DISTRIBUTION OF DIRECT DEPARTMENTAL EXPENSES
FOR INPATIENTS PER PATIENT DAY BY MAJOR DE-
PARTMENTAL GROUPING FOR UNITED HOSPITAL
FUND MEMBER GENERAL HOSPITALS,
NEW YORK CITY, 1949 AND 1958

Major Departmental Grouping	Amount (in Dollars)		*Increase, 1949–58*		
	1949	1958	Rate	Amount (in Dollars)	Percent Distribution
All departments	18.45	31.60	71	13.15	100.0
Professional	9.29	17.46	88	8.17	62.1
General	6.55	11.64	78	5.09	38.7
Nursing, including school	4.32	7.43	72	3.11	23.6
Other	2.23	4.21	89	1.98	15.1
Special	2.74	5.82	112	3.08	23.4
Nonprofessional	9.16	14.14	54	4.98	37.9
Nutrition	3.52	4.43	26	.91	6.9
Housekeeping, laundry, and maintenance	3.41	4.98	46	1.57	12.0
Administrative, general, and other	2.23	4.73	112	2.50	19.0

SOURCE: United Hospital Fund of New York, "Analysis of Direct Departmental Expenses, Year 1958." its *Bulletin,* No. 234 (July 1, 1959).

services, including drugs, medical records, social work, and house
staff, contributed 15 percent. This is not much more than was contributed by housekeeping, laundry, and maintenance.

Allocated Cost. Data on cost by major departmental grouping
after the allocation of indirect costs are available from the United
Hospital Fund and the New York City Department of Hospitals.
The former have been published [6] and need not be reproduced
here. It should be noted that the Fund's shift in allocation methods
in 1953 (see Chapter 14) did serve to alter the distribution of inpatient day cost by major departmental grouping, thereby impair-
ing comparability over time. The data reported by the Department
of Hospitals are undoubtedly affected by the improvement in accounting procedures that took place in 1951. Moreover, whereas
some of the departmental groupings are fine, the cost of medical,
surgical, and nursing services could not be subdivided.

The largest increase took place in housekeeping, laundry, and
linen. Partly responsible is the transfer of some functions from
nursing to housekeeping.

Table 19.3. DISTRIBUTION OF PATIENT DAY COST BY MAJOR
DEPARTMENTAL GROUPING FOR MUNICIPAL
GENERAL HOSPITALS, NEW YORK CITY,
1948 AND 1958

Major Departmental Grouping	Amount (in Dollars)		Increase, 1948–58		
	1948	1958	Rate	Amount (in Dollars)	Percent Distribution
All departments	10.38	28.04	170	17.66	100.0
Medical, surgical, and nursing services	6.12	15.42	152	9.30	52.7
Dietary	1.79	4.51	152	2.72	15.4
Plant operation and maintenance	1.27	2.91	129	1.64	9.3
Housekeeping, laundry, and linen	0.33	2.75	733	2.42	13.7
Administration	0.39	1.29	231	.90	5.1
Other	0.48	1.16	142	.68	3.8

source: New York City Department of Hospitals, Distribution of Cost of Inpatient
Services in General Hospitals, 1948 and 1958, two charts (photostats).

The major differences between Table 19.3 (for municipal hospitals) and Table 19.2 (voluntary hospitals) are two: the municipal system shows a higher patient day cost than the voluntary in
housekeeping, laundry, and plant maintenance, and a much lower
cost in administration. In part, these differences in cost are explained by the difference between the two hospital systems in salary
structure. Municipal hospitals have traditionally paid better than
other hospitals in lower job classifications (most of which are found
in housekeeping, laundry, maintenance, as well as in dietary) and
not so well in higher ones; [7] in the 1950s there was a narrowing in salary differentials between lower and higher job classifications in the municipal system. In administration there may be a
combination of factors: (1) voluntary hospitals pay better than municipal hospitals in the higher job classifications; (2) owing to the
difference in accounting concepts, Table 19.2 (direct expenses) is
very likely to show a higher cost of administration than Table 19.3
(allocated cost); (3) municipal hospitals require a smaller administrative structure than voluntary hospitals, because the former serve
only ward patients and do not maintain machinery at the local
level for collecting patients' bills; and (4) municipal hospitals receive certain services from other departments of the City, such as

Comptroller's Office, Corporation Counsel, and Department of Purchasing, for which no cost figure is entered.

EXPLANATORY FACTORS

In a recent study reference is made to three explanations of the increase in hospital cost during the postwar era.[8] The increase may be attributed chiefly to: (1) closing the gap in wages and working conditions between hospitals and other industries; (2) the impact of medical advances; and (3) the inability of hospitals to match other industries in productivity gains. The three explanations are not mutually exclusive.

Closing the Gap in Wages and Working Conditions. In the late 1940s the belief was widespread that the postwar rise in hospital cost was the result of pressures to improve wages and working conditions of hospital employees sufficiently to catch up with other industries. It seemed reasonable, therefore, that the increase in hospital wages would temporarily exceed increases in other industries. In 1948 it seemed that the rate of increase in hospital cost was slowing down and might soon cease. It was expected that by 1950 patient day cost would stabilize, provided that the rate of occupancy did not decline.[9] The possibility that as more registered nurses became available hospitals would hire more of them was considered a potentially disturbing factor. If there were no overbuilding of hospital beds, if the proportion of registered nurses did not increase, and if there were no general inflation, hospital cost would remain stable.

Impact of Medical Advances. As more precise and more specific methods of medical treatment are developed, there arises a parallel need for more precise diagnosis. The latter furnishes the basis for selecting the most appropriate treatment from the array of available treatment measures. The various procedures are time consuming and expensive,[10] at least initially. In hospitals there is increasingly rapid obsolescence of equipment and the need to support some items of equipment on a stand-by basis, however infrequently they may be used.

Lag in Productivity. In most industries increases in wages and salaries are absorbed in part by increased productivity. Hospitals are a personal service industry in which there are few possibilities for achieving gains in productivity through the introduction of labor-saving machines. The New York State Board of Charities (now Social Welfare) recognized this more than thirty years ago.[11]

Closing the Gap. The first explanation, that the increase in hospital cost is attributable chiefly to closing the gap in wages and working conditions between hospitals and other industries, can help to explain developments in the middle and late 1940s. Before World War II hospitals had a longer work week than other industries and paid lower wages. During the war increasing competition from industry for female workers compelled hospitals to raise wages and improve working conditions. The tendency toward higher hospital cost was aggravated by the simultaneous elimination of the split shift, which had enabled hospitals in the past to staff for two peak loads with one complement of employees. Furthermore, changes in working conditions affected not only paid employees but also student nurses (see below).

By now the split shift without extra remuneration is gone. The average work week of the hospital employee declines slowly, if at all, though some costs are entailed in the expansion of fringe benefits for employees. Wages for comparable occupations remain lower in hospitals than in other industries. Early in 1959 thousands of employees of voluntary hospitals in New York City were still receiving less than $1.00 an hour.[12] Despite the stability shown by these factors, the increase in hospital cost has continued. The view that the increase in hospital cost reflects the closing of a gap that once existed in wages and working conditions between hospitals and other industries is not consistent with the long-term evidence.

It seems reasonable to suppose that hospital cost is affected by the numerous factors that make up the hospital environment and that this environment includes the economy as a whole. Within the hospital the influence of medical advances is obvious. Outside the hospital are a host of developments that impinge on it and influence the direction and level of cost.

Medical Progress. Advances in medical knowledge or technique usually lead to higher cost, as more can be—and is—done for the patient. The criteria of what constitutes good medical care are constantly being reappraised and revised, usually upward. Seldom do medical advances result in a cost reduction, as when a procedure is simplified and standardized, permitting the elimination of duplicate tests.

The reduction in average length of patient stay is one manifestation of medical progress. It need not entail any direct outlays, as, for example, early ambulation after surgery or child birth. However, associated with the reduced stay is a concentration of certain diagnostic and major therapeutic services over a shorter period. The more intensively used hospital is more costly to operate (see pages 460–61). Where the shorter average stay results in a lower rate of occupancy—which may readily occur, in the absence of an intensive effort by management to prevent it—patient day cost is further increased.

It may be that the pressures toward higher cost generated by medical advances are more intense and appear earlier in a major teaching and research center than in a community hospital. It is interesting that since 1954 the proportion of wages and salaries to total expenditures in the member general hospitals of the United Hospital Fund has been constant at 65.5 percent, terminating an upward trend that had persisted throughout the postwar era. (In part, the rise in the proportion of wages and salaries reflected the commutation or conversion of employee maintenance into cash payments.) [13] In the large teaching and research hospitals a peak of 66 percent was reached in 1954, when a decline set in. In the small hospitals the proportion of wages and salaries to expenditures is still climbing; it reached 67 percent in 1958, compared with 64 percent in the large centers.[14] The greater importance of the non-wage component in large hospitals may reflect the greater impact of medical advances in these hospitals—an impact they would feel ahead of others.

A study of costs in manufacturing in this country shows that payments to nonproduction workers were a major factor in causing the compensation of all workers in manufacturing to increase almost twice as fast as payrolls for production workers alone. Thousands of workers have been added who perform administrative, research, and other overhead tasks.[15] The extent to which these phenomena apply to hospitals is not known. The data for voluntary general hospitals in New York City are suggestive, however. The patient-day dollar increase in expenditures for administration, fringe benefits, and so forth, was only $0.58 less than the dollar increase in special hospital services.

Lag in Productivity. When working hours of hospital employees are reduced or a new method of diagnosis or treatment is introduced, it is usually necessary to hire additional employees. Improved or more automatic machinery does not replace them. Although hospitals are not fully competitive with other industries for employees, they must—and ultimately do—compete for some additional employees and replacements. As other industries raise wages and salaries with the growth of the economy, hospitals must follow suit. For them, unlike manufacturing firms, an increase in wages is equivalent to an increase in cost. One student has said: "Any improvement in the productivity of labor in general will adversely affect hospitals costs." This is apart from general inflation, a condition in the economy to which hospitals are also "extremely allergic." [16]

This is confirmed by one of the few studies of productivity comparing trends in hospitals and in other fields. Among eight agencies or major components of agencies of the federal government only one—the hospitals operated by the Veterans Administration—failed to show an increase in productivity for the twelve-year period, 1947–58. In various activities, such as the Post Office Department, Internal Revenue Service, and Social Security Administration, respectable gains in productivity were achieved. In hospitals productivity (defined as the inverse of the ratio of staff to patients) declined by 11 percent—the result of a loss of 16 percent between 1947 and 1954 and a recovery of 5 percent between 1954 and 1958.[17]

Additional Factors. Another factor to consider is the cost of medical and nursing education. A school of nursing was once a source of profit to the hospital and is now a source of loss (see Chapter 7; however, one recent study does not find an association between patient day cost in a hospital and the presence of a nursing school.) [18] In medical education it is still possible to recall when interns received no stipend (see Chapter 6). Today the requirements of medical education and research are leading to the employment of paid, full-time chiefs of clinical service in an increasing number of hospitals (see Chapter 9).

It has been said that the trend toward increased use of hospitals reflects in part a rise in the standard of living of the American people.[19] It is not unreasonable to suppose that the same rise in the standard of living would raise the public's expectations of hospitals, both as to quality of care and the amenities and comforts of life.

There is need for systematic knowledge about the major forces that have influenced hospital cost during the postwar period and about their relative importance. One useful, and almost essential, research undertaking would be a series of cost histories of individual institutions which would record the decisions that resulted in cost increases.

IMPLICATIONS FOR POLICY

Tentative as the above discussion may be, it contains some implications for future policy, particularly in the field of hospital staffing.

Continuing pressures toward higher cost are in part acceded to by hospitals and in part resisted. One way in which hospitals resist the pressures is to lower the qualifications required of applicants for certain positions. Frequently these recruits cannot be used flexibly and require considerable supervision. In a service industry such as hospitals, effective supervision is difficult to provide, since standards of output cannot easily be set.[20] It is more efficient to hire persons who know their jobs, require little supervision, and can be held responsible for their performance.[21] A recent finding that hospitals with low ratios of registered nurses have higher cost than those with high ratios suggests that the former may supplement their staffs with large numbers of technical and nonprofessional personnel.[22]

The matter of flexibility in the use of personnel is important. For example, the operations research group at a major teaching hospital has found that significant gains in efficiency are obtained in the outpatient department if the clerical and administrative personnel are given more than one task.[23] To do this, persons must be hired with higher initial qualifications and greater training potential than are required to perform a single task.

This operations research group has developed criteria for adjusting staffing on the nursing unit to changes in the work load, taking account of the degree of illness of patients. This means that some people will be required to shift from one hospital area to another. To do this, standardized procedures throughout the hospital are helpful.[24]

Despite the rise in hospital cost, increases in total expenditures for medical care can be restrained through substituting other, less expensive, types of medical care. Care of patients on an ambulatory basis, whenever possible, becomes an economic necessity. It would also seem essential to control the possible oversupply of beds,[25] both to avoid the wasteful cost of maintaining vacant beds and to reduce the use of hospitals in cases of marginal medical necessity. The second of these two objectives is receiving increasing attention.

PROJECTIONS OF COST

Despite the large increase in patient day cost that has already taken place, there are indications that expenditures for hospital care in New York City may be inadequate. In the first place, the characteristic that most distinguishes voluntary hospitals with net deficits is their above-average patient day cost; by contrast, hospitals with operating surpluses have below average cost (see Chapter 14). A hospital without access to supplementary sources of income and dependent almost exclusively on income from patients cannot afford to operate at high cost. Second, stabilization in the proportion of wages and salaries to total expenditures in voluntary hospitals, when coupled with a relatively low salary level, suggests that pressing demands for new equipment and supplies may have been met at the expense of other unmet needs. Moreover, when a major voluntary hospital recently offered to staff certain clinical departments in a municipal hospital, a prerequisite condition was that the City appropriate more than $250,000 to expand and improve the latter's laboratory and x-ray services (see Chapter 11).

The outlook for future increases in cost in New York City is examined separately for voluntary and municipal hospitals.

Voluntary Hospitals. Two projections of cost were recently prepared for voluntary hospitals. One forecasts an increase in patient day cost of at least 50 percent in ten years; [26] another, for a smaller group of hospitals, expects an increase of 50 percent within five years.[27] The former estimate projects into the future the same *amount* of increase that took place in the decade 1947–57; the latter projects the same *rate* of increase that took place in the period 1952–57 and adds an extra allowance for raising employee salaries. On an annual basis the difference between the two projections is wide—an average (geometric mean) rate of increase of 4 percent compared with one of 8.5 percent.

Annual data for the general hospital members of the United Hospital Fund show an average (median) increase in patient day cost of 7 percent a year in the decade 1947–57. More recently, for the period 1952–57 or 1953–58, the average annual rate of increase was 6 percent. There was a cost increase of 9 percent between 1956 and 1957 and one of 7 percent between 1957 and 1958.[28] With pay raises given in early 1960 and with more in the offing, unusually high increases in cost may be anticipated.

In the next few years increases in cost in voluntary hospitals are likely to be above average. On the assumptions that (1) cost increases will return to the average experience of the past decade after two years and (2) there will be no significant change in rate of occupancy, it is projected that over a five-year period patient day cost in voluntary general hospitals will increase between 39 and 45 percent. The midpoint, 42 percent, is the most probable figure.

Municipal Hospitals. Annual increases in patient day cost fluctuate more widely in municipal hospitals than in voluntary hospitals. One reason is that in the former wages and salaries are raised simultaneously throughout the system. Although voluntary hospitals consult one another regarding employee salaries, they operate as autonomous institutions. In municipal hospitals control over wage rates and salary schedules is exercised at a single point. Wide fluctuations in the past make projections of cost uncertain.

The increase in cost in municipal general hospitals has apparently slowed down. For the period 1953–58 the average annual rate of increase was 7 percent, compared with 14 percent in the period 1948–53. Between 1956 and 1957 patient day cost increased 10 percent, but between 1957 and 1958 only 3 percent.[29]

The most important single factor favoring a modest, rather than a large, increase in cost in the foreseeable future is that the pay scale for lower grade positions is not being questioned. Certain changes in program that were initiated within the past year or two point, however, to appreciable increases in cost in municipal hospitals. Among them is the alignment of the salary scale for registered nurses with that for practical nurses; another increase in stipend for interns and residents; new positions in the Budget for preventive plant maintenance at several hospitals; and a decision to appoint full-time chiefs of clinical service in some unaffiliated hospitals. A continuing influence toward increased expenditures in the municipal system is the growing number of paid sessions in the outpatient department. Another factor is the provision for larger periodic pay increments under the Career and Salary Plan than were formerly granted.

In light of these contingencies a projection of patient day cost in municipal hospitals must have a wide range. A lower limit of 5 percent a year and an upper limit of 8 percent seem not unreasonable. At the end of five years these figures yield an increase in cost of 28 to 47 percent.

Comparability of Cost

So far in this chapter cost data have been presented as reported, without any attempt to appraise them—and adjust them—for comparability. It is recognized, however, that reported cost figures derive from different sources and are calculated by methods that differ in concept and technique.

In the remainder of this chapter comparisons are made between pertinent patient day cost figures calculated on alternative bases, as follows:

1. *Cost in voluntary and in municipal hospitals.* One policy proposal that has been advanced is for the City of New York to pay voluntary hospitals at, or in relation to, their individual costs; another is that the City pay voluntary hospitals at, or in relation to, cost in its own hospitals (see Chapter 21). What is patient day

cost in each hospital system when calculated according to the same criteria?

2. *Reported cost and more complete cost, inclusive of capital charges.* As the Hospital Survey for New York pointed out, interest on debt and depreciation represent the current use of resources invested in hospitals.[30]

3. *Cost after recognition of certain additional items.* The Hospital Survey determined the value of the exemptions from real estate taxes and water charges enjoyed by voluntary hospitals and compared it with the value of free care rendered.[31] If similarly calculated for municipal hospitals, the value of the tax exemptions may be regarded as an element of cost to the community that should be recognized in comparing the cost of hospital care with that of alternative ways of providing medical care. Also calculated here is cost per patient day of private-duty nursing in voluntary hospitals.

4. *Cost in New York City and in other parts of the country.* Patient day cost in one area, such as New York City, is often compared with average unit cost in the nation. In recent years comparisons have also been made between New York City and California, with the latter offered as an example of a high cost area and perhaps as a forerunner. The cost data for the United States and for the State of California are taken from the annual "Guide Issue" of *Hospitals,* the official publication of the American Hospital Association (AHA); [32] the figures for New York City are usually obtained from the United Hospital Fund of New York. Since government hospitals reported in the "Guide Issue" include both local and state hospitals and are otherwise not comparable to municipal hospitals in New York City, the geographic comparison in this chapter is limited to hospitals under voluntary ownership.

PATIENT DAY COST IN THE TWO HOSPITAL SYSTEMS

Unlike the United Hospital Fund, the New York City Department of Hospitals did not until recently isolate the costs of the emergency department, emergency ambulance service, and newborn infant service. These remained imbedded in expenditures for inpatient care, after expenditures for the outpatient department and home care were removed. In addition, all expenditures incurred for employees' meals and lodgings, some of which are reimbursed, remain in the cost figures. Such miscellaneous receipts are not processed through the regular accounts of the Department and are regarded as income to the City Treasury.

For the year 1958 patient day cost in municipal general hospitals is reported at $28.04. If the items listed above are isolated, patient day cost is reduced by more than $2.50, as follows (see Appendix 19.B for the calculations):

Patient day cost, as reported		$28.04
Less exclusions (expenditures divided by patient days)		
Emergency department	$1.32	
Emergency ambulance service	.56	
Reimbursed meals and lodgings of employees	.21	
Total exclusions		2.09
Subtotal		$25.95
Less: Cost of newborn care		.49
Cost, on basis comparable to UHF		$25.46

Expenditures by the Department of Hospitals do not encompass all the costs incurred in municipal hospitals. Accordingly, the Department has for almost a decade included in its cost statement certain cash expenditures incurred in behalf of its institutions and employees by other City agencies. Among them are pension contributions, employer contributions for social security, and the cost of gas, electricity, and steam.

The Department's cost statement still does not reflect the cost of services furnished to municipal hospitals by other agencies of the City, such as central purchasing, some legal advice, and the processing of disbursements. To this extent patient day cost in municipal hospitals is not so complete as cost in voluntary hospitals, which receive few contributions of services that others pay for.

In 1934 and 1948 the Hospital Survey for New York and the New York State Hospital Study, respectively, estimated the value of services furnished to municipal hospitals by other City agencies. When gas, electricity, and steam are included the value of such services furnished amounted to 4.5 percent of total expenditures in 1934 [33] and to 5 percent in 1948.[34] For 1958 the proportion should be appreciably lower, and the value of the services furnished by other City agencies is estimated at $0.52 per patient day.

When this item is added, adjusted patient day cost in municipal general hospitals in 1958 was $26. This is $2.00 less than the originally reported figure and $1.50 less than the figure of $27.60 reported for the member general hospitals of the United Hospital Fund.

The cost figure for municipal hospitals is for general hospitals, exclusive of psychiatric units, whereas that for voluntary hospitals includes the expenditures of several psychiatric units of general hospitals. The import of this difference is difficult to assess, because the relationship between patient day cost in a psychiatric unit and in the general hospital as a whole is not uniform. Sometimes cost is higher in the former and sometimes in the latter. Fortunately for this report, the number of patient days involved is small.

INTEREST ON DEBT AND DEPRECIATION

Interest on debt was calculated for this report and included in hospital expenditures in New York City in 1934, 1948, and 1957. It is not, however, included in the reported figures on patient day cost. For the year 1958 this item is estimated at $0.08 and $0.96 for the voluntary and municipal general hospitals, respectively. The difference between the figures reflects a difference in policy in financing capital expenditures—pay as you go, as far as possible, by the former and exclusive reliance on borrowing by the latter.

The two hospital systems follow the same policy in omitting a charge for depreciation in their reported figures on patient day cost. In municipal hospitals expenditures for capital purposes are kept separate from operating expenditures and appear in different budgets. In voluntary hospitals some members of the United Hospital Fund report a charge for depreciation. In calculating patient day cost the Fund deletes this item when it appears. The Fund does, however, recognize expenditures for extraordinary repairs and replacement as an element of cost.

The hospital literature contains many discussions of the propriety and desirability of voluntary hospitals' charging depreciation. The essential distinction between capital expenditures—for building and equipment—and operating expenditures—for wages and salaries and supplies—is that the latter are for goods and services that are consumed in the year in which expenditures are incurred, whereas the former are for goods that continue to render service in future years.[35]

In recent years this point has received acceptance, and more hospitals tend to record a depreciation charge. Purchasers of large volumes of hospital care, such as government and insurance plans, are increasingly willing to recognize depreciation as an item of cost and to pay hospitals accordingly. Usually payment for depreciation takes the form of a percentage allowance on expenditures. This is a simpler procedure than calculating a charge on the value of the investment in physical plant. It also provides a measure of built-in protection against inflation, to the extent that increases in operating cost and in building cost are of similar magnitude. Payment of the depreciation charge may be conditioned upon funding by the hospital, that is, setting the receipts aside and spending them only for capital purposes.

If certain simplifying assumptions are made, it is possible to calculate a rate of depreciation for each hospital system. In 1958 this rate came to 5 percent of expenditures for voluntary hospitals and to 7.5 percent for municipal hospitals (see Table 19.7). There are two reasons for the difference: (1) municipal hospitals have a higher cost of construction; and (2) their buildings and equipment probably have a shorter life, because of poorer maintenance of plant.

Per patient day depreciation amounts to $1.40 in voluntary hospitals and $1.95 in municipal hospitals. The former should be reduced by $0.22, the cost of extraordinary repairs and replacement, which is already represented in patient day cost.

In summary, patient day cost compared as follows between the two hospital systems in 1958:

Patient Day Cost	Voluntary Hospitals	Municipal Hospitals
Adjusted inpatient cost	$27.60	$25.98
Add: interest on debt	.08	0.96
Adjusted cost, prior to depreciation	$27.68	$26.94
Add: depreciation charge	1.18	1.95
Adjusted cost, including depreciation	$28.86	$28.89

The final figures are almost identical.

VALUATION OF OTHER ELEMENTS OF COST

The value of the exemptions from the real estate tax and water charge in 1958 is estimated according to the procedures outlined in Appendix 19.B.

	Voluntary Hospitals	Municipal Hospitals
Real estate tax	$1.39	$1.66
Water charge	0.08	0.09
Total	$1.47	$1.75

The value of the exemption is greater for municipal hospitals than for voluntary hospitals, because the former have relatively newer, therefore more costly, buildings (see Chapter 8).

It has been suggested that one source of difference in cost between voluntary and municipal hospitals is that the former exclude expenditures for private-duty nurses.[36] Per patient day these amount to $2.67. It is, of course, recognized that only part of this sum represents expenditures in lieu of staff nurses.

COST IN NEW YORK CITY, CALIFORNIA, AND UNITED STATES

California is frequently mentioned as a state with high hospital cost, which may be setting the pace for other parts of the country. For the years 1957 and 1958 reported patient day cost in voluntary general-care hospitals in New York City compared as follows with patient day cost in California and in the United States:

Geographic Area	1957	1958
New York City	$26.05	$27.80
United States	26.81	29.24
California	37.29	40.86

These figures show that patient day cost in New York City is approximately two thirds that in California and less than patient day cost in the nation. That New York City ranks below the United States may seem surprising, since patient day cost in New York State, as reported in the "Guide Issue" of the AHA's *Hospitals,* consistently exceeds the nation's.

The explanation lies in certain differences in timing and in concept between the local and other data that should be clarified. Two differences are major.

1. In a period of rising cost the data in the AHA *Guide* lag behind true cost. (The AHA inventory form requests that hospitals furnish financial data for the year ending September 30, if possible. Some hospitals, especially government hospitals, submit financial data for the fiscal year ending June 30 and some do so for the year ending December 31 preceding. A few hospitals submit financial data for other fiscal years. In the absence of more complete information it is not unreasonable to assume an average filing date of June 30.) Patient day cost for a calendar year can be computed for the United States and California by averaging the published data for two successive years.

2. The AHA *Guide* computes patient day cost by dividing the total expenditures of hospitals by the number of patient days.[37] This procedure yields a correct inpatient cost figure for a hospital that provides inpatient services only and overstates cost for any hospital that provides services to ambulatory patients as well. Since the ratio of services for ambulatory patients to services for inpatients varies among geographic regions, the relationship between reported patient day cost and true patient day cost also varies.

The availability of detailed information on expenditures in New York City hospitals makes it possible to calculate several patient day cost figures, based on alternative assumptions. They follow for calendar year 1957, along with computed figures for California and the United States for the same year.

Area and Type of Cost	Patient Day Cost
United States	$28.02
California	39.07
New York City:	
Inpatient care	26.05
All care (operating cost)	33.40
Total expenditures, excluding depreciation	35.60
Total expenditures, including depreciation	37.40

Four patient day cost figures are shown for New York City. The divisor is the same, the number of patient days. The dividend in the first or lowest figure is expenditures for the care of inpatients; in the second, all operating expenditures; in the third, operating expenditures plus nonoperating expenditures; and in the fourth, operating expenditures plus nonoperating expenditures plus depreciation. Depending on which of the three latter concepts is considered most comparable with that employed in the AHA *Guide,* the difference between patient day cost in New York City and in California is between $1.65 and $5.65, not $13.00. The ratio of cost in New York City to California is not two thirds, as appeared at first impression, but between 85 and 95 percent.

The available data do not permit a determination of the true difference. On the one hand, services for ambulatory patients probably constitute a smaller proportion of hospital care in California than in New York City. On the other hand, the United Hospital Fund is known to exclude depreciation from its patient day cost, whereas the AHA *Guide* has no fixed policy on this and has no knowledge of the extent to which reported hospital expenditures may include an allowance for depreciation.[88]

In 1953 four fifths of the voluntary short-term hospitals responding to a nation-wide questionnaire stated that they calculate depreciation; and one fourth of this group, in turn, funded it.[39] No information was submitted as to the size of the depreciation charge or the amount included in the expenditures reported annually to the American Hospital Association.

Summary

1. The chief factor in the increase in hospital expenditures in New York City has been the increase in patient day cost.

2. Three explanations are generally offered for the increase in patient day cost: (*a*) hospitals formerly lagged in wages and working conditions and have been trying to catch up with other industries; (*b*) the impact of medical advances is to raise cost; (*c*) because hospitals are personal service institutions and cannot achieve appreciable gains in productivity, pay raises and improvements in working conditions result in an increase in unit cost.

3. These explanations are not mutually exclusive. Nevertheless, the evidence is no longer consistent with the correction of lag hypothesis. Medical advances, in so far as they are reflected in the ancillary services of the hospital, account for less than one fourth of the dollar increase in patient day cost in the 1950s. Their future role may be larger, however. The third explanation, that of lag in productivity gains, seems to account for a larger fraction of

the increase in cost. Research is needed in individual hospitals to focus on specific decisions that led to increases in cost.

4. Understanding of the factors underlying increases in hospital cost is important for projecting future cost, improving the efficiency of hospital operations, and guiding changes in the payment formulas employed by large purchasers of hospital care.

Examples are offered of the flexible use of personnel with higher qualifiications and requiring less supervision, and these suggest that efforts to limit increases in cost by reducing the qualifications of employees may be expensive.

5. For voluntary general hospitals in New York City an increase in patient day cost of 39–45 percent is projected for the five-year period beginning in 1960. For municipal hospitals the number of contingencies affecting cost is considerably greater, and the range of projection is estimated between 28 and 47 percent.

6. The annual charge for depreciation is estimated at 5 percent of operating cost for voluntary hospitals and at 7.5 percent for municipal hospitals. Reasons for the difference are higher cost of construction in the municipal system and poorer plant maintenance.

7. The reported patient day cost in general hospitals in New York City in 1958 was $27.60 in the voluntary system and $28.04 in the municipal system. After adjustments for comparability, prior to interest on debt and depreciation, the respective cost figures were $27.60 and $26.00. After allowances for depreciation and interest—both of which are higher in municipal hospitals—patient day cost in the two systems was the same.

8. For some purposes it is useful to have the value of the exemption from taxes. The combined value of the exemptions from the real estate tax and the water charge is estimated at $1.47 per patient day in voluntary general hospitals and $1.75 in municipal general hospitals.

9. Patient day expenditures for private-duty nurses in voluntary general hospitals amounted to $2.67. Some part represents expenditures in lieu of staff nurses.

10. Patient day cost is higher in California than in New York City. However, the difference between them is closer to 5–15 percent than to the 33 percent usually reported.

Appendix 19.A

DISTRIBUTION OF INCREASE IN EXPENDITURES
FOR GENERAL HOSPITAL INPATIENT CARE
BETWEEN VOLUME OF SERVICES AND
UNIT COST, NEW YORK CITY,
1934, 1948, AND 1957

The problem is to divide the increase in hospital expenditures during a time interval between the increase in volume of services and the increase in patient day cost.

The first step was to calculate the number of patient days, patient day cost, and expenditures for inpatients in the years selected—1934, 1948, and 1957. For each of these years the number of patient days in each hospital ownership group was multiplied by the corresponding cost per patient day. The product is the amount spent for inpatient care (Table 19.4). The division of the increase in expenditures between patient days and cost was accomplished by the following method:

Let: P_0 = patient day cost in the base year

        P_1 = patient day cost in the terminal year

        ΔP = increase in patient day cost between the base and terminal years

        Q_0 = number of patient days in the base year

        Q_1 = number of patient days in the terminal year

        ΔQ = increase in number of patient days between the base and terminal years

        $P_0 Q_0$ = expenditures for inpatients in the base year

        $P_1 Q_1$ = expenditures for inpatients in the terminal year

Then: $P_1 Q_1 = (P_0 + \Delta P)(Q_0 + \Delta Q)$

        $P_1 Q_1 = P_0 Q_0 + \Delta Q P_0 + \Delta P Q_0 + \Delta P \Delta Q$

        $P_1 Q_1 - P_0 Q_0 = \Delta Q P_0 + \Delta P Q_0 + \Delta P \Delta Q$

$P_1 Q_1 - P_0 Q_0$ is the increase in expenditures between the base and terminal years. The term $\Delta Q P_0$ in the equation accounts for part of the increase, that due to the increase in patient days; the term $\Delta P Q_0$ accounts for another part of the increase, that due to the increase in patient day cost; and the term $\Delta P \Delta Q$ accounts for the remainder of the increase, that due to the interaction of the increases in patient days and in cost. The third term cannot be attributed to either patient days or cost and is disregarded here in the percentage distribution of the increase in expenditures by source.[40]

COMPUTATIONS, WITH INCREASED ACTIVITY IN HOSPITALS NEGLECTED

If the data are accepted as reported, the figures required to compute the terms of the equation are given in Table 19.5.

Table 19.4. DERIVATION OF PATIENT DAYS, PATIENT DAY COST,
AND EXPENDITURES FOR INPATIENTS IN
GENERAL HOSPITALS, NEW YORK CITY,
1934, 1948, AND 1957

Year and Hospital Ownership	Patient Days (in Thousands)	Patient Day Cost (in Dollars)	Inpatient Expenditures (in Thousands of Dollars)
1934			
All hospitals	8,035	5.26	42,250
Voluntary	3,899	6.04	23,550
Municipal	3,601	3.38	12,150
Proprietary	535	12.24	6,550
1948			
All hospitals	9,649	13.18	127,100
Voluntary	4,850	14.62	71,000
Municipal	3,918	10.38	40,550
Proprietary	881	17.65	15,550
1957			
All hospitals	9,983	26.40	263,200
Voluntary	5,663	25.77	145,900
Municipal	3,046	27.51	83,900
Proprietary	1,274	26.18	33,400

SOURCE: 1934: Patient days, voluntary and municipal hospitals—Hospital Survey for New York, Report, II (New York, 1937), p. 175; patient days and patient day cost, proprietary hospitals—Arthur W. Jones and Francisca K. Thomas, Report of the Hospital Survey for New York, III (New York, 1938), p. 353; patient day cost, voluntary and municipal hospitals—ibid., pp. 343, 348. 1948: Voluntary hospitals—United Hospital Fund of New York, Financial and Statistical Information Relating to Member Hospitals and Hospital Statistics for Greater New York, Year 1948 (New York, 1949); municipal hospitals—New York City Department of Hospitals, Statement of the Cost of Maintaining and Operating the Department of Hospitals for the Year Ended December 31, 1948 (New York, 1949); proprietary hospitals—for patient days, Hospital Council of Greater New York, unpublished data; for expenditures, Eli Ginzberg, A Pattern for Hospital Care (New York, 1949), Chapter 19; and unpublished data, New York State Hospital Study. 1957: Voluntary hospitals—same as 1948; municipal hospitals—patient days, same as voluntary hospitals; patient day cost, same as 1948; proprietary hospitals—Hospital Council, unpublished data, with patient day cost based on "Guide Issue" of Hospitals.

Table 19.5. VALUES OF TERMS IN EQUATION FOR DISTRIBUTING
INCREASE IN EXPENDITURES FOR INPATIENTS IN
GENERAL HOSPITALS, NEW YORK CITY,
1934, 1948, AND 1957

Year or Period	P (in Dollars)	Q (in Thousands of Dollars)	PQ (in Thousands of Dollars)
1934	5.26	8,035	42,250
1948	13.18	9,649	127,100
1957	26.40	9,983	263,200
1934–48	7.92	1,614	84,850
1948–57	13.22	334	136,100
1934–57	21.14	1,948	220,950

SOURCE: Table 19.4.

The distribution of the increase in expenditures among the three terms of the equation is shown in Table 19.6.

Table 19.6. DIVISION OF INCREASE IN EXPENDITURES FOR INPA-
TIENTS BETWEEN INCREASE IN PATIENT DAYS AND
INCREASE IN PATIENT DAY COST IN GENERAL HOS-
PITALS, NEW YORK CITY, 1934–48, 1948–57, AND 1934–57
(IN THOUSANDS OF DOLLARS)

Term in Equation	1934–48 Amount	Per-cent	1948–57 Amount	Per-cent	1934–57 Amount	Per-cent
1. Increase in expenditures	84,850		136,100		220,950	
2. ΔQP_0	8,500	11.8	4,400	3.3	10,250	5.7
3. ΔPQ_0	63,550	88.2	127,500	96.7	169,500	94.3
4. Subtotal (item 2 plus item 3)	72,050	100.0	131,900	100.0	179,750	100.0
5. $\Delta P\Delta Q$ (item 1 minus item 4)	12,800		4,200		41,200	

SOURCE: Table 19.5.

The third term or interaction (item 5) increases with the length of the time interval.

COMPUTATIONS, WITH ALLOWANCE FOR INCREASED ACTIVITY IN HOSPITALS

To take account of the increased activity in hospitals owing to shorter patient stay, the following figures were obtained:

Length of stay, 1934	14.3 days
Length of stay, 1957	10.8 days
Percent decline, 1934–57	24.5 percent
Proportion of cost of ancillary services to total cost, 1957 [41]	29.4 percent

There were 9,983,000 patient days in general hospitals in New York City in 1957 (Table 19.4). When higher intensity of care is taken into account, this figure is equivalent to 10,800,000 patient days (9,983,000 patient days/92.8 percent; 92.8 percent = 100.0 percent − 7.2 percent; 7.2 percent is the product of 24.5 percent by 29.4 percent, above). Patient day cost in 1957 is, therefore, no longer $26.40 (Table 19.4) but $24.35 ($263,200,000/10,800,000 patient days). The increase in patient day cost between 1934 and 1957 is $19.09, instead of $21.14 (Table 19.5).

The recomputed values of the three terms of the equation for the period 1934–57 are as follows:

		Amount	Percent
1.	Increase in expenditures	$220,950,000	
2.	ΔQP_0	14,750,000	8.8
3.	ΔPQ_0	153,500,000	91.2
4.	Subtotal (item 2 plus item 3)	$168,250,000	100.0
5.	$\Delta P \Delta Q$ (item 1 minus item 4)	52,700,000	

Another study estimates that the volume of services per patient day in general-care hospitals in this country increased by one fourth between 1946 and 1952.[42] Part of the difference between this figure and the 7 percent figure for New York City is attributable to the smaller reduction in duration of patient stay in New York City than in the nation. Most of the difference results, however, from differences in the techniques of estimation.

Appendix 19.B

CALCULATION OF ELEMENTS OF PATIENT DAY COST ON ALTERNATIVE BASES

Reported patient day cost serves as a point of departure. What happens when (1) reported cost for each hospital system is recalculated according to uniform criteria; (2) reported cost is made more complete; (3) and reported cost in New York City is made more comparable with reported cost elsewhere?

ADJUSTMENTS TO MAKE MUNICIPAL GENERAL HOSPITALS COMPARABLE TO VOLUNTARY HOSPITALS, 1958

Unlike the United Hospital Fund of New York, which is the source of data for voluntary general hospitals, the New York City Department of Hospitals did not until 1959 segregate expenditures for the emergency department and newborn infants. These, as well as expenditures for the emergency ambulance service, remained in expendiitures for inpatients, after deduction of expenditures for the out-patient department and home care.

The elements of cost required to make patient day cost in munic-ipal general hospitals in 1958 comparable to cost in voluntary hospitals were calculated as follows:

Emergency Ambulance Service. The value of this item is available directly from the Department's special analysis of cost for 1948 and 1958.[43] The cost per patient day is $0.56.

Emergency Department. The number of visits is available from the Hospital Council's annual inventory (968,500). Cost per visit was set at $4.00 for these calculations. The basis for so doing was as fol-lows: for United Hospital Fund member general hospitals cost per emergency department visit can be calculated ($3.15); at the same time cost per outpatient department visit was $6.50.[44] There is reason to believe that the former is understated and the latter overstated. Since cost per visit in municipal hospital outpatient departments was $5.81,[45] a figure of $4.00 for the emergency department did not seem unreasonable.

Total expenditures of the emergency departments of municipal general hospitals are, therefore, estimated at $3,874,000 ($4.00 times 968,500); these were divided by 2,929,000, the number of patient days in municipal general hospitals.[46] Per patient day the value, therefore, is $1.32.

Income from Employees' Meals and Lodgings. The United Hos-pital Fund deducts such revenue from expenditures for patients. For the purpose of separating the income of short-term and long-term mu-nicipal hospitals (see Chapter 15), miscellaneous revenues of the for-mer were estimated at $750,000. The ratio of inpatient expenditures to total in general-care hospitals was 84 percent; the number of pa-tient days in these hospitals, 3,076,000. Per patient day the value is $0.21.

Newborn Infants. The above three deductions total $2.09 per pa-tient day; subtracted from the reported cost of $28.04, adjusted cost is $25.95. The allowance for newborn can be taken at one third of the latter figure, or $8.65. There were 166,800 newborn patient days in 1958, yielding total expenditures for newborn of $1,443,000. Divided by 2,929,000 patient days in general hospitals, the value is $0.49.

Contributed Services by Other Departments of the City. This was estimated with precision at 4.5 percent of total expenditures in 1934 [47] and more roughly at 5 percent in 1948.[48] For total departmental ex-penditures of $158.8 million, the 4.5 percent figure yields a value of contributed services of $7.1 million. From this subtract $1.3 million already included in 1958 expenditures for the cost of gas, electricity, steam, and operation of central headquarters.[49] For general hospitals expenditures for inpatients, ($82.1 million), are 52 percent of $158.8 million. Divided by 2,929,000 patient days, the value per patient day is $1.03. This is on the high side and fails to reflect such changes as the appointment of counsel to the Department of Hospitals. Similarly, the increased proportion of wages and salaries to total expenditures reduces the relative importance of the contribution to the Department by central purchasing. The Department of Hospitals also renders off-setting services to other agencies of the City, such as filing claims for public charges in voluntary hospitals. The value of contributed services to the Department is arbitrarily set at one half of the figure based on the 1934 proportion, or $0.52.

INTEREST ON DEBT, DEPRECIATION, AND OTHER ITEMS, BOTH HOSPITAL
SYSTEMS, 1958

Interest on Debt. For voluntary hospitals the amount is available from the United Hospital Fund—$513,000. The proportion if inpatient to total expenditures for patient care was 88 percent ($153.1 million divided by $174.3 million), and the number of patient days in general hospitals 5,360,000. Per patient day the value is $452,000 divided by 5,360,000, or $0.08.

For municipal hospitals the amount of interest for the entire system was calculated by multiplying the amount of debt outstanding in behalf of the Department of Hospitals by the average rate of interest. This came to $5.4 million ($169.1 million times 3.195 percent).[50] The share of the inpatient services of general hospitals was 52 percent, as above, or $2.8 million. Divided by 2,929,000 patient days, the value is $0.96.

Allowance for Depreciation. Neither hospital system includes depreciation in patient day cost. The United Hospital Fund does, however, allow certain expenditures for extraordinary repairs and replacement.

From a practical standpoint the simplest way to calculate depreciation is as a percentage of annual expenditures, rather than of assets. To do this the following must be specified: (1) cost of construction per bed; (2) the proportions of total cost devoted to building and to equipment; (3) estimated lives of the building and of equipment; (4) cost of operation per patient day; and (5) rate of occupancy.

For example, if the cost of construction is taken as $25,000; the proportion of the cost devoted to the building (including some fixed equipment), as 90 percent and to equipment, as 10 percent; and the prevailing rate of occupancy, as 80 percent, then the allowance for depreciation as a proportion of expenditures varies with the estimated lives of the building and of equipment and with patient day cost. Table 19.7 presents illustrative computations.

Table 19.7. DEPRECIATION AS PROPORTION (PERCENT) OF EX-
PENDITURES, WITH VARIATION IN PATIENT DAY
COST AND IN LIVES OF BUILDING AND OF EQUIP-
MENT, UNDER SPECIFIED ASSUMPTIONS

Lives of Building and of Equipment (in Years)	Patient Day Cost			
	$24	$26	$28	$30
50 and 10	6.4	5.9	5.5	5.1
50 and 15	5.7	5.3	4.9	4.6
40 and 10	7.4	6.8	6.3	5.9
40 and 15	6.7	6.2	5.8	5.4

SOURCE: Hypothetical computations based on specified assumptions, as follows: cost per bed, $25,000; proportion of cost for the building, 90 percent; proportion of cost for equipment, 10 percent; rate of occupancy, 80 percent.

For voluntary general hospitals the most likely assumptions seemed to be lives of 50 and 14 years for the building and equipment, respectively,[51] and $28 a day. These give a depreciation rate of 5 percent (Table 19.7) and a patient day cost of $1.40. However, the cost of extraordinary repairs and replacement should be subtracted. Per patient day this was reported by the United Hospital Fund [52] at $0.22. The net additional value of the depreciation charge for voluntary general hospitals is, therefore, $1.18.

For municipal general hospitals the cost of construction per bed was taken as $27,500 (see Appendix 8.B). Because plant maintenance is poorer than in voluntary hospitals, estimated lives of building and equipment are taken as 40 and 10 years, respectively. Patient day cost, adjusted above, is $26.00. On the basis of these assumptions, the depreciation rate is 7.5 percent. Per patient day this amounts to $1.95.

Exemption: Real Estate Tax. The assessed value of voluntary general hospital members of the United Hospital Fund was $200.5 million in fiscal year 1959.[53] The city-wide real estate tax rate was $4.25 per $100. The value of the exemption is, therefore, $8.5 million; the proportion attributable to inpatients, 88 percent; and the number of patient days 5,360,000. The patient day cost for this is $1.39.

For municipal general hospitals the assessed value was $200.4 million.[54] The value of the exemption is also $8.5 million. Included for this purpose are the psychiatric and tuberculosis facilities of municipal hospital centers. For these hospitals inpatient expenditures constituted 83 percent of the total; and the number of patient days was 4,245,000. The patient day cost is, therefore, $1.66.

Exemption: Water Charge. Collections for the entire city were 5.7 percent of the real estate tax levy ($49.7 million compared with $875.2 million in fiscal year 1958). Per patient day the amount for voluntary hospitals is $0.08. For municipal hospitals the value is $0.09.

Expenditures for Private-Duty Nurses. In municipal hospitals expenditures for private-duty nurses are included in cost, and in voluntary hospitals they are not. There were 2,195 private-duty nurses in United Hospital Fund member general hospitals in 1958.[55] At $6,500 per year (360 sessions at $18 a day), total expenditures amount to $14.3 million. Divided by 5,360,000 patient days, the value per patient day is $2.67.

(The figure of $6,500 is based on prevailing relationships between the number of private-duty nurses on a given day and annual expenditures for them, as reported by several member hospitals of the United Hospital Fund which compile such expenditures data.)

ALTERNATIVE COMPUTED COSTS, GENERAL-CARE HOSPITALS, NEW YORK CITY, 1957

For United Hospital Fund member general-care hospitals patient day cost in 1957 amounted to $26.05 (slightly above the reported cost of $25.77 for general hospitals only). The number of patient days involved was 5,597,000.[56]

Alternative computations were made on these bases:

	Amount	Patient Day Cost
1. Operating expenditures	$187,000,000	$33.40
2. All expenditures	199,000,000	35.60
3. All expenditures plus depreciation at 5 percent	209,000,000	37.40

Table 19.8. DISTRIBUTION OF DIRECT DEPARTMENTAL EXPENSES
(IN DOLLARS) FOR INPATIENTS PER PATIENT DAY
BY MAJOR DEPARTMENTAL GROUPING FOR
VOLUNTARY GENERAL-CARE HOSPITALS,
NEW YORK AREA, 1947 AND 1957

| Major Departmental Grouping | 1947 | 1957 | Increase, 1947–57 | | |
			Rate	Amount	Percent Distribution
All departments	15.50	29.51	90	14.01	100.0
Professional	7.29	16.05	120	8.76	62.5
General	5.25	10.93	108	5.68	40.5
Payroll	3.95	8.60	117	4.65	33.2
Other expenses	1.30	2.33	79	1.03	7.3
Special	2.04	5.12	155	3.08	22.0
Payroll	1.38	3.61	161	2.23	15.9
Other expenses	0.66	1.51	129	.85	6.1
Other	8.21	13.46	64	5.25	37.5
Dietary	3.14	3.75	20	0.61	4.4
Housekeeping, laundry, and maintenance	2.97	4.72	59	1.75	12.5
Administrative and general expenses	2.10	4.99	138	2.89	20.6

NOTE: There are 108 hospitals in this sample, of which 101 are voluntary. These hospitals' primary Blue Cross affiliation is with Associated Hospital Service of New York. Each of them cares for public-charge patients and files an annual financial report with the New York State Department of Social Welfare.

SOURCE: Ray E. Trussell and Frank van Dyke, *Prepayment for Hospital Care in New York State* (Albany, N.Y., 1960), p. 142.

20 COMPARISONS WITH OTHER AREAS

There is no simple and easy way to judge the fairness of the existing pattern of financing hospital care in New York City. Reasonable men may differ on what is an equitable distribution of the financial burden among consumers (with or without hospital care insurance), government, and philanthropy. The facts on the existing distribution in New York City do not in themselves convey a judgment. They can, however, contribute to the forming of an informed judgment, if viewed (1) as an historical trend, reflecting the peculiar experience and traditions of this city, and (2) in comparison with similar facts for other localities, where various patterns of financing have been found to be practicable.

In this chapter it will be shown that the pattern of financing hospital care in New York City differs from that in the country as a whole and from patterns prevailing in most large cities in the nation: the relative importance of tax funds is substantially greater here than elsewhere and the relative importance of income from philanthropy is somewhat greater; and, correspondingly, the relative importance of private payments is smaller here than elsewhere. Moreover, the difference between New York City and the nation in the proportion of private payments, which had been narrowing at one time, has widened in recent years.

All comparisons are made for short-term hospitals, with federal hospitals excluded. There are three major reasons for excluding federal hospitals and long-term hospitals. (1) Federal hospitals and state mental hospitals typically draw patients from large geographic areas. Their presence in a city does not mean that the local population has exclusive access to them; conversely, their location outside the city does not mean that the local population is deprived of access to them. (2) Long-term hospitals vary greatly in their range of services and in cost. In addition, more needs to be known about the volume and range of services offered by nursing homes and by infirmary sections of homes for the aged before any conclusions may be drawn from a geographic comparison of long-term institutions listed as hospitals. (3) There are valid technical grounds for excluding federal and long-term hospitals from the nation-wide estimates. For the former there is the problem of classification into short-term and long-term hospitals, with many falling into the latter category by reason of the long average stay of patients in their psychiatric and tuberculosis units. For long-term hospitals under other ownership, methods for allocating total income by source are highly uncertain.[1]

New York City versus United States

The distribution of hospital income by source of payment is available for the United States for the years 1935, 1950, and 1958. The first estimate was prepared by the United States Public Health Service on the basis of data collected by the United States Bureau of the Census; and the second and third estimates were developed for this study on the basis of data on income and expenditures given in the "Guide Issue" of Hospitals[2] and ratios for distributing totals employed by the Social Security Administration of the United States Department of Health, Education, and Welfare (see Appendix 20.A, including Table 20.9).

In fiscal year 1958 civilian short-term hospitals in this country, other than federal, received $4.8 billion. Private payments consti-

Table 20.1. DISTRIBUTION OF INCOME BY SOURCE FOR NON-FEDERAL SHORT-TERM HOSPITALS, UNITED STATES, 1935, 1950, AND 1958 (IN MILLIONS OF DOLLARS)

	1935		1950		1958	
Source of Income	Amount	Percent	Amount	Percent	Amount	Percent
All sources	430	100.0	2,220	100.0	4,782	100.0
Private payments	266	61.9	1,645	74.1	3,867	80.8
Tax funds	105	24.4	440	19.8	715	15.0
Income from philanthropy	59	13.7	135	6.1	200	4.2

SOURCE: Elliott H. Pennell, Joseph W. Mountin, and Kay Person, Business Census of Hospitals, 1935 (Washington, D.C., 1939), p. 24; Appendix 20.A, including Table 20.9.

tuted more than four fifths of the total. Income from philanthropy contributed 4 percent of the total and tax funds the remaining 15 percent.

Private payments rose steadily from 1935 to 1958. During this period tax funds and income from philanthropy increased in amount but declined as a proportion of the total. The decline in the proportion of tax funds was shared almost equally between the periods 1935–50 and 1950–58, whereas the greater part of the decline in the proportion of income from philanthropy was concentrated in the first period.

Table 20.2 shows income by source for the hospitals in New York City in 1934, 1948, and 1957. The data for 1957 do not agree with those presented in Table 12.3. To further comparability between the financial data for New York City and the United States, the income of municipal general-care hospitals has been augmented by the income of tuberculosis and psychiatric units of municipal hospital centers.

Table 20.2. DISTRIBUTION OF INCOME BY SOURCE FOR GENERAL-CARE HOSPITALS, NEW YORK CITY, 1934, 1948, AND 1957 (IN THOUSANDS OF DOLLARS)

	1934		1948		1957	
Source	Amount	Percent	Amount	Percent	Amount	Percent
All sources	54,833	100.0	180,840	100.0	380,590	100.0
Private payments	27,451	50.1	110,184	61.0	203,279	53.4
Tax funds	18,579	33.9	55,099	30.4	139,382	36.7
Philanthropy	8,803	16.0	15,557	8.6	27,185	7.1
Other	0	0	0	0	10,744	2.8

SOURCE: Table 12.3; 1957 was raised by inclusion of certain units of municipal hospital centers, as given in New York City Department of Hospitals, *Statement of Cost of Maintaining and Operating the Department of Hospitals for the Year Ended December 31, 1957* (New York, 1958; mimeographed).

In New York City in 1957 private payments constituted 53 percent of total hospital income. The proportion of income from philanthropy was greater than in the United States—7 percent compared with 4 percent. Far greater is the difference in the proportion of tax funds, with New York City's two and one half times as high—37 percent compared with 15 percent.

Even twenty-five years ago a sizable difference existed between New York City and the United States in the proportion of hospital income met by private payments—50 percent compared with

62 percent. At that time the proportions of income from philanthropy were close, so that the offsetting difference was largely in the proportion of tax funds. By 1948 private payments in New York City had increased to 61 percent of total income. In the nation the increase in the proportion of private payments between 1935 and 1950 was of similar magnitude—12 percentage points. In both areas a large part of the offsetting decline took place in income from philanthropy. By 1957 the proportion of private payments had declined in New York City to 53 percent but continued to rise in the nation. The difference between the two areas was, therefore, much larger than ever before—27 percentage points.

As of 1957–58 the major difference between New York City

Table 20.3. PERCENTAGE DISTRIBUTION OF INCOME OF SHORT-TERM HOSPITALS BY HOSPITAL OWNERSHIP AND SOURCE OF INCOME, NEW YORK CITY AND UNITED STATES, 1957 AND 1958

Source of Income	New York City	United States	Difference
All hospitals			
All sources	100.0	100.0	
Private payments	53.4	80.8	− 27.4
Tax funds	36.7	15.0	+ 21.7
Income from philanthropy	7.1	4.2	+ 2.9
Other	2.8	0	+ 2.8
Voluntary hospitals			
All sources	56.5	74.1	− 17.6
Private payments	41.7	65.5	− 23.8
Tax funds	4.9	4.4	+ 0.5
Income from philanthropy	7.1	4.2	+ 2.9
Other	2.8	0	+ 2.8
State * and local hospitals			
All sources	34.1	20.9	+ 13.2
Private payments	2.5	10.4	− 7.9
Tax funds	31.6	10.5	+ 21.1
Income from philanthropy	0	0	0
Other	0	0	0
Proprietary hospitals			
All sources	9.4	5.0	+ 4.4
Private payments	9.2	4.9	+ 4.3
Tax funds	0.2	0.1	+ 0.1
Income from philanthropy	0	0	0
Other	0	0	0

* There are short-term state hospitals in the United States but not in New York City.
SOURCE: Table 20.9.

and the nation were in the proportions of private payments and of tax funds to total income. Most of the difference in private payments occurred in voluntary hospitals (24 of 27 percentage points) and most of the difference in tax funds occurred in government hospitals (21 of 22 percentage points).

The next largest difference (8 percentage points) is in the proportion of private payments in government hospitals. In the United States many patients in government hospitals pay for their care in full, whereas in New York City relatively few do. The third largest difference (4 percentage points) is in the proportion of private payments in proprietary hospitals. Their role in New York City is almost twice as large as in the nation.

Smaller differences (3 percentage points) occur in income from philanthropy and in "other income" (mostly for research and undergraduate medical education), both of them in voluntary hospitals.

Relations between Government and Voluntary Hospitals in Other Cities

For this study the Hospital Council set out to compare the patterns of financing hospital care for the indigent (recipients of public assistance) and medically indigent (those who normally pay their own way but are unable to finance their medical care) in New York City and in other large cities. In the spring of 1959 a questionnaire was mailed to nineteen large cities that have a hospital council (or hospital association) with permanent staff. They were requested to furnish detailed information on hospital use and finances in their area. Each hospital council also received a completed questionnaire for New York City to serve as a guide. Telephone contact was established before the mailing and was maintained afterwards. The response was gratifying. Despite the pressures of their regular work, seventeen hospital councils or associations returned questionnaires, namely; Baltimore, Boston, Buffalo, Chicago, Cincinnati, Cleveland, Columbus, Detroit, Los Angeles, Philadelphia, Pittsburgh, Rochester, St. Louis, San Francisco, Scranton, Syracuse, Washington D.C.

Gaps in the data were filled in some instances by recourse to the "Guide Issue" of *Hospitals*. The Hospital Council is also indebted to the Research and Statistics Department of the United Community Funds and Councils of America for offering access to unpublished data for a number of cities on the philanthropic income of hospitals in the year 1955. In several instances it was possible to draw on published hospital surveys [3] and on unpublished results of earlier studies.[4] As a result, all seventeen questionnaires were usable for some purposes and fifteen furnished financial data.

CERTIFICATION, RATE OF PAYMENT, AND RELATED POLICIES IN
OTHER LARGE CITIES

A number of questions can be answered from the questionnaire concerning existing relations between government and voluntary hospitals. No attempt is made here to distinguish among the levels of government—state, county, or city—that deal with hospitals.

1. *Does government pay voluntary hospitals in your city for the care of some inpatients?*

The answers for 17 cities are: "Yes"—13; "No"—4. (In 2 of the 13 cities with affirmative replies there is no government hospital.)

The negative answers should be qualified. Two cities pay voluntary hospitals for the care of indigent and medically indigent patients who could not be admitted to the county hospital for lack of a bed; one city pays voluntary hospitals for the care of obstetrical patients; and the fourth city is moving to institute payment to voluntary hospitals, but the method of payment has not yet been determined.

2. *In cities in which voluntary hospitals are paid for the care of some inpatients, what is the basis for computing government's rate of payment?*

Three broad bases are employed by the 13 cities:

Basis of Payment	Number of Cities
Cost of individual voluntary hospital	9
Uniform rate for all voluntary hospitals	3
Cost of local government hospital	1

The uniform rate is, of course, also New York City's method of payment.

Among the 3 cities in which voluntary hospitals receive infrequent payment, 1 pays at the cost of the individual hospital,

1 at the cost of the county hospital, and 1 city's formula was not reported.

Payment in relation to cost does not necessarily mean full cost. The 9 cities in which payment is related to the cost of the individual voluntary hospital pay varying proportions of patient day cost.

Percent of Cost Met	Number of Cities
100	3
92	2
90	2
80	1
75	1

In discussions and letters it was reported that the elements of reimbursable cost—what is allowed and what is excluded—may be as controversial a subject of negotiation between voluntary hospitals and government as is the proportion of total cost met.

In at least 7 of the 9 cities a ceiling governs the rate paid to an individual hospital. For one city there is no information. Another city, which has just changed from a uniform to an individualized rate, does not set a ceiling. Ceilings are calculated in relation to all hospitals in 3 cities and in relation to a hospital's peers in 4. The latter means that hospitals in an area are grouped according to some criterion, say, bed size or scope of educational program. The city that pays voluntary hospitals infrequently but at cost imposes a ceiling that is calculated separately for four classes of hospitals.

In one city the rate paid by government is related to the individual hospital's Blue Cross rate. In another the government rate is computed from data developed in the process of calculating a hospital's Blue Cross rate.

The 3 cities in which hospitals are paid at a uniform rate are located in the same state. Here the government program is that of state aid, rather than of purchase of care. Varying with the prevailing level of hospital cost in a city, the daily payment by government is approximately 40 to 50 percent of average patient day cost.

The hospital council located in the city in which payment to voluntary hospitals is related to the cost of operating the municipal hospital points out that such cost may be unfairly low. One reason is failure to allow for services contributed to the municipal hospital by other agencies of government. Another reason is inclusion in the cost calculation of long-term facilities, which operate at lower cost than general-care hospital units.

3. *Does government pay voluntary hospitals in your city for the care of outpatients?*

The first—simple—answers are: "Yes"—10; "No"—7. The number of negative answers is larger than for inpatients. The affirmative answers cover, however, a wide range, from payment for all visits by indigent and medically indigent persons to payment limited to visits by recipients of public assistance, to payment of token lump sums unrelated to the volume of care rendered. A more realistic set of answers would be:

Pay for Outpatient Care	Number of Cities
Yes, unqualified	3
Yes, for indigents only	4
Yes, small sums	3
No	7

In 3 cities the community chest plays a major role in paying voluntary hospitals for care to outpatients.

4. *In cities in which government pays voluntary hospitals for outpatient care, what is the basis of payment?*

The 10 cities which make some payment are distributed as follows:

Basis of Payment	Number of Cities
Individual hospital visit rate	0
Uniform visit rate for all hospitals	8
Lump sum payment	2

The 8 uniform rates show a wide range:

Rate per Visit (in Dollars)	Number of Cities
1.50	2
2.00	1
2.50	1
3.00	1
3.01–4.00	1
4.01–5.00	1
6.00	1

Sometimes the visit rate is negotiated between hospitals and government, and sometimes it is promulgated by government. When negotiated, the cost of service may or may not be taken into account.

The impact of government's failure to pay for outpatient care is sometimes cushioned by a reduction in the amount deducted as the cost of outpatient care when the inpatient rate is calculated. Such cushioning is partial, since the higher rate for inpatients applies only to that fraction of patient days paid for by government.

5. *Does the government hospital in your city care for private patients?*

An important issue in the relations between government and voluntary hospitals is whether a short-term hospital operated by government should care for all classes of patients, including patients able to pay the hospital and physician. Two of the 17 cities have no government hospital. The distribution of the other 15 by their policies on admitting private patients to government hospitals follows:

Admit Private Patients	*Number of Cities*
No	10
Yes	2
Yes and No	3

A city for which the answer is given as "Yes" and "No" has two or more government hospitals. One city reports a university hospital owned by the state (Yes) and a city hospital (No); one reports a university hospital (Yes), suburban community hospitals owned by local units of government (Yes), and a metropolitan county hospital (No); and one reports a suburban community hospital (Yes) and a city hospital (No). Of the two instances in which the answer is "Yes," one is a state university hospital. The other is a community hospital that the state has continued to operate for historical reasons; here an effort is being made to transfer the institution to voluntary ownership.

On the other hand, in two of the cities in which government hospitals do not now admit private patients, the policy is being reviewed. In one the hospital council has recently recommended that the city hospital plan to admit private patients, in order to use the plant with greater flexibility.[5] Further qualifications to the answer "No" are in order. In several instances it is reported that the local government hospital accepts all patients with acute communicable disease, regardless of income. In one city municipal employees injured on the job receive care in the government hospital.

It is evident that, with the exception of university hospitals, the prevailing pattern in the large cities covered by this survey is to limit government hospitals to the care of the indigent and medically indigent.

6. *On what basis does the community chest in your city allocate funds to hospitals?*

The United Community Funds and Councils reports a doubling between 1950 and 1958 in the amount of money distributed to hospitals and clinics by community chests and united funds.[6] In part, the increase in centrally raised funds is a substitute for moneys that previously were contributed directly to hospitals.

The role of the community chest or united fund in financing hospital care is usually supplementary to that of tax funds and private payments. Occasionally it may serve as a replacement for tax funds. The basis for allocating available moneys to hospitals may be the relative size of deficit, volume of free care rendered, or the purchase of specified services. All of these methods are in use, as well as others that cannot be readily classified. Three of the 17 questionnaires had no information on this score.

The distribution of 14 cities according to the basis employed by community chests to allocate funds to hospitals follows:

Basis of Allocation	Number of Cities
Deficit financing	2
Volume of free care	7
Simple formula	4
Refined formula	3
Purchase of care	4
For outpatients	3
For inpatients	1
Other (negotiated)	1

Where the free-care formula is refined, it contains two or more elements. In one city three fourths of the moneys contributed by the community chest to hospitals are distributed in accordance with their respective shares of the total volume of free care rendered, and one fourth in a manner that gives weight to the amount of free care a hospital renders in relation to its own total volume of care.

SOURCES OF HOSPITAL INCOME

In a study of hospital care in New York State in 1948 it was found that general-care hospitals in New York City had a higher proportion of income from tax funds and from philanthropy than those in other large cities in the state.

Table 20.4. PROPORTION (PERCENT) OF TAX FUNDS AND INCOME FROM PHILANTHROPY TO TOTAL FOR GENERAL HOSPITAL CARE IN SELECTED LARGE CITIES IN NEW YORK STATE, 1948

City	Tax Funds	Income from Philanthropy
New York City	25.5	8.9
Buffalo	15.2	2.7
Rochester	13.5	3.6
Syracuse	12.4	2.4
Albany	8.6	3.7

SOURCE: Eli Ginzberg, A Pattern for Hospital Care (New York, 1949), p. 160.

The proportions for New York City differ slightly from those shown in Table 20.2, above, because payments for psychiatric and tuberculosis patients in general hospitals are excluded here.

For 1957–58 questionnaires provide financial data for 15 large cities in the nation. In some the data refer to hospitals within city limits, whereas in others they pertain to a metropolitan area. This introduces an element of incomparability that was aggravated by other intercity differences, including patient day cost, hospital use per capita, the proportion of nonresidents using local hospitals, and the pay status of nonresident patients.

Accordingly, it was deemed best to present the analysis of sources of hospital income in terms of percentages, that is, the percentage of income from philanthropy to total, of tax funds, and of private payments. Table 20.5 lists the cities by code letter and shows for each the distribution of hospital income by source. Since it was thought that the pattern of financing hospital care may vary geographically, the 15 cities were classified into two groups: East and West. East embraces all cities in states touching on the Atlantic Ocean.

Table 20.5. PERCENTAGE DISTRIBUTION OF INCOME BY SOURCE
FOR SHORT-TERM HOSPITALS IN FIFTEEN LARGE
CITIES CLASSIFIED BY REGION AND IN
NEW YORK CITY, 1957–58

City	Income from Philanthropy	Tax Funds	Private Payments
East Coast			
A	2.0	27.2	70.8
B	1.7	28.5	69.8
C	1.8	9.3	88.9
D	1.8	13.3	84.9
E	2.8	4.4	92.8
F	3.6	14.3	82.1
G	4.5	20.8	74.7
H	7.2	17.9	74.9
All cities in region	4.3	16.7	79.0
Midwest and Far West			
I	1.3	15.8	82.9
J	2.5	22.7	74.8
K	3.1	18.2	78.7
L	3.4	11.5	85.1
M	3.7	17.3	79.0
N	4.9	12.2	82.9
O	1.8	19.5	78.7
All cities in region	2.8	18.0	79.2
All cities in nation	3.4	17.5	79.1
New York City *	7.6	33.0	56.5

* In addition, 2.9 percent in "other income," not traced to source, for medical education and research.
SOURCE: Hospital Council of Greater New York, inter city Survey.

Table 20.5 shows:

1. The proportion of income from philanthropy, 3.4 percent, is lower than the 4.2 percent estimated for the nation in Table 20.1. The latter includes the value of donated services of Sisters and probably includes some contributions and investment income for designated purposes. Table 20.5 may reflect a downward bias in investment income for general purposes, since several of the cities reported that sizable amounts of income from philanthropy accrue to a small number of hospitals but did not give a figure.

2. There is an interregional difference of 1.5 percentage points in income from philanthropy, with the East Coast showing the higher figure.

3. The proportion of income from tax funds, 17.5 percent, is above the 15 percent estimated for the nation in Table 20.1. Hospitals in large cities may receive a higher proportion of support from this source than hospitals in other urban and rural areas.

4. The interregional difference in tax funds is the same as in income from philanthropy, with the East Coast's figure lower. The two cities with the lowest proportions of income from tax funds (C and E) do not have a government hospital.

5. There is no difference between the regions in the proportion of private payments.

6. The important differences in sources of income are not between regions but within them. The range of variation is greater among the cities in the East.

7. For each source of income New York City, which ranks third among the 16 cities in per capita income, falls oustide the range of variation shown by the 15 large cities.

Source of Income	Percent of Source to Total Income	
	Range (15 Cities)	New York City
Income from philanthropy	1–7	8
Tax funds	4–28	33
Private payments	70–93	56

ANALYSIS OF CORRELATIONS

The above findings raise certain questions that can be examined by statistical methods.

1. Is the proportion of income from philanthropy high where the proportion of tax funds to total hospital income is high, or does the one tend to offset the other? A direct correlation would support the notion that income from philanthropy and tax funds meet the same type of need and are perhaps fed by the same springs. An inverse correlation would be consistent with the view that one source fills the gap left by the other.

2. In the absence of a government hospital the proportion of

tax funds to total hospital income in the community is low. Is there a tendency for the proportion of tax funds to be high where a large share of tax funds is spent in government hospitals? A direct correlation would be consistent with the view that government hospitals are not effective collectors of revenue from patients. An inverse correlation would be consistent with the view that the availability of tax funds to voluntary hospitals may diminish their collection effort.

3. Fourteen of the cities submitted estimates of the proportion of population enrolled by hospital-care insurance plans. Does the proportion of private payments vary directly with the percentage of the population insured?

Relationship between Philanthropy and Tax Funds. Table 20.6 shows a distribution of the 15 cities by two variables. Along the vertical axis is the proportion of income from philanthropy and along the horizontal axis, the proportion of tax funds. What would be significant is the presence of a clearly discernible linear or curvilinear pattern and its direction or slope. Departures from the theoretical line of best fit—scatter—are always to be expected. The question is whether the departures are so many as to suggest the absence of such a line; if so, there is no correlation. A line sloping downward to the right would represent a positive correlation, and a line sloping upward to the right would represent an inverse correlation.

Table 20.6. JOINT DISTRIBUTION OF FIFTEEN LARGE CITIES BY
PROPORTION OF INCOME FROM PHILANTHROPY
AND BY PROPORTION OF TAX FUNDS TO
TOTAL HOSPITAL INCOME, 1957–58

Percent Phi-lanthropy to Total Income	*Percent Tax Funds to Total Income*				
	Total	*0–9.9*	*10.0–14.9*	*15.0–19.9*	*20.0–29.9*
All cities	15	2	4	5	4
1.0–1.9	5	1	1	2	1
2.0–2.9	3	1	0	0	2
3.0–3.9	4	0	2	2	0
4.0 and over	3	0	1	1	1

SOURCE: Table 20.5.

The scatter in Table 20.6 is so random as to reveal no association, either positive or inverse, between the proportion of income from philanthropy and the proportion of tax funds. Whatever the relationship may be in a given city, it is the result of local traditions and practices.

Relationship between Tax Funds and Expenditures in Government Hospitals. Table 20.7 distributes the 13 cities with government hospitals by the proportion of tax funds to total income (vertical axis) and the proportion of such funds spent in government hospitals (horizontal axis).

Table 20.7. JOINT DISTRIBUTION OF THIRTEEN CITIES BY PROPORTION OF TAX FUNDS TO HOSPITAL INCOME AND BY PROPORTION OF SUCH INCOME SPENT IN GOVERNMENT HOSPITALS, 1957–58

Percent Tax Funds to Total Income	*Percent Tax Funds Spent in Government Hospitals*				
	Total	60.0–69.9	70.0–79.9	80.0–89.9	90.0–99.9
All cities	13	3	3	4	3
10.0–14.9	4	2	1	0	1
15.0–19.9	5	0	1	3	1
20.0–24.9	2	1	0	0	1
25.0–29.9	2	0	1	1	0

SOURCE: Hospital Council of Greater New York, inter city survey.

There is no evidence of correlation in Table 20.7. The data suggest that it is possible for a city's hospital system to derive a moderate proportion of income from tax funds, if government does not pay a great deal of money to voluntary hospitals. It is also possible to have a moderate proportion of tax funds to total hospital income if government pays substantial amounts of money to voluntary hospitals. Finally, it is possible to have a high proportion of tax funds to total hospital income whether government pays little or much money to voluntary hospitals.

Relationship between Private Payments and Hospital Care Insurance. In general, one might expect that the higher the percentage of the population that is insured, the higher would be the proportion of private payments to total hospital income. This has not been the experience in New York City over the years. The proportion of tax funds rose during a period (1948–57) when the proportion of the population with hospital care insurance also rose.

Table 20.8. JOINT DISTRIBUTION OF THIRTEEN CITIES BY PRO-
PORTION OF PRIVATE PAYMENTS TO HOSPITAL
INCOME, 1957–58, AND BY PROPORTION OF POPULA-
TION INSURED FOR HOSPITAL CARE, 1959

Percent Private Payments to Total Income	*Percent of Population Insured*				
	Total	*50–59*	*60–69*	*70–79*	*80–89*
All cities	13	1	3	5	4
70–74	2	0	1	1	0
75–79	4	0	1	1	2
80–84	3	1	1	1	0
85–89	3	0	0	2	1
90–94	1	0	0	0	1

SOURCE: Hospital Council of Greater New York, inter city survey.

There is no evidence of correlation in Table 20.8. Once again, local factors seem to exercise a predominant influence.

Summary

1. The differences between New York City and the nation in sources of hospital income, which were always sizable, have widened in the past decade. The proportion of private payments to total income has declined in New York City, while increasing in the United States; the proportion of tax funds has followed the opposite course in both areas; and the proportion of income from philanthropy has declined at a lower rate in New York City than in the nation.

2. Most of the difference in the proportion of tax funds is accounted for by (a) the greater importance of government hospitals in New York City than in the United States and (b) the even greater difference in the proportion of tax funds to income in government hospitals.

3. New York City is unique in having both high proportions of hospital income from tax funds and from philanthropy and a low proportion of private payments.

4. Beyond this, the analysis of fifteen other large cities may be summarized as follows:

(a) It fails to show regional differences in the role of private payments. Differences within a region are greater than those between regions.

(*b*) The relationship in a city between the proportion of income from philanthropy and the proportion of tax funds appears to be random.

(*c*) In the absence of a government hospital, tax funds constitute a small proportion of hospital income. In the presence of a government hospital, tax funds can be moderate or large. Restrictions on the use of voluntary hospitals (and of payment to them) do not insure a low proportion of tax funds to total hospital income.

5. Contrary to expectations, there is no clear, direct correlation between the proportion of private payments in a city and the proportion of its population enrolled in hospital care insurance plans. This finding is consistent with the experience of New York City over the years.

6. The policies and practices of fifteen other large cities in this country in certifying and paying for public charge patients are as follows:

(*a*) There are two cities without a government hospital. In both instances government pays voluntary hospitals for the care of indigent and medically indigent inpatients.

(*b*) Government also pays voluntary hospitals for the care of inpatients in 11 of the other 15 cities.

(*c*) In 9 of the 13 cities where voluntary hospitals are paid, the rate of payment is related to the cost of the individual voluntary hospital. The proportion of cost met ranges between 75 and 100 percent.

(*d*) In 7 of the 9 cities with individualized rates of payment a ceiling is imposed on the rate paid to a hospital.

(*e*) Payment by government to voluntary hospitals is less common for the care of outpatients. Of 17 cities reporting, 7 pay nothing, 3 pay small sums, 4 pay only for public assistance recipients, and only 3 pay for medically indigent patients as well.

(*f*) Where payment for outpatient care exists, it tends to take the form of a uniform rate per visit. There is a wide range—from $1.50 to $6.00 per visit.

(*g*) Government hospitals in large cities, except for university hospitals, do not admit and care for private patients.

Appendix 20.A

ESTIMATES OF INCOME BY SOURCE FOR NON-
FEDERAL SHORT-TERM HOSPITALS, UNITED
STATES, 1950 AND 1958

Estimates derived by distributing totals through the application of
ratios leave much to be desired. The ratios derived in one year may
not apply several years hence. Nor are the totals themselves beyond
question.

For this report an attempt was made to develop a set of estimates
on hospital income in the United States for a recent year that would
permit a cross classification of source of income by hospital ownership
and by type of hospital. Such a table has the virtue of completeness;
it also permits checks for internal consistency. The data for 1958 were
derived in this manner.

For the estimates developed for 1950 the procedure was not nearly
so refined. Here the goal was to obtain as expeditiously as possible a
distribution of hospital income by source for some year intermediate
between 1935 and 1958. For 1950 there exist sufficient data in accessible form to permit the development of an approximate set of figures.

CALENDAR YEAR 1950

1. The income of short-term hospitals is based on data in the "Guide
Issue" of *Hospitals,* with calendar year 1950 representing the average
of fiscal years 1950 and 1951. For voluntary and proprietary hospitals
total income was taken; and for government hospitals expenditures
were taken.

2. Payments from tax funds were derived as follows:

(*a*) Total expenditures of state and local governments for hospitals are given in a report by the President's Commission on the
Health Needs of the Nation.[7]

(*b*) From this figure, expenditures for construction were subtracted.[8]

(*c*) In addition, expenditures for long-term hospital care were
subtracted. Total expenditures of governmental long-term hospitals
are given in the "Guide Issue" of *Hospitals.* This figure is reduced by
private payments to these hospitals (8.5 percent of income) and raised
by government payments to long-term hospitals under voluntary and
proprietary ownership (25 percent of income). The several ratios for
allocating given totals between public and private payments were
either furnished the Hospital Council by the Social Security Administration,[9] which employs them in estimating private expenditures for
hospital care in the United States, or are derived from its estimates.[10]

3. Income from philanthropy is based on data prepared by the Social Security Administration, reduced both for health activities outside the hospital and for philanthropic contributions to long term hospitals. For basic data see Thomas Karter in the *Social Security Bulletin*.[11] Cognizance was taken of the amount estimated for 1958, below.

4. Private payments are equal to total income less tax funds and less income from philanthropy.

FISCAL YEAR 1958

1. Total hospital income is taken from the "Guide Issue" of *Hospitals* for 1959, in the same manner as in paragraph 1 above. The distribution of income by source was determined in another way, however, with a separate distribution prepared for each hospital ownership group.

2. Voluntary hospitals.

(a) Income from tax funds. Income from patients was first converted into billings, by taking account of billings not collected. The proportion of billings to government was applied to total estimated billings and the result was treated as income from government.

(b) Philanthropy. This was the most difficult area, and several methods were employed. Method 1: Other operating income was subtracted from nonpatient income. When the former was set at 2 percent of income from patients (somewhat lower than for proprietary hospitals), the estimate for philanthropy was $196 million. Method 2: Philanthropic contributions were estimated at 4 percent of income;[12] investment income was estimated at a 4 percent return on two thirds of the non-plant assets of these hospitals;[13] and an allowance was made for the donated services of Sisters; the result was an estimate of $206 million. Method 3: Another set of figures[14] yielded a projected value of $230 million, inclusive of long-term hospitals. Method 4: A comparison was made with the findings of the Hospital Council's survey of large cities. The figure of $200 is midway between the results of Methods 1 and 2; it is above the results of Method 4 and below those of Method 3.

(c) Private payments. This is the difference between total income and the sum of income from tax funds and from philanthropy.

3. State and local hospitals. Private payments have been, and still are, estimated by the Social Security Administration at 58 percent of total income. This was arbitrarily reduced to 50 percent, on the ground that it is more consistent with (a) the estimate for 1950, derived independently, (b) with the results of the Hospital Council's survey of large cities, and (c) with the known revenue sources of some government hospitals, which tend to treat and report the purchase of

services by certain agencies of government as no different from purchases by patients. The difference between total income and private payments is income from tax funds.

4. Proprietary hospitals. There is a small item of income from tax funds in behalf of services rendered to patients. This was set at 2 percent, based on the Survey of Hospital Rates in 1955.[15] All other income is attributed to private payments.

Table 20.9. INCOME OF SHORT-TERM HOSPITALS BY SOURCE OF INCOME AND HOSPITAL OWNERSHIP, NEW YORK CITY AND UNITED STATES, 1957 AND 1958

Source of Income	New York City (in Thousands of Dollars)	United States (in Millions of Dollars)
All hospitals		
All income	380,590	4,782
Private payments	203,279	3,867
Tax funds	139,382	715
Income from philanthropy	27,185	200
Other	10,744	0
Voluntary hospitals		
All income	215,009	3,538
Private payments	158,722	3,130
Tax funds	18,483	208
Income from philanthropy	27,060	200
Other	10,744	0
Government hospitals		
All income	130,031	1,003
Private payments	9,631	501
Tax funds	120,275	502
Income from philanthropy	125	0
Other	0	0
Proprietary hospitals		
All income	35,550	241
Private payments	34,926	236
Tax funds	624	5
Income from philanthropy	0	0
Other	0	0

SOURCE: Hospital Council of Greater New York.

21 A PATTERN FOR FINANCING HOSPITAL CARE IN NEW YORK CITY

It is appropriate to conclude the analysis of hospital finances in New York City with a discussion of policy recommendations and possible implementing mechanisms. There is a need for interim, as well as long-range, adjustments, for deep-seated historical patterns cannot be changed overnight.

Background for Proposals

It is worth stating that drastic changes in policies are not justifiable if they merely promise modest improvements upon the existing pattern. Rather, they should promise important improvements upon the pattern likely to exist in the foreseeable future. Moreover, the proposed new pattern should be sufficiently superior to offset the costs attached to change. Costs of change are not exclusively monetary, and it is often difficult to determine whether the net advantages of change outweigh possible disadvantages. One way to cope with these difficulties is to try to spell out the considerations that enter into the analysis of alternative proposals.

REASONS FOR PROPOSING MAJOR CHANGES

Why is it appropriate at this time to contemplate major changes in the pattern for financing hospital care?

The financial position of voluntary hospitals in New York City has deteriorated in recent years to the point where several are incurring deficits of a size they cannot afford (see Chapter 14). This development antedates the large increases in hospital cost that are currently taking place and are likely to continue (see Chapter 19).

In the municipal system the proportion of income from private payments is low. More than 90 percent of the income of municipal general-care hospitals still derives from tax funds (see Chapter 15).

With tax funds constituting two fifths of the income of all hospitals in New York City and one third of the income of its general-care hospitals (see Chapter 12), there rests a heavy residual responsibility on local funds. The role of federal funds in financing hospital care has been negligible; and, although the amount of State aid has increased, the proportion of such moneys to total tax funds is still low (see Chapter 16).

Compared with fifteen other large cities surveyed during this study, the proportion of private payments to total income of general-care hospitals is by far lowest in New York City (see Chapter 20). Yet New York City ranks third among the sixteen cities in the ability of residents to pay for hospital care, as measured by per capita income. The proportion of private payments in New York City hospitals is also low in comparison with the nation as a whole. Furthermore, whereas the proportion of private payments has been rising in the United States, it has declined in New York City. These comparisons suggest that (1) the pattern of financing hospital care in New York City differs significantly from that in other cities and (2) the local pattern is not attributable to lack of ability on the part of New York City's residents to pay for hospital care. There is leeway to change the pattern for financing hospital care in New York City, if that is desired.

Voluntary hospitals in New York City have a higher proportion of income from philanthropy than do hospitals in other cities (see Chapter 20). Here income from philanthropy kept up much better with rising hospital cost in the period 1948–57 than in the earlier period, 1934–48 (see Chapter 13). Availability of such income for the support of free care tends to be limited, however, by an increasing tendency to earmark gifts and by the continued concentration of certain types of contribution and investment income among a few hospitals (see Chapter 18).

Some trustees of voluntary hospitals believe that income from philanthropy should continue to play a part in financing the care of patients unable to pay for it. Important as medical education and medical research are, they should not become the sole objects of philanthropic support, to the exclusion of care of patients. In New York City income from philanthropy is relatively large and can play a useful role in all three areas.

PRESERVATION OF TRADITIONAL VALUES

An important objective is to preserve the worth-while characteristics of the existing pattern. Thus, a high value may be attached to the tradition of partnership between voluntary and municipal hospitals in caring for the sick poor. In recent years a shift has occurred from voluntary to municipal hospitals in the distribution of general-care ward, outpatient department, and emergency department patients (see Chapter 2). If these trends persist, the partnership pattern of caring for the sick poor will be weakened and perhaps endangered.

The partnership policy presupposes that a patient would receive equally good care in either hospital system. Historically the Hospital Council of Greater New York has distinguished among hospitals in range of services and scope of educational program but not in quality of care.

Owing to certain developments in the past generation, which have been accentuated during the postwar period, some municipal hospitals are experiencing increasing difficulty in staffing their facilities and, therefore, in providing care of good quality. It is shown in this report that municipal hospitals not affiliated with medical schools have been unable to attract graduates of American medical schools as interns and residents, a weakness they share with a large number of voluntary hospitals (see Chapter 6). Most of the same municipal hospitals face an attrition in visiting staff that may be irreversible (see Chapter 5). Staffing of the nursing service is weak throughout the municipal system and in many voluntary hospitals (see Chapter 7). Finally, the quality of top management is declining in the municipal system (see Chapter 9).

With the expansion of formal programs of medical education, the availability of patients for clinical teaching has assumed increasing importance. Although private and semiprivate patients can be—and are—used for teaching, they seldom serve as the nucleus of a teaching program unless the medical staff of the hospital functions as an organized medical group. Special difficulties arise in training surgical residents and in entrusting ultimate responsibility to a chief resident in medicine (see Chapter 6). Ultimately, if ward or service patients did not exist, some solution would have to be found. It is by no means true, however, that a solution is here or imminent. As long as there are ward patients in sizable numbers in New York City, medical education and training must be centered around them.

In the absence of a change in the pattern for financing hospital care on a national scale, it is not unreasonable to expect that private payments should constitute a higher proportion of hospital income in New York City than they currently do. Benefits from voluntary health insurance plans are, of course, included under private payments.

In short, the following goals seem important: (1) perpetuating the tradition of partnership between voluntary and municipal hospitals in caring for the sick poor; (2) providing equally good care in each hospital system; and (3) making the utmost use of ward patients for teaching purposes, while also exerting efforts to use more private and semiprivate patients for this purpose. In the distribution of hospital income by source, the objectives are: (1) to increase the proportion of private payments to total hospital income; (2) to share the remainder between philanthropy and tax funds in equitable fashion; and (3) to avoid undue reliance on local tax funds. At the same time efforts must continue to obtain a good return for every dollar spent on hospital care, regardless of whose dollar it is.

FINANCIAL PROPOSALS

It is easier to state the broad objectives of a sound pattern for financing hospital care in New York City than to give the means of achieving them. In the course of this study many suggestions for improving hospital care were explored, among them proposals with important financial implications. A number of such proposals are discussed below.

To Limit Certification of Public Charges in Voluntary Hospitals to Emergency Admissions. Criteria for certifying patients as public charges in voluntary hospitals are the same as in municipal hospitals (see Chapter 16). Since many patients who were not emergencies at the time of admission are approved as public charges, the certification policy may be called a liberal one. The daily rate paid by the City is, however, below patient day cost in most voluntary hospitals, as well as below average cost in its own hospitals. This may be called a conservative policy. The combined effect of the two policies on the income of voluntary hospitals in New York City is more favorable than the combined effect of certification and rate policies pursued by adjacent suburban counties, which pay a higher daily rate in behalf of a small number of patients.

Nevertheless, once a patient is certified as a public charge, the voluntary hospital is precluded from earning for his care anything above the City's payment. If the daily rate for public-charge patients is below a hospital's average cost, the latter's financial viability depends on access to earnings from other patients and on income from philanthropy.

Conceivably a voluntary hospital might enjoy greater flexibility in financing if the daily rate approached average cost, even if the number of patients paid for were reduced by limiting certification to emergency admissions. This combination of policies would, however, signify a retrogression in the relations between government and voluntary hospitals in New York City, since it would signify an intention to concentrate the sick poor in municipal hospitals. Only a few voluntary hospitals could then afford to care for patients unable to pay for hospital care but denied certification as public charges.

To Concentrate Care for the Sick Poor in Municipal Hospitals. A more extreme variant of the above proposal is to provide all (or almost all) hospital care for the sick poor in municipal hospitals. There would then be little concern over the daily rate the City pays to voluntary hospitals.

This proposal has a number of defects. They include: violation of the tradition of partnership between voluntary and municipal hospitals; additional outlays for capital purposes to expand municipal hospitals; imposing additional responsibilities on a hospital system that is already hard pressed; probable weakening of voluntary hospitals as teaching institutions; operation of voluntary hospitals at a reduced rate of occupancy, at least during the period of transition; and heavy, perhaps increasing, reliance on tax funds—in this case, mostly local tax funds—to finance hospital care. Each of these consequences would be a backward step.

To Affiliate Municipal Hospitals with Medical Schools or Major Voluntary Hospitals. This proposal is essentially not a financial one but has financial implications in two respects. In the first place, since it calls on a medical school or a major voluntary hospital to assume responsibility for medical staffing and medical education in one or more services of a municipal hospital currently without university affiliation, it implies increased expenditures to strengthen the laboratory, x-ray, and other ancillary services of the hospital. Such additional expenditures should, of course, rest on the City of New York and not on the voluntary institution offering to help. In the second place, affiliation between physically distant institutions is usually regarded as an interim arrangement, pending relocation of the municipal hospital on the campus of the voluntary hospital. Ultimately, it implies a different, more basic, set of financial questions, discussed elsewhere (see Chapter 11).

To Establish Private Services in Municipal Hospitals. Under this proposal, which may or may not be coupled with the first or the one that follows, certain municipal hospitals would set aside a number of beds to which members of the attending staff might admit private and semiprivate patients. The justification is that members of the attending staff would be enabled to spend more time at municipal hospitals if they did not have to go elsewhere to care for their private and semiprivate patients. Furthermore, it is claimed, the City treasury would receive additional revenues. This proposal is discussed in another chapter (see Chapter 11). Suffice it to state here that private payments to the City Treasury are likely to fall short of the additional expenditures for the care of private and semiprivate patients.

To Set the City's Daily Rate of Payment to Voluntary Hospitals at the Average Cost of Municipal Hospitals or in Relation to Such Cost. With income from tax funds playing a significant but varied role in the income of voluntary hospitals in New York City, a uniform rate of payment is no longer tenable. In the most recent appeal by the trustees of voluntary hospitals for higher payments in behalf of public charges, it was suggested that the City pay the hospitals at a rate related to the average patient day cost of the municipal system. There would be different rates—100, 90, and 80 percent of the cost figure—assigned to classes of hospitals, in accordance with the amount of community service rendered and the scope of teaching program.[1]

This method of payment by government is not sufficiently geared to meet the revenue needs of the individual hospital, and these should be met if the hospital is rendering essential community services at economical cost. To be of maximum value to hospitals with a high proportion of public-charge patients, the criteria for classifying hospitals would have to be closely related to cost and the number of hospital classes would have to be large. There is, moreover, reason to believe that a misapprehension may exist as to the prevailing level of patient day cost in municipal hospitals in comparison with voluntary hospitals (see Chapter 19).

To Establish Dual Rates of Payment. Under this proposal the City might pay voluntary hospitals a higher rate for indigent than for medically indigent patients. It could be argued that the City can afford to pay more for the former, since its expenditures in behalf of indigent patients are reimbursed by the State, whereas expenditures in behalf of the medically indigent are not. Furthermore, if the City's rate for medically indigent patients were somewhat lower, it might be less likely to embark on a strict certification policy in voluntary hospitals at times of financial stringency or in the event of a large decline in the occupancy rate in municipal hospitals.

The principal, and conclusive, disadvantage of this proposal is that at the prevailing ratio of medically indigent to indigent patient days reimbursed by the City (3 to 1), any appreciable difference between the two rates would be too costly for the voluntary hospitals to absorb (see Chapter 16).

To Offset the Value of Tax Exemptions. Under this proposal the City would, in calculating its payments to voluntary hospitals, take cognizance of the value of the exemptions from the real estate tax and the water charge. The value of the exemptions might be treated as an initial payment in behalf of public charges.

For all voluntary hospitals in New York City the value of the two exemptions is estimated at $11.6 million—$11 million for the real estate tax and $0.6 million for the water charge.

For the member general hospitals of the United Hospital Fund the value of the real estate tax exemption in 1958 is estimated at $8.5 million and the value of the exemption from the water charge at $0.5 million (see Appendix 19.B). The computed value of the free care rendered by these hospitals is $20.0 million—$12.5 million for inpatients and $7.5 for outpatients.

Upon reflection, it is clear that hospitals with public-charge and other ward patients are in no position to apply the tax exemptions against the cost of care rendered to such patients, as long as voluntary hospitals without corresponding responsibilities also enjoy tax exemptions. To do so would mean a higher level of charges to private and semiprivate patients in hospitals with public charges than in hospitals without them.

Proposed Relationships

The following pattern of financing is intended to reflect the objectives of a sound program as previously outlined. It is derived from elements of the preceding proposals and from the experience of other cities.

BASIC PATTERN

The desirable combination of policies is an adequate daily rate of payment to voluntary hospitals coupled with uniform criteria in the two hospital systems for certifying patients as public charges. It is recognized that such a combination of policies would entail larger expenditures by the City.

For inpatient care the relations between the City and voluntary hospitals might take the following form.

1. The City's liability to a hospital would be, as now, the product of the daily rate of payment and the number of days of care rendered to public charges. A contractual arrangement for the sale of specified services to the City by a voluntary hospital or medical school would constitute an exception.

2. The daily rate would be set to approximate cost in the individual voluntary hospital. The preferred way of doing this

would be for the City to become a party to the joint rate-making mechanism established by the hospitals in this area and Associated Hospital Service. The new formula recognizes that a patient day on the ward represents a lower revenue potential than a patient day on the semiprivate or private service.

3. The number of days paid for would be determined, as now, by criteria for financial eligibility applied uniformly to patients in voluntary and in municipal hospitals. An infant born to a mother who is a public charge would be counted as an appropriate fraction (one fourth or one third) of the adult patient day.

4. Voluntary hospitals would be less selective than formerly in admitting patients and would refrain from referring or transferring to municipal hospitals patients in need of hospital care merely because they are expected to have a prolonged stay. It is recognized that related facilities in ample supply and of good quality would be required (see Chapter 3).

5. The City would discontinue one of its present practices, under which it sometimes fails to pay for all the days of care incurred by a public-charge patient. This can happen when a patient is accepted as a public charge in the course of his hospital stay, rather than at the beginning. The rule is that the City deducts from its payments any sum that the hospital may have received from or in behalf of the patient that exceeds the amount computed by applying the City's daily rate to the patient's entire stay. (Realistic safeguards may, however, be indicated.)

Some of the reasoning underlying the proposed pattern follows.

It is no longer tenable for the City to pay voluntary hospitals at a uniform daily rate. With hospital cost so high today and still rising, a large number of voluntary hospitals lack the supplementary resources to help them finance the care of public-charge patients.

The experience of the local Blue Cross plan is ample precedent for a shift by a major purchaser of hospital care from a uniform rate to individual hospital rates, when its payments to hospitals become large and increasingly important (see Chapter 17). In other large cities government has shifted to individual hospital rates, subject to a ceiling for each class of hospitals (see Chapter 20).

A further advantage of the proposed pattern, it is believed, is that the calculation of hospital rates for one large group of patients would become closely related to the calculation of rates for another large group of patients. The total revenue requirements of the hospital would receive due consideration, and the usual difficulties attached to allocating cost among private, semiprivate, and ward accommodations would be avoided.

Application of uniform criteria of certification to patients in both hospital systems means that the City could not unilaterally decide to restrict payments to emergency admissions when it chose to do so. There is no implication here that the uniform criteria for determining medical indigency should be liberal. Ultimately, the type of certification policy followed in this city will depend on the attitude of the community, on its wishes concerning the future role of local tax funds in financing hospital care, and on the degree of success achieved in devising practicable mechanisms for altering the prevailing pattern of financing hospital care. An important fact of which the public must be made aware is the much lower proportion of private payments in New York City than in the nation or in other large cities and the much higher proportion of tax funds.

To a voluntary hospital that demonstrably has no resources to contribute toward financing free care, the sum paid by the City must be no less than the liability computed by multiplying the daily rate by the number of public-charge patient days.

Where a hospital can make a contribution to free care, it might be afforded an opportunity to do so. It has been suggested that in these instances hospitals may choose to make a stated contribution toward the cost of free care, thereby reducing the role of tax funds. It seems reasonable to anticipate that the community would respond with generosity to appeals for funds to help defray the cost of free care in the hospital. If this proved to be the case, the traditional relationship of partnership between tax funds and income from philanthropy in financing free care in New York City would be reaffirmed and strengthened. A major difference between the suggested relationship and the present one is that the contribution of each party would be made more explicit, with the financial contribution of each voluntary hospital set annually in advance.

An obvious criticism of this suggestion is that it may not be realistic to expect an individual hospital to make a voluntary contribution of appreciable size to help finance the care of public charges, for whom the City is otherwise prepared to assume financial responsibility. Nor is it apparent how the amount of such a contribution might be determined.

Under the formula recently negotiated between the local hospitals and Associated Hospital Service, the deduction for outpatient care in calculating reimbursable expenditures for inpatients is the income from such services rather than the expenditures allocated to them. This proviso reduces the deficit attributable to the care of outpatients and lessens the urgency, though not the necessity, of securing more income from the care of outpatients.

In the absence of any change in payment for services to ambulatory patients, the above proposals for inpatients imply an increase in annual expenditures by the City of $10–12 million (above the daily rate of $24 for medical or surgical patients prevailing in fiscal year 1960–61). Although this estimate was developed for short-term voluntary hospitals, it is not increased appreciably when psychiatric and tuberculosis hospitals are taken into account.

IMPLEMENTING MECHANISMS

The proposed pattern cannot be separated from the development of means to help attain the basic objectives. Three sets of means are in the forefront: (1) to increase the amount and relative importance of private payments in financing hospital care in New York City; (2) to control the total supply of hospital beds; and (3) to assist voluntary hospitals in obtaining capital funds for building, where indicated.

Increasing the Amount of Private Payments. In New York City large numbers of persons with hospital care insurance receive care in the ward. Although the reasons for this are not known precisely, a number of explanations were encountered in the course of this study. These fall into three broad groups: financial, physician-patient relationships, and organizational. If the financial limitations of the benefits provided by voluntary health insurance are the principal factor, the volume of ward care can be reduced only by improving benefits. If the other factors, which derive from habit and custom, are important, an intensive, widespread, and varied educational effort will also be required (see Chapter 4).

Within the field of voluntary health insurance a number of steps are indicated to increase the amount and proportion of private payments. Among them are promotion of enrollment among groups still uninsured and among those currently with insurance who are most likely to lose it; increasing benefits, particularly for long term patients; fostering of subscriber understanding of the general purposes and specific provisions of health insurance plans; and adjusting hospital policies and medical practices to the opportunities afforded by voluntary health insurance.

For self-paying patients it is important, on the one hand, to limit the facilities available for free care, especially in municipal hospitals, and, on the other hand, to charge patients—and to try to collect from them—in accordance with rising hospital cost. Perhaps it is time to devise and experiment with improved organized mechanisms for postpaying for hospital care over an extended period, as a counterpart to the mechanisms that have been developed for prepayment. This is not meant to be an improved collection mechanism for accounts that have already become delinquent.

Accomplishment of these objectives is complicated by the presence of other objectives that are certainly no less, and perhaps even more, important. No person in need of hospital care should be deprived of it for lack of ability to pay; and no person or family should be impoverished in the course of getting and paying for hospital care. This is an area in which the risks of hurting and antagonizing people are great, so that methods must be devised that will be effective when applied tactfully and in humane fashion.

It is reasonable to ask why an enterprise fraught with such risks and uncertainties should be undertaken. The answer is that if the effort is not made, private payments will within a decade fall to one half of total income in general-care hospitals in New York City and to a lower proportion in all hospitals. Moreover, the residual burden on local tax funds will continue to be heavy. It is probable that such tax funds will prove unequal to the task, both because the total amount may be insufficient and because the claims of hospital care must compete at the City Treasury with other uses, such as education, transportation, and so forth.

Limiting the Number of Hospital Beds. At current and prospective levels of hospital cost, it is highly important that all expenditures for hospital care be justifiable on medical grounds. Regardless of what other gains in efficiency and economy may be achieved through new knowledge, improvement in management practices, or regional organization of hospital services, the foremost source of saving currently visible is avoidance of an excessive number of hospital beds.

A community's total expenditures for hospital care tend to reflect the number of beds in operation. Obviously the vacant hospital bed is too costly a bed to build. It is also too costly a bed to operate, since a large proportion of a hospital's expenditures is independent of the daily patient census. An abundance of beds also creates an opportunity to prolong patients' stay. The temptation to overuse hospitals is greatest where a third party, rather than the patient or his family, pays the bill.

There is no effective control today over the total number of hospital beds in New York City. In undertaking new construction the City of New York is, of course, subject to the limitations imposed by the availability of capital funds within the constitutional debt limit; existing voluntary hospitals need approval of their building plans from the New York State Department of Social Welfare, whereas applicants for a charter for a new voluntary hospital are required to obtain approval from the Board of Social Welfare; and owners of proprietary hospitals, both existing and new, must comply with the City's Hospital Code (see Chapter 10). However, owners of proprietary hospitals have not been required to meet the test of the community's need for additional facilities. Presumably the test of the market place—profits or losses on the contemplated investment—is deemed to be a sufficient deterrent to overbuilding. Although the State inquires into the community's need for a new voluntary hospital, this is only one of several factors it takes into consideration in granting or withholding a charter. Review of plans to build at existing voluntary hospitals is concerned with physical layout and function, not with community need.

A major endeavor of the Hospital Council since its establishment in 1938 has been the study of hospital bed need in local areas in the city and the submission of recommendations to individual hospitals for meeting such need. For practical purposes proprietary hospitals have been outside the purview of the Hospital Council's recommendations, if not outside the scope of its studies. Moreover, voluntary hospitals and municipal agencies have sometimes been unable to carry out the Hospital Council's recommendations not to build (or to build) for reasons that seemed compelling to them.

Experience suggests that it may take the support of governmental authority to bring the total supply of hospital facilities under control, just as in the public utility field. Increasingly the modern hospital is being compared to a public utility, in the sense that it is a necessary facility with a large capital investment, much of which is operated on a stand-by basis. In deciding whether or not to issue a certificate of necessity to a hospital, an official agency can avail itself of the advice of voluntary organizations with experience in planning the development of hospital facilities and services. One model for such a relationship is provided by the role of the Hospital Council as local agent of the State in administering the Hill-Burton program in New York City.

Building Loans for Voluntary Hospitals. In 1957 the Hospital Council completed an evaluation of the physical plants of the member hospitals of the United Hospital Fund. It found that it would take $180 million to raise these hospitals to satisfactory condition, without any expansion of program (see Chapter 8).

So large a need was found after these hospitals had already spent $150 million for capital purposes during the postwar period. In the Hospital Council's experience only a small number of voluntary hospitals have financed their construction programs without strain. Most voluntary hospitals, particularly those without backing from a central agency, have arranged their financing with considerable difficulty and by assuming sizable debts for a short or long period. Some voluntary hospitals have been unable to raise the necessary funds and have refrained from building.

Two sources of capital funds that have not hitherto been tapped in New York City might be considered: (1) a joint campaign by voluntary hospitals and (2) loans from government at a low rate of interest.

The Hospital Council has encouraged a coordinated drive by the voluntary hospitals of New York City to raise a substantial fraction of the capital fund need as determined by its survey.[2] Similar drives have succeeded in other large cities.

Consideration might also be given to establishing a revolving fund for lending public moneys for capital purposes to voluntary hospitals whose building programs are designed to meet community need. If federal funds do not become available for this purpose, the feasibility of State or local government auspices might be explored.[3]

Consideration might also be given to the desirability of enacting a State and local version of the Hill-Burton program. If such a program is found to be desirable, it should be studied for conformity to the State Constitution.

PROVISION OF IMMEDIATE FINANCIAL ASSISTANCE

The persistence of financial deficits saps the vigor of hospitals and impairs their ability to provide adequate care. Since such hospitals cannot be identified by means of general characteristics, they must be dealt with in terms of their own special circumstances (see Chapter 14).

Several voluntary hospitals have an urgent need for financial assistance. Accordingly, consideration might be given to additional measures.

1. Supplementary financial support for individual hospitals that incur losses beyond their ability to bear in providing essential community services.

2. Creation of a fund, perhaps $1 million annually, jointly from tax funds and philanthropy to finance such supplementary support. Among the possible sources of tax funds for this purpose could be the approximately $0.5 million annually that the City now contributes to voluntary hospitals toward salaries of custodians (special policemen). Among the possible sources of income from philanthropy for this purpose, amounting perhaps to another $0.5 million, could be the annual increment in contributions to hospitals by the Greater New York Fund and a portion of the dis-

tribution by the United Hospital Fund allocated to direct benefit payments. If established, such a fund should be administered by
a committee of leading citizens conversant with the affairs of the
City and of voluntary hospitals but not representative of either.

There are precedents for supplementary grants to hospitals
to meet financial need. In the 1930s the United Hospital Fund
distributed $250,000 a year on the basis of demonstrated indi-
vidual need (see Chapter 18). In one large city the community
chest takes into consideration not only a hospital's share of the
total volume of free care, but the proportion of free to total care
in the individual institution (see Chapter 20).

There is no known precedent for financial participation by
the City in such a joint endeavor. It should be borne in mind,
however, that a good part of the financial need in question arises
from the care of public charges (see Chapter 14).

Redirection to this purpose of the City's contribution toward
custodians in voluntary hospitals might be temporary. It becomes
increasingly difficult to justify this contribution as the City's daily
rate of payment for the care of inpatients approaches cost.

Summary

1. A short summary of the data on sources of income and on
the financial position of hospitals in New York City, now and in
the past and in comparison with hospitals elsewhere, serves as
background for a discussion of alternative financial proposals.

2. The financial aspects of the following proposals are considered and criticized:

(a) To limit certification of public charges in voluntary hospitals to emergency admissions

(b) To concentrate care for the sick poor in municipal hospitals

(c) To affiliate municipal hospitals with medical schools or
major voluntary hospitals

(d) To establish services for private and semi-private patients
in municipal hospitals

(e) To relate the City's daily rate of payment to voluntary
hospitals to the average cost in municipal hospitals

(*f*) To establish different rates of payment for indigent and medically indigent patients

(*g*) To offset the value of a hospital's exemption from the real estate tax against the City's computed obligation

3. A proposed pattern of financing is presented that consists of the following elements:

(*a*) The City's daily rate of payment to voluntary hospitals would be an individualized rate, geared to cost.

(*b*) The rate would be calculated by the same process that produces the Blue Cross rate. This would be practicable if the City of New York became a party to the rate-making mechanism established by Blue Cross and the hospitals.

(*c*) The certification policy, which determines the number of patient days the City pays for, would continue to be uniformly applied in both hospital systems. Such a policy may be liberal or conservative.

(*d*) In return, voluntary hospitals would be less selective in admitting patients.

(*e*) The City would abandon one of its rules governing payment that reduces payments to voluntary hospitals: payment for a patient's care would begin as of the date of his certification.

4. The additional cost to government of the proposed pattern of financing is estimated at $10–$12 million a year.

5. It is suggested that individual hospitals may wish to make a voluntary contribution toward the cost of free care, budgeting it in advance every year.

6. As important as the proposed pattern of financing hospital care are certain implementing mechanisms. Suggestions are made to increase the role of private payments. However, no person in need of hospital care should be deprived of it for lack of financial ability, and no person or family should be impoverished in the course of getting and paying for hospital care.

7. At current and prospective levels of hospital cost, expenditures for hospital care should be justifiable on medical grounds. This means that surplus hospital beds must be avoided. It may take the support of governmental authority to bring the total supply of hospital facilities under control. The official agency

may, of course, avail itself of the advice of voluntary organizations with experience in planning.

8. Voluntary hospitals require assistance for building. Suggested are a joint campaign for contributions to a capital fund and loans from a revolving fund established by government.

9. Consideration is given to possible sources of moneys for immediate financial assistance to hospitals providing essential community services. One million dollars a year could be obtained by diverting certain distributions by the United Hospital Fund and the Greater New York Fund and by eliminating the City's subsidy of custodians (special policemen) in voluntary hospitals.

NOTES

INTRODUCTION

1. Hospital Council of Greater New York, *New York City and Its Hospitals: A Study of the Roles of the Municipal and Voluntary Hospitals Serving New York City* (New York, 1960).

1. POPULATION, INCOME, AND HEALTH INSURANCE

1. C. Morris Horowitz and Lawrence J. Kaplan, *The Jewish Population of the New York Area, 1900–1975,* prepared for Demographic Study Committee of Federation of Jewish Philanthropies (New York, 1959), p. 7.

2. Raymond Vernon, *The Changing Economic Function of the Central City* (Supplementary Paper, Committee for Economic Development, New York, 1959), p. 40.

3. New York City Department of City Planning, "Population Changes in New York City," its *Bulletin,* November 22, 1954, Table III.

4. *Ibid.*

5. *Ibid.;* New York City Planning Commission, *New York City: A Study of Its Population Changes* (New York, 1951), p. 11.

6. Oscar Handlin, *The Newcomers* (Cambridge, Mass., 1959), pp. 68–69.

7. Anthony M. Lowell, *Tuberculosis in New York City, 1958* (New York, 1959), p. 10.

8. Sam Shapiro, Harold Jacobziner, Paul M. Densen, and Louis Weiner, *Further Observations on Prematurity and Perinatal Mortality in a General Population and in the Population of a Prepaid Group Practice Medical Care Plan,* paper read before American Public Health Association, October 20, 1959 (mimeographed), Appendix Table B.

9. Eleanor M. Snyder, *Public Assistance Recipients in New York State, January–February 1957* (Albany, N.Y., 1958), p. 36.

10. Horowitz and Kaplan, p. 9.

11. New York City Department of City Planning, "Population Changes in New York City," Table V.

12. New York City Office of the Mayor, *Final Report on Fourth Migration Conference, May 31–June 4, 1960* (New York, 1960; mimeographed), p. 2.

13. Commonwealth of Puerto Rico Department of Labor, Migration Division, *A Summary in Facts and Figures,* January, 1959, edition (New York, 1959), p. 15.

14. *Ibid.,* p. 16.

15. New York City Office of the Mayor, *Final Report on Fourth Migration Conference,* p. 3.

16. New York City Board of Education, *The Puerto Rican Study, 1953–1957* (New York, 1959), p. 176.

17. New York State Commission against Discrimination, *Nonwhites in New York's Four Suburban Counties* (New York, 1959; mimeographed), p. 2.

18. Henry Cohen, *Where Is New York Going?,* paper delivered at Upper Manhattan YMCA Workshop, April 18, 1958 (mimeographed), p. 6.

19. Regional Plan Association, *Population, 1954–1975* (Bulletin No. 85; New York, 1954), p. 27.

20. New York City Department of City Planning, "Population Changes in New York City," Table V.

21. Regional Plan Association, *People, Jobs and Land, 1955–1975* (Bulletin No. 87; New York, 1957), p. 3.

22. New York City Planning Commission, *Rezoning New York City* (New York, 1959), p. 7.

23. Cohen, p. 2.

24. Horowitz and Kaplan, p. 9.

25. Regional Plan Association, *People, Jobs, and Land, 1955–1975.*

26. Daniel Creamer, *Low Income Families in New York State in 1949* (New York, New York State Interdepartmental Committee on Low Incomes, 1957), p. 14.

27. Harvey H. Segal, *Personal Income of the New York Metropolitan Region* (New York Metropolitan Region Study; New York, 1958; mimeographed), p. 10.

28. New York State Department of Commerce, "Personal Income in New York State," *New York State Commerce Review,* XII, No. 12 (December, 1958), p. 9, and XIV, No. 2 (February, 1960), p. 4; and *Sales Management,* May 10, 1959, pp. 192, 506, 510, 512, 514.

29. Herman P. Miller, *Income of the American People* (New York, 1955), p. 15.

30. Horowitz and Kaplan, p. 69.

31. *Sales Management,* May 10, 1959.

32. New York State Interdepartmental Committee on Low Incomes, *Family Income in New York State: 1956* (Bulletin No. 1, Pt. 1; New York, 1958), Table 11.

33. Miller, p. 102.

34. Creamer, pp. 79–82.

35. Gladys Engel Lang, *Minority Groups and Economic Status in New York State* and *Working Tables,* prepared for State Commission against Discrimination (New York, 1958; mimeographed), p. 23.

36. Elmo Roper and Associates, *The Public's Attitudes toward Hospitals in New York City and Their Financing in May, 1958*, II (New York, 1959), p. 217.

37. Health Insurance Council, *The Extent of Voluntary Health Insurance Coverage in the United States, 1958* (New York, 1959), p. 8.

38. Committee for Special Research Project in the Health Insurance Plan of Greater New York, *Health and Medical Care in New York City* (Cambridge, Mass., 1957), p. 34.

39. Wharton School of Finance and Commerce, *Study of Consumer Expenditures, Income and Savings*, VIII (Philadelphia, 1956), pp. 30–31.

40. Hospital Council of Greater New York, "Hospital Care Insurance in New York City," its *Bulletin*, XIV, No. 1 (1959).

41. Elmo Roper and Associates, p. 225; Health Information Foundation, unpublished data for year 1955; and New York State Department of Labor, Division of Research and Statistics, *Health Benefit Coverage of the Labor Force in New York State* (New York, 1960), p. 6.

42. New York State Department of Labor, *Health Benefit Coverage of the Labor Force*, pp. 45, 47.

43. *Ibid.*, p. 6.

44. Elmo Roper and Associates, p. 213.

45. Health Insurance Council, *The Extent of Voluntary Health Insurance Coverage*, pp. 13, 21.

46. New York State Department of Labor, *Health Benefit Coverage of the Labor Force*, pp. 6, 8.

47. Health Insurance Council, *The Extent of Voluntary Health Insurance Coverage*, pp. 13, 21.

48. Agnes W. Brewster, "Independent Plans Providing Medical Care and Hospital Insurance: 1957 Survey," *Social Security Bulletin*, XXI, No. 4 (April, 1958), p. 4; and letter from A. W. Brewster to Herbert E. Klarman, with data on independent plans in New York State outside New York City.

49. New York City Department of Commerce and Public Events, *Statistical Guide for New York City* (New York, 1958), p. 14.

50. Elmo Roper and Associates, p. 217.

2. PATTERNS OF HOSPITAL USE

1. Letters from Veterans Administration Hospitals to Herbert E. Klarman, giving unpublished data for three hospitals in New York City: Bronx, May 21, 1958; Brooklyn, June 16, 1958; and New York, June 20, 1958.

2. Letter from Robert E. Patton, New York State Department of Mental Hygiene, to Herbert E. Klarman, June 26, 1959.

3. Hospital Council of Greater New York, "Emergency Department Services in Hospitals in New York City," its *Bulletin*, XIV, No. 2 (1959).

4. Hospital Council of Greater New York, *Emergency Ambulance Service in New York City* (New York, 1950), p. 4.

5. The 1920 data were derived from several sources, chiefly, American Medical Association, "Hospital Service in the United States," its *Bulletin,* XV, No. 3 (Hospital Number; May 12, 1921), pp. 263-65, and Edward H. L. Corwin, *The Hospital Situation in Greater New York* (New York, 1924), pp. 20-24, 34-35, 39.

6. Hospital Council of Greater New York, *Master Plan for Hospitals and Related Facilities for New York City* (New York, 1947).

7. *Ibid.,* pp. 29, 31.

8. United Hospital Fund of New York, unpublished information.

9. *Ibid.*

10. Hospital Council of Greater New York, "Emergency Department Services."

11. Federation of Jewish Philanthropies, Subcommittee on Hospitals and Health Agencies of the Study Committee, *Outpatient Services in Federation Hospitals,* (Information Memorandum No. 37; New York, 1959; mimeographed), p. 17.

12. Letter from Hospital Council of Greater New York to Charles F. Preusse, City Administrator, July 5, 1956.

13. Hospital Council of Greater New York, "Emergency Department Services."

14. Hospital Council of Greater New York, "Diagnostic Services for Ambulatory Patients Considered Important Activity of General Hospitals," its *Bulletin,* VII, No. 4 (April, 1951).

15. Letter from Martin R. Steinberg to Dr. Hayden C. Nicholson, December 15, 1958.

16. Hospital Council of Greater New York, *Emergency Ambulance Service,* p. 9.

17. New York City Department of Hospitals, *Regulations Governing the Emergency Ambulance Service in the City of New York* (New York, 1957), para. 81.

18. Hospital Council of Greater New York, *Emergency Ambulance Service,* p. 3.

19. Hospital Council of Greater New York, *Organized Home Medical Care in New York City* (Cambridge, Mass., 1956).

20. *Ibid.,* p. 266.

21. David Littauer, I. Jerome Flance, and Albert F. Hessen, *Home Care* (Chicago, 1961), p. 70.

22. Hospital Council of Greater New York, *Organized Home Medical Care,* p. 334.

23. Associated Hospital Service of New York, *Report of a Study Concerning the Feasibility of Providing Visiting Nurse Service Following Hospitalization for Blue Cross Subscribers* (New York, 1957), p. 26.

24. Greenwich Hospital Association, *The Home Care Program: Three-Year Pilot Study Report* (Greenwich, Conn., 1959; mimeographed), p. 3.

25. Health Information Foundation, "Hospitalized Mental Illness in the U.S.," *Progress in Health Services,* IX, No. 8 (October, 1960).

26. Joint Information Service of the American Psychiatric Association and the National Association for Mental Health, *Psychiatric Patients in General Hospitals 1954–1958*, (Fact Sheet No. 13; Washington, D.C., November, 1960).

27. Hospital Council of Greater New York, *Master Plan for Hospitals and Related Facilities*, p. 41.

28. Hospital Council of Greater New York, "Recent Developments in General Hospitals in New York City," its *Bulletin*, XI, No. 1 (March–April, 1956).

29. Joint Information Service of the American Psychiatric Association and the National Association for Mental Health, *List of General Hospitals Surveyed and Appendices to Psychiatric Patients in General Hospitals* (Washington, D.C., 1960), pp. 22–23.

30. National Tuberculosis Association and U.S. Public Health Service, *The Arden House Conference on Tuberculosis* (Washington, D.C., 1960), p. 3.

31. Anthony M. Lowell, *Tuberculosis in New York City* (New York, annually).

32. National Tuberculosis Association and U.S. Public Health Service, *The Arden House Conference*.

33. Carl Muschenheim and others, *Report of the 1958 Tuberculosis Hospital Survey in New York City*, I (New York, 1959; mimeographed), p. 14.

34. National Tuberculosis Association and U.S. Public Health Service, *The Arden House Conference*, p. 5.

35. Hospital Council of Greater New York, "Ten Years of Hill-Burton Program in New York City," its *Bulletin*, XII, No. 2 (March–April, 1957).

36. *Ibid.*

37. Magda G. Pendall, *Convalescence and Institutional Convalescent Care* (New York, 1959), pp. 10–14.

38. *Ibid.*, p. 2.

39. Alvin I. Goldfarb, *Report to the Commissioner of Mental Hygiene of New York State, Summarization of Activities for the Year 1958 from the Office of the Consultant on Services for the Aged* (New York [1959]; mimeographed), p. 8.

40. Herbert E. Klarman, *Background, Issues and Policies in Health Services for the Aged in New York City* (New York, 1962).

41. United Hospital Fund of New York, *Financial and Statistical Information Relating to Member Hospitals of the United Hospital Fund of New York and Hospital Statistics for Greater New York* (New York, annually).

42. American Medical Association, "Hospital Service in the United States," its *Journal*, CXVI, No. 11 (March 15, 1941).

43. Lowell.

44. New York City Department of Hospitals, *Annual Report*, 1940 (New York, 1941), p. 12.

45. American Medical Association, "Hospital Service in the United States," 1941.

46. Lowell.

47. *Ibid.*

48. New York City Department of Hospitals, *Annual Report*, 1940, p. 12.

49. American Medical Association, "Hospital Service in the United States," 1941.

3. CHARACTERISTICS OF PATIENTS IN SHORT-TERM HOSPITALS

1. Sadie Zuchovitz and William Kaufman, *Hospital Utilization by Recipients in the Aid to Dependent Children Program in New York City, 1958* (Special Research and Statistical Reports, No. 14; Albany, N.Y., New York State Department of Social Welfare, 1960); and their *Hospital Utilization by Recipients in the Adult Public Assistance Programs in New York City, 1957* (Special Research and Statistical Reports, No. 15; Albany, N.Y., New York State Department of Social Welfare, 1960).

2. Eleanor M. Snyder, *Public Assistance Recipients in New York State, January–February 1957* (Albany, N.Y., 1958), p. 36.

3. Marta Fraenkel, New York City Department of Hospitals, unpublished information.

4. New York City Department of Health, special tabulations for Hospital Council of Greater New York on births and deaths by ethnic status, by hospital, and by Health Area of residence.

5. Letters from New York State Department of Health to Hospital Council of Greater New York.

6. Neva R. Deardorff and Marta Fraenkel, *Hospital Discharge Study*, 2 vols., New York, 1942; and unpublished summary books in custody of Hospital Council of Greater New York.

7. C. Morris Horowitz and Lawrence J. Kaplan, *The Jewish Population of the New York Area, 1900–1975* (New York, 1959), p. 9.

8. New York City Department of Hospitals, *Annual Report, 1946* (New York, 1947), p. 13.

9. Federation of Jewish Philanthropies, Subcommittee on Hospitals and Health Agencies of the Study Committee, unpublished tabulations of one-day patient census, April 15, 1959.

10. Hospital Morbidity Reporting, Joint Project of the New York City Departments of Health and Hospitals, *Bulletins*, 1–11, special reports, and tabulations, prepared by Marta Fraenkel (New York, 1957–58; mimeographed).

11. Horowitz and Kaplan.

12. Dorothy F. Holland and Marion E. Altenderfer, *Sickness in a Metropolitan Community—The Results of a Health Survey of New York City* (Washington, D.C., 1946; mimeographed), p. 79.

13. Deardorff and Fraenkel, unpublished summary books in custody of Hospital Council of Greater New York.

14. Sam Shapiro, Harold Jacobziner, Paul M. Densen, and Louis Weiner, *Further Observations on Prematurity and Perinatal Mortality in a General Population and in the Population of a Prepaid Group Practice Medical Care Plan*, paper read before American Public Health Association, October 20, 1959 (mimeographed), Figure 1.

15. Hospital Council of Greater New York, *Report on the Hospitalization Needs of Lower Manhattan* (New York, 1956), p. 38.

16. *Ibid.*, unpublished data from this study.

17. Federation of Jewish Philanthropies, Subcommittee on Hospitals and Health Agencies of the Study Committee, unpublished tabulations of one-day patient census, April 15, 1959.

18. Deardorff and Fraenkel, unpublished summary books in custody of Hospital Council of Greater New York.

19. Hospital Morbidity Reporting, Joint Project of the New York City Departments of Health and Hospitals, *Bulletins* 1–11, special reports, and tabulations, prepared by Marta Fraenkel.

20. Frank G. Dickinson, *Age and Sex Distribution of Hospital Patients* (Bulletin 97, Bureau of Medical Economic Research, American Medical Association; Chicago, 1955).

21. Herbert E. Klarman, *Background, Issues and Policies in Health Services for the Aged in New York City* (New York, 1962).

22. United Hospital Fund of New York, "Average Length of Stay, Voluntary Non-Profit Hospitals in New York City, 1951–1958," its *Bulletin, No. 231* (April 1, 1959).

23. Ray E. Trussell and Frank van Dyke, *Prepayment for Hospital Care in New York State* (Albany, N.Y., 1960), pp. 243–46.

24. Floyd L. Wergeland, *The Medicare Program*, paper delivered at meeting of Dependents' Medical Care Advisory Committee Meeting, April 29, 1960, Washington, D.C. (mimeographed), p. 19.

25. Frank G. Dickinson and James Raymond, *Some Categories of Patients Treated by Physicians in Hospitals* (*Bulletin 102*, Bureau of Medical Economic Research, American Medical Association; Chicago, 1956).

26. Associated Hospital Service, *Report of the Average Length of Stay of Cases Paid by AHS to Member Hospitals during the Last Six Months of 1959* (New York, 1960).

27. Hospital Survey for New York, unpublished memoranda in files of Hospital Council of Greater New York.

28. Hospital Council of Greater New York, "Long-Term Illnesses Seen as a Major Community Problem Requiring Extension of Medical Services," its *Bulletin*, III, No. 8 (August, 1947).

29. Hospital Council of Greater New York, *Organized Home Medical Care in New York City* (Cambridge, Mass., 1956), pp. 333–35.

30. Howard M. Rusk, John E. Silson, Joseph Novey, and Michael M. Dasco, *Hospital Patient Survey* (New York, 1956), p. 26.

31. Carl Muschenheim and others. *Report of the 1958 Tuberculosis Hospital Survey in New York City*, I (New York, 1959; mimeographed), p. 10.

32. Zuchovitz and Kaufman (Special Research and Statistical Reports Nos. 14 and No. 15).

33. Snyder, p. 141.

34. Federation of Jewish Philanthropies, Subcommittee on Hospitals and

Health Agencies of the Study Committee, unpublished tabulations of one-day patient census, April 15, 1959.

35. Hospital Morbidity Reporting, Joint Project of the New York City Departments of Health and Hospitals, *Bulletins* 1–11, special reports, and tabulations, prepared by Marta Fraenkel.

36. Marta Fraenkel and Carl L. Erhardt, *Morbidity in the Municipal Hospitals of the City of New York* (New York, 1955).

37. Deardorff and Fraenkel, *Hospital Discharge Study.*

38. Fraenkel and Erhardt.

39. Muschenheim and others, II, Table 4.

4. USE OF WARD SERVICE BY HOSPITAL INSURANCE SUBSCRIBERS

1. Committee for Special Research Project in the Health Insurance Plan of Greater New York, *Health and Medical Care in New York City* (Cambridge, Mass., 1957), p. 34.

2. Elmo Roper and Associates, *The Public's Attitudes toward Hospitals in New York City and Their Financing in May, 1958*, II (New York, 1959), p. 219.

3. Hospital Council of Greater New York, "Changing Factors in Determining Requirements for Maternity Beds," its *Bulletin*, May–June 1957. For year 1958, unpublished data from annual inventory of hospitals.

4. Odin W. Anderson and Jacob J. Feldman, *Family Medical Costs and Voluntary Health Insurance: A Nationwide Survey* (New York, 1956), p. 66.

5. U.S. Veterans Administration and U.S. Bureau of the Budget, *Current and Projected Veteran Patient Load through 1986* (Washington, D.C., 1958; mimeographed), p. IV–9, figure for United States. New York City figure was obtained from special tabulation performed for Hospital Council by Department of Medicine and Surgery, Veterans Administration.

6. Elmo Roper and Associates, p. 213.

7. Paul M. Densen, Eva Balamuth, and Sam Shapiro, *Prepaid Medical Care and Hospital Utilization* (Chicago, 1958) p. 55.

8. Baltimore Hospital Survey Committee, *General Hospital Facilities for the Baltimore Area* (Baltimore, 1958), pp. 69–70.

9. Committee for Special Research Project in the Health Insurance Plan of Greater New York, *Health and Medical Care in New York City*, p. 59.

10. Anderson and Feldman, p. 39.

11. Hospital Council of Greater New York, "Changing Factors in Determining Requirements for Maternity Beds."

12. *Ibid.*

13. Martin Segal and Company, *Union Family Fund of the Hotel Industry of New York City* (Report on Studies Nos. 1 and 2; New York, 1958), p. 53.

14. Federation of Jewish Philanthropies, Subcommittee on Hospitals and Health Agencies of the Study Committee, unpublished tabulations of one-day patient census, April 15, 1959.

15. Hospital Council of Greater New York, *Twenty First Annual Report* (New York, 1959), p. 18.

16. *Ibid.*, pp. 18–19.

17. Hospital Council of Greater New York, *Report on Hospital Care for Staten Island* (New York, 1956), p. 50.

18. *Ibid.*, p. 8.

5. ATTENDING STAFF

1. Hospital Council of Greater New York, *Hospital Staff Appointments of Physicians in New York City* (New York, 1951).

2. William Weinfeld, "Income of Physicians, 1929–49," reprinted from *Survey of Current Business*, July 1951, p. 21.

The difference persisted in 1955. See *Medical Economics*, XXXIV, No. 1 (October, 1956), p. 119.

3. Health Insurance Institute, *Source Book of Health Insurance Data* (New York, 1959), p. 53.

4. Health Information Foundation, "The Increased Use of Medical Care," *Progress in Health Services*, VII, No. 8 (Oct. 1958).

5. Medical Society of the State of New York, *Medical Directory of New York State*, 1959, Vol. XLVIII (New York, 1959). Earlier volumes published biennially.

6. American Medical Association, Directory Department, *Survey of Number of Physicians in the United States by County, Dependencies and Canada, March 1, 1950* (Chicago, 1950), pp. 64–65.

7. Frank G. Dickinson, *Distribution of Physicians by Medical Service Areas* (Bulletin 94, Bureau of Medical Economic Research, American Medical Association; Chicago, 1954), pp. 20–21.

8. Maryland Y. Pennell and Marion E. Altenderfer, *Health Manpower Source Book, Section 4, County Data* (Washington, D.C., 1954), p. 125.

9. Hospital Council of Greater New York, *Hospital Staff Appointments of Physicians*.

10. American Medical Association, *American Medical Directory, 1958* (20th Edition; Chicago, 1958).

11. Hospital Council of Greater New York, *Hospital Staff Appointments of Physicians*, p. 25.

6. INTERNS AND RESIDENTS

1. Leland S. McKittrick, "Objectives of Medical Education," *Journal of American Medical Education*, CLXXIII, No. 12 (July 23, 1960), pp. 1289–90.

2. American Medical Association, Council on Medical Education and Hospitals, *Essentials of an Approved Internship* (Chicago, 1958), p. 7.

3. Victor Johnson and others, "Report of the Advisory Committee on

Internships to Council on Medical Education and Hospitals," *Journal of American Medical Association*, CLI, No. 6 (February 7, 1953), p. 509.

4. John C. Leonard, in Beverly Hospital, *Report on Seminar on Graduate Medical Education in Non University Hospitals* (Beverly, Mass., 1959), p. 70.

5. Hospital Council of Greater New York, *Master Plan for Hospitals and Related Facilities for New York City* (New York, 1947), p. 11.

6. *Ibid.*, pp. 31, 34.

7. Jean Alonzo Curran (for the Committee on the Study of Hospital Internships and Residencies), *Internships and Residencies in New York City, 1934–1937; Their Place in Medical Education* (New York, 1938), pp. 34–35.

8. *Ibid.*, p. 85.

9. James E. McCormack, *Graduate Medical Education*, reprinted from *Seminar* (Sharp and Dohme), XVI, No. 4, p. 2.

10. *Ibid.*

11. Curran, *Internships and Residencies in New York City*, p. 59.

12. Jean Alonzo Curran, "Internships and Residencies, Historical Backgrounds and Current Trends," *Journal of Medical Education*, XXXIV, No. 9 (September, 1959), pp. 873–74, 879.

13. Hospital Council of Greater New York, *Emergency Ambulance Service in New York City* (New York, 1950), pp. 38–39.

14. John McK. Mitchell, in University of Pennsylvania, Graduate School of Medicine, First Annual Conference on Graduate Medical Education, *Report of Proceedings* (Philadelphia, 1959), pp. 12–13.

15. Curran, "Internships and Residencies, Historical Backgrounds and Current Trends."

16. Maryland Y. Pennell and Marion E. Altenderfer, *Health Manpower Source Book, Section 1, Physicians* (Washington, D.C., 1952), p. 24.

17. Curran, "Internships and Residencies, Historical Backgrounds and Current Trends."

18. American Medical Association, Council on Medical Education and Hospitals, *Directory of Approved Internships and Residencies, 1960*, reprinted from *Journal of American Medical Association*, CLXXIV, No. 6 (October 8, 1960), p. 583.

19. Hospital Council of Greater New York, *Emergency Ambulance Service*, pp. 38–39.

20. McCormack, p. 6.

21. American Medical Association, *Directory of Approved Internships and Residencies, 1960*, p. 583.

22. I. S. Ravdin, in University of Pennsylvania, Graduate School of Medicine, First Annual Conference on Graduate Medical Education, *Report*, pp. 42–43.

23. House of Representatives, Committee on Interstate and Foreign Commerce, Staff Report, *Medical School Inquiry* (Washington, D. C., 85th Congress, First Session, 1957), p. 258.

24. Curran, *Internships and Residencies in New York City*, pp. 22–23.

25. New York Academy of Medicine Institute on Medical Education, *Trends in Medical Education*, Mahlon Ashford, editor (New York, 1949), p. 124.

26. Association of American Medical Colleges, *Datagrams*, I, No. 5 (November, 1959), p. 2.

27. American Medical Association, *Directory of Approved Internships and Residencies, 1960*, p. 548.

28. U.S. Public Health Service, Division of Public Health Methods, *Health Manpower Source Book, Section 9* (Washington, D.C., 1959), p. 9.

29. Frank Bane and others, *Physicians for a Growing America* (Washington, D.C., 1959), p. 9.

30. American Medical Association, *Directory of Approved Internships and Residencies, 1960*, p. 583.

31. John M. Weir, "Obstacles to Medical Education at the International Level," *Journal of American Medical Association*, CLXXIII, No. 13 (July 30, 1960), pp. 1451–52.

32. Educational Council for Foreign Medical Graduates, *Summary of Examination Results* (Chicago, November 23, 1960; mimeographed).

33. American Medical Association, Council on Medical Education and Hospitals, *Consolidated List of Approved Internships, 1914–1955, revised to November 1, 1955* (Chicago, 1955), pp. 9–11.

34. American Medical Association, Council on Medical Education and Hospitals, *Medical Education in the United States and Canada, 1934–35*, reprinted from *Journal of American Medical Association*, CV, No. 9 (August 31, 1935), p. 699.

35. American Medical Association, Council on Medical Education and Hospitals, *Directory of Approved Internships and Residencies, 1959*, reprinted from *Journal of American Medical Association*, CLXXI, No. 6 (October 6, 1959), p. 666.

36. American Medical Association, *Medical Education in the United States and Canada, 1934–35*, p. 709.

37. American Medical Association, *Directory of Approved Internships and Residencies, 1959*, p. 671.

38. Curran, *Internships and Residencies in New York City*, pp. 166–67.

39. *Ibid.*, p. 85.

40. New York Committee on the Study of Internships and Residencies, unpublished data in files of Hospital Council of Greater New York.

41. American Medical Association, *Medical Education in the United States and Canada, 1958–1959*, reprinted from *Journal of American Medical Association*, CLXXI, No. 11 (November 14, 1959), p. 1551.

42. Curran, *Internships and Residencies in New York City*, p. 86.

43. New York Committee on the Study of Internships and Residencies, unpublished data.

44. Hospital Council of Greater New York, questionnaire survey of house staff in hospitals in New York City, April 20, 1959.

45. American Medical Association, *Directory of Approved Internships and Residencies, 1960*, p. 583.

46. Myron Rose, "State Survey Sketches Intern-Resident Picture," *Hospitals*, XXXIV, No. 23 (December 1, 1960), p. 66.

47. American Medical Association, Council on Medical Education and Hospitals, *Medical Education in the United States and Canada, 1959–60*, reprinted from *Journal of American Medical Association*, CLXXIV, No. 12 (November 12, 1960), p. 1476.

48. National Intern Matching Program, *1959 Results: Number of Interns Sought and Number Matched for Each Participating Hospital* (Chicago, 1959), pp. 7–8.

49. Rose, p. 60.   50. Johnson and others, p. 499.

51. Letter from National Intern Matching Program to Herbert E. Klarman, April 9, 1959.

52. Federation of Jewish Philanthropies, Subcommittee on Hospitals and Health Agencies of Study Committee, *Characteristics of Interns and Residents in Federation Hospitals, 1958–59* (Information Memorandum No. 28; New York, 1959; mimeographed), p. 24.

53. Institute of International Education, unpublished data.

54. Federation of Jewish Philanthropies, *Characteristics of Interns and Residents in Federation Hospitals*, p. 31.

55. American Medical Association, *Consolidated List of Approved Internships, 1914–1955*, pp. 9–11.

56. Henry T. Heald and others, *Meeting the Increasing Demand for Higher Education in New York State* (Albany, N.Y., 1960), p. 37.

57. American Medical Association, *Directory of Approved Internships and Residencies, 1960*, p. 581.

58. Dean P. Smiley in University of Pennsylvania, Graduate School of Medicine, First Annual Conference on Graduate Medical Education, *Report*, p. 65.

59. Nathan Smith and Harris Blinder, "The Critical Problem of Obtaining House Staff and Visiting Staff in the Non University Municipal Hospital," *New York State Journal of Medicine*, LIX, No. 9 (May 1, 1959), p. 1780.

60. American Medical Association, *Essentials of an Approved Internship*, pp. 27–28.

61. Otto C. Brantigan, "The Purpose of a Hospital: Good Patient Care or House Officer Training," *The American Surgeon*, XXV, No. 6 (June, 1959), p. 441.

62. Smith and Blinder, pp. 1780–81.

63. Saran Jonas (for the Committee of Interns and Residents of the New York City Municipal Hospitals), *The Crisis in the New York City Hospital System* (New York, 1959; mimeographed), pp. 8–9.

64. David M. Heyman and others, *Report of the Commission on Health Services of the City of New York, Adopted July 20, 1960* (New York, 1960;

mimeographed), pp. 13–14; Herbert G. Vaughn, Jr. (for the Committee of Interns and Residents of the New York City Municipal Hospitals), *Hospital Organization and Patient Care: A Survey of the New York Municipal Hospital System with Proposals for Increased Efficiency of Service* (New York, 1959; mimeographed), pp. 13–14.

65. Johnson, p. 503.

66. Letter from John C. Nunemaker, American Medical Association, Council on Medical Education and Hospitals, to Dr. Hayden C. Nicholson, September 9, 1959.

67. American Medical Association, *Essentials of an Approved Internship*, p. 12.

68. American Medical Association, *Directory of Approved Internships and Residencies, 1960*, pp. 363, 368.

69. *Ibid.*, p. 582.

70. Vaughn, p. 16.

71. American Medical Association, *Essentials of an Approved Internship*, p. 25.

72. Ralph E. Dolkart, Joan McJoynt Brossard, and John A. D. Cooper, "Hospitals Which Do and Do Not Fill Their Intern Quotas," *Journal of Medical Education*, XXXIII, No. 10 (October, 1958), p. 721.

73. Jonas, p. 3.

74. Joan R. McJoynt and Edwin L. Crosby, "The Fifth National Intern Matching Program," *Journal of Medical Education*, XXXI, No. 9 (September, 1956), p. 594.

75. Jonas, p. 2.

76. Letter from Saran Jonas to Herbert E. Klarman, November 17, 1959.

77. Jonas, pp. 8–9.

78. Weir, p. 1453.

79. Bane, pp. 34–35.

80. Russell A. Nelson, "Foreign Medical Graduates," *Hospitals*, XXXIV, No. 15 (August, 1960), Pt. 1, p. 52.

81. American Medical Association, *Directory of Approved Internships and Residencies, 1960*, p. 583.

82. Dean P. Smiley, in Beverly Hospital, *Report on Seminar*, p. 48.

83. Harold S. Diehl, Edwin L. Crosby, and Paul K. Kaetzel, *Hospital House Staff, 1950–1955*, reprinted from *Hospitals*, May 16, 1957, Table 3.

84. James E. McCormack, *The Problem of the Foreign Physician*, p. 6, reprinted from *Journal of the American Medical Association*, CLV (1954), pp. 818–23.

85. U.S. Public Health Service, *Health Manpower Source Book, Section 9*, p. 24.

86. National Science Foundation, *Scientific Manpower Bulletin* (NSF 58–4, No. 8, Washington, D.C., 1958).

87. Letter from National Science Foundation to Herbert E. Klarman, August 18, 1959.

88. American Medical Association, *Medical Education in the United States and Canada, 1959–60*, pp. 1455 and 1459; U.S. Public Health Service, *Health Manpower Source Book, Section 9*, p. 24.

89. Diehl, Crosby, and Kaetzel.

90. U.S. Public Health Service, *Health Manpower Source Book, Section 9*, p. 9.

91. Bane, p. 9.

92. Curran, *Internships and Residencies in New York City*.

93. Hospital Survey for New York, *Report*, II (New York, 1937), p. 247.

94. Curran, *Internships and Residencies in New York City*, p. 86.

95. *Ibid.*, p. 23.

96. Hospital Survey for New York, *Report*, II, p. 247.

7. NURSING PERSONNEL

1. American Nurses' Association, *Facts About Nursing, 1955–56* (New York, 1956), p. 20; Dorothy E. Reese and Stanley E. Siegel, "Vacancies for Professional Nurses in Non-Federal Hospitals, 1958," *Hospital Management*, LXXXVIII, No. 5 (November, 1959), p. 100.

2. Margaret Arnstein, "Setting the Record Straight," *Nursing Outlook*, II, No. 6 (June, 1954); Margaret D. West and Edwin L. Crosby, *Nursing Students in the Future*, reprinted from *Hospitals*, January 16, 1956.

3. U.S. Public Health Service, Division of Public Health Methods, *Health Manpower Source Book, Section 9* (Washington, D.C., 1959), p. 63.

4. Helen G. Tibbits and Eugene Levine, *Health Manpower Source Book, Section 2, Nursing Personnel* (Washington, D.C., 1953), p. 84; American Hospital Association, *Hospitals*, XXXIII, No. 15 (August 1, 1959), Pt. 2 (Guide Issue), p. 424.

5. Arnstein.

6. United Hospital Fund of New York, special questionnaire on working conditions of nursing personnel, 1940, unpublished.

7. Appollonia Adams, *Nursing Resources* (Washington, D.C., 1958), Chart 17.

8. University of the State of New York, *Needs and Facilities in Professional Nursing Education in New York State* (Albany, N.Y., 1958; mimeographed), p. 17.

9. New York State Hospital Association, "Nurse Study Reports More Facilities Needed," *Hospital Forum*, XXVI, No. 10 (October, 1958), p. 9.

10. American Public Health Association, *Public Health and Hospitals in the St. Louis Area* (New York, 1957), p. 285.

11. American Hospital Association, *Hospitals*, XXXIII, 426–27.

12. Tibbits and Levine, p. 71.

13. American Hospital Association, *Hospitals*, XXXIII, 430.

14. American Nurses' Association, *Spot Check of Current Hospital Nursing Employment Conditions, February, 1959* (New York, 1959; mimeo-

graphed), p. 32; confirmed by completed questionnaires submitted to American Hospital Association by hospitals in New York City.

15. Tibbits and Levine, pp. 71-72.

16. Hilda M. Torrop, *Today's Practical Nurse: Concepts behind Her Education*, reprinted from *Hospitals*, August 16, 1959.

17. Adams.

18. Albert W. Snoke and Richard B. Ogrean, *Nursing Service and Education*, reprinted from *Hospitals*, January 1 and 16, 1956, p. 5.

19. Mark S. Blumberg, *Men, Machines and Hospitals*, reprinted from *Hospital Progress*, November, 1959; Snoke and Ogrean, p. 8.

20. Committee on the Function of Nursing, *A Program for the Nursing Profession* (New York, 1948), p. 86.

21. Stewart T. Hamilton, "The Future Nurse: Her Place and Preparation," *Hospitals*, XXXIII, No. 5 (March 1, 1959), p. 36.

22. Sister Charles Marie, *The Utilization of Nursing Personnel*, paper delivered at National League for Nursing, Philadelphia, 1959 (typewritten); New York State Hospital Association, "Nurse Study Reports More Facilities Needed," p. 8.

23. University of the State of New York, *Professional Nurses Registered in New York State during the First Four Months of the Biennium, September 1, 1955–August 1, 1957* (Albany, N.Y., 1956; mimeographed), Table 9A.

24. American Public Health Association, *Public Health and Hospitals in the St. Louis Area*, pp. 294–95.

25. Newport Hospital, *Comparative Analysis of Net Cost of Nursing Education for the Year Ended September 30, 1957* (Newport, R.I., 1957), Exhibits C and C3.

26. New York City Department of Hospitals, *Nursing Personnel Budget Preparation Formulae* (New York, 1956; mimeographed).

27. Interview with staff of New York State Employment Service, from files of New York State Hospital Study, unpublished memorandum, August 8, 1949.

28. Letter from Louis S. Reed to Herbert E. Klarman, November 3, 1959.

29. U.S. Bureau of Labor Statistics, *Earnings and Supplementary Benefits in Hospitals, February, 1957* (Washington, D.C., 1957), p. 4; University of State of New York, *Needs and Facilities in Professional Nursing Education in New York State*, p. 71.

30. Hospital Council of Greater New York, *Report of Study of Kings County Hospital* (New York, 1952), p. 82.

31. Lily Mary David, *The Economic Status of Registered Professional Nurses, 1946–47* (Washington, D.C., 1948), p. 24.

32. City Hospital Visiting Committee, *Annual Reports to the New York State Department of Social Welfare, 1958–59* (New York, 1959), Report on Morrisania City Hospital, p. 2.

33. U.S. Bureau of Labor Statistics, *Earnings and Supplementary Benefits*, p. 10.

34. *Ibid.*, p. 11.

35. U.S. Public Health Service, *Health Manpower Source Book, Section 9*, p. 68.

36. Louis Block, *The Nursing School—Its Cost*, reprinted from *Hospital Progress*, September, 1947, p. 8.

37. William K. Turner, "Financing Nursing Education—An Unfair Burden for 1100 Hospitals," *Hospitals*, XXXIII, No. 19 (October 1, 1959), p. 42; Illinois Hospital Association, *Report on 1958 School of Nursing Cost Study*, I (Chicago, 1959), p. 3.

38. State University of New York, Advisory Committee on Nursing Education, *Facts Bearing on Nursing Education in New York State* (Albany, N.Y., 1951; mimeographed), p. 7.

39. Letter from University of the State of New York to Herbert E. Klarman, March 23, 1959.

40. National League for Nursing, *Schools of Professional Nursing, 1958–1959* (New York, 1959), pp. 24–25.

41. Arnstein.

42. U.S. Public Health Service, *Health Manpower Source Book, Section 9*, p. 70.

43. Tibbits and Levine, p. 11.

44. U.S. Public Health Service, *Health Manpower Source Book, Section 9*, p. 70.

45. Marion Cleveland, *New Plans for Providing Nursing Care for Acutely Ill Patients*, paper delivered at Conference on Prepaid Financing for Nursing Service, Community Council of Greater New York, September, 1958.

46. Roberta R. Spohn, *A Study of Private Duty Nurses* (New York, 1954), p. 27.

47. Harriet Stamback, *Private Duty Nursing in Prepaid Medical Care Plans*, paper delivered at Conference on Prepaid Financing for Nursing Service, Community Council of Greater New York, September, 1958.

48. University of the State of New York, *A Survey of Nursing Personnel Resources in Hospitals in New York State* (Albany, N.Y., 1956), Appendix V, Table 17.

49. United Hospital Fund of New York, *Analysis of Hospital Personnel, December 31, 1953*, Supplement V: Financial and Statistical Analysis (New York, 1954); also annually.

50. Letter from University of the State of New York to Herbert E. Klarman, March 23, 1959.

51. United Hospital Fund of New York, *Analysis of Hospital Personnel*.

8. CONDITION OF PLANT AND EXPENDITURES FOR CONSTRUCTION

1. Hospital Council of Greater New York, *The Master Plan for Hospitals and Related Facilities for New York City* (New York, 1947), p. 55.

2. Hospital Council of Greater New York, "A Method of Estimating Hospital Capital Needs," its *Bulletin*, XIII, No. 1 (January–February, 1958).

3. Hospital Council of Greater New York, "Did You Know?" its *Bulletin*, V, No. 1 (January, 1949).

4. Paul A. Lembcke, David R. Hermansen, and Eleanor Poland, "A Proposed Standard Method of Measuring Hospital Capacity," *Public Health Reports*, LXXIV, No. 8 (August, 1959), p. 682.

5. Hospital Council of Greater New York, "Measurement of Hospital Bed Capacity," its *Bulletin*, XV, No. 1 (1960).

6. Hospital Council of Greater New York, "A Method of Estimating Hospital Capital Needs."

7. Hospital Council of Greater New York, "Changes in General Care Hospitals and Beds in New York City, 1946–1953," its *Bulletin*, IX, No. 6 (June, 1953).

8. Hospital Council of Greater New York, *Master Plan*, p. 31.

9. Hospital Council of Greater New York, *Twentieth Annual Report* (New York, 1958), pp. 10–20.

10. Hospital Council of Greater New York, *Master Plan*, p. 27.

11. Hospital Council of Greater New York, "A Method of Estimating Hospital Capital Needs."

12. *Ibid.*

13. Hospital Council of Greater New York, "Post War Construction Program of the Department of Hospitals, City of New York," its *Bulletin*, VIII, No. 11 (November, 1952).

14. New York City Office of the City Administrator, *Property Maintenance in the Department of Hospitals* (New York, 1958; mimeographed), p. 1.

15. U.S. Public Health Service, Division of Hospital and Medical Facilities, *Principles for Planning the Future Hospital System* (Washington, D.C., 1959), p. 222.

16. *Ibid.*, p. 221.

17. Hospital Council of Greater New York, "The Hill-Burton Program with Emphasis on Financial Requirements of Applicants," its *Bulletin*, XIII, No. 5 (November–December, 1958).

18. Hospital Council of Greater New York, "Ten Years of Hill-Burton Program in New York City," its *Bulletin*, XII, No. 2 (March–April 1957).

19. Ray E. Trussell and Frank van Dyke, *Prepayment for Hospital Care in New York State* (Albany, N.Y., 1960), p. 151.

20. United Hospital Fund of New York, *Analysis of Financial Statements Submitted by UHF Voluntary General Hospital Members* (New York, 1947–58), Table II.

21. New York State Joint Hospital Survey and Planning Commission, *Cost of Construction of Selected Hospital and Related Facilities in New York State Receiving Federal Aid for Which Principal Contracts Were Awarded between August 1, 1952 and July 1, 1957* (Albany, N.Y., 1957).

9. PROBLEMS IN HOSPITAL MANAGEMENT

1. Edith M. Lentz, *Hospital Administration—One of a Species*, mimeographed from *Administrative Science Quarterly*, I, No. 4 (March, 1957), p. 10.

2. Frederick C. LeRocker and Kenneth S. Howard, *What Decisions Do Trustees Actually Make?* reprinted from *The Modern Hospital*, April, 1960.

3. American Hospital Association, *Hospitals*, XXVI, No. 6 (June, 1952), Pt. 2 (Guide Issue), p. 29, Table I.

4. American Hospital Association, *Model Constitution and Bylaws for a Voluntary Hospital* (Chicago, 1957), p. 8.

5. Columbia University, *The Role of the Trustees of Columbia University* (New York, 1957), p. 9.

6. George Bugbee, *The Physician in the Hospital Organization*, reprinted from *The New England Journal of Medicine*, October 29, 1959.

7. New York City, *Charter, Effective January 1, 1938 (as amended to November 1, 1951)* (New York, 1953), pp. 50–51.

8. Jacob Levine, *Lecture on Budgeting: Pre-Examination Course for Promotion to Administrative Assistant, Department of Hospitals* (New York, 1960; mimeographed), pp. 11–13.

9. Citizens' Committee for Children, *Why Children's Services Suffer* (New York, 1960), p. 7.

10. Hospital Council of Greater New York, *Report of Study of Kings County Hospital* (New York, 1952), p. 23.

11. Letter from Daniel I. Rosen, U.S. Veterans Administration, to Herbert E. Klarman, June 7, 1960.

12. American Hospital Association, *Hospitals*, XXVII, No. 6 (June, 1953), Pt. 2 (Guide Issue), p. 40, Table J.

13. Citizens' Committee for Children, p. 29.

14. Hospital Council of Greater New York, *Full-Time System of Medicine* (New York, 1950), p. 7.

15. St. Luke's Hospital, *Annual Report, 1958* (New York, 1959), p. 22.

16. American Medical Association, Council on Medical Education and Hospitals, *Essentials of an Approved Internship*, reprinted from the *Journal of the American Medical Association*, CLXXIV, No. 6 (October 8, 1960), pp. 669–70.

17. Beverly Hospital, *Report on Seminar on Graduate Medical Education in Nonuniversity Hospitals* (Beverly, Mass., 1959), p. 9.

18. New York University, *The Regional Hospital Plan of New York University-Bellevue Medical Center* (New York, 1952), p. 7.

19. American Hospital Association, *Workshop-Conference on the Role of the Director of Medical Education in the Hospital* (Chicago, 1959), p. 13.

20. *Ibid.*, p. 8.

21. Isidore Snapper, "Research and the Teacher of Medicine," *Journal of the American Medical Association*, CLXX, No. 4 (May 23, 1959), p. 445.

22. Hospital Council of Greater New York, *Report of Committee on Full-Time Salaried Directors of Service in Unaffiliated Municipal Hospitals* (New York, June 6, 1960; mimeographed).

10. QUALITY OF CARE

1. New York State Board of Social Welfare, *By-Laws*, Article IV, paragraph 3.

2. New York City Board of Hospitals, *Hospital Code and Regulations*, Article III.

3. Joint Commission on Accreditation of Hospitals, *Standards for Hospital Accreditation* (Chicago, 1957), p. 1.

4. Leonard S. Rosenfeld, "Quality of Medical Care in Hospitals," *American Journal of Public Health*, XLVII, No. 7 (July, 1957), pp. 856–57.

5. Milton C. Maloney, Ray E. Trussell, and Jack Elinson, *Physicians Choose Medical Care*, paper delivered at American Public Health Association, October 20, 1959 (mimeographed), p. 1.

6. Paul M. Densen, *Approaches to the Problem of Measuring the Quality of Medical Care*, paper delivered at Group Health Institute, New York, May 27, 1959 (mimeographed), p. 4.

7. David P. Barr, *Principles Relating to the Success of a Medical Care Plan*, paper delivered at Group Health Institute, New York, May 26, 1959 (mimeographed), p. 8; Joint Commission on Accreditation of Hospitals, "Analysis, Review, and Evaluation of Clinical Practice in the Hospital," its *Bulletin*, No. 24 (August, 1960), p. 3; and Willard C. Rappleye, *Responsibility of Hospital Trustees in the Future*, paper delivered at Greater Detroit Hospital Council, November 18, 1958, p. 2.

8. Paul A. Lembcke, "Medical Auditing by Scientific Methods," *Journal of American Medical Association*, CLXII, No. 7 (October 3, 1956).

9. U.S. Veterans Administration, Department of Medicine and Surgery, *Report of the Committee on Measurement of the Quality of Medical Care* (Washington, D.C., 1959), p. 8.

10. Robert S. Myers, "Hospital Statistics Don't Tell the Truth," *Modern Hospital*, LXXXIII, No. 1 (July, 1954), pp. 53–54.

11. Robert S. Myers and Vergil N. Slee, *Basic Ingredients of a Medical Audit*, reprinted from *Modern Hospital*, April, 1956.

12. Lembcke, "Medical Auditing by Scientific Methods."

13. Vergil N. Slee, The Internal Medical Audit, paper delivered at American Public Health Association, October 20, 1959, p. 1.

14. Myers and Slee, "Basic Ingredients of a Medical Audit"; and their "Audit Shows Hospitals Where They Stand," *Modern Hospital*, LXXXVIII, No. 6 (June, 1957), pp. 57–62.

15. Paul M. Lembcke, "Regional Organization of Hospitals," *The Annals of the American Academy of Political and Social Science*, CCLXXIII (January, 1951), p. 56.

16. Paul M. Lembcke, *A Scientific Method for Medical Auditing*, reprinted from *Hospitals*, XXXIII (July 1, 1959), p. v.

17. Barr, p. 10.

18. Slee, p. 4.

19. Rosenfeld, p. 861.

20. Beverly Hospital, Department of Medical Education, *Report on Seminar on Graduate Medical Education in Nonuniversity Hospitals* (Beverly, Mass., 1959), p. 20.

21. Myers, "Hospital Statistics Don't Tell the Truth," p. 54.

22. Rosenfeld, p. 862.

23. U.S. Veterans Administration, *Report of the Committee on Measurement*, p. 2.

24. Joint Commission on Accreditation of Hospitals, "Analysis, Review, and Evaluation of Clinical Practice in the Hospital," p. 2.

25. Rosenfeld, p. 858.

26. Edwin F. Daily and M. A. Morehead, *A Method of Evaluating and Improving the Quality of Medical Care*, paper delivered at American Public Health Association, November 15, 1955 (mimeographed), p. 4.

27. Myers and Slee, "Basic Ingredients of a Medical Audit."

28. U.S. Veterans Administration, *Report of the Committee on Measurement*, p. 4.

29. Esther Everett Lape and associates, for the American Foundation, *Medical Research: A Midcentury Survey*, I (Boston, 1955), pp. 563–73.

30. *Ibid.*, p. 561.

11. AFFILIATION, REGIONALIZATION, AND COORDINATION

1. David M. Heyman and others, *Report of the Commission on Health Services of the City of New York, Adopted July 20, 1960* (New York, 1960; mimeographed), pp. 14–15.

2. New York University, *The Regional Hospital Plan of New York University–Bellevue Medical Center* (New York, 1952), p. 2.

3. U.S. Public Health Service, *Preliminary Report on Survey of Regional Organization of Health Services* (Washington, D.C., 1952), p. 9.

4. Heyman.

5. Milton I. Roemer and Robert C. Morris, "Hospital Regionalization in Perspective," *Public Health Reports*, LXXIV, No. 10 (October, 1959), p. 916.

6. U.S. Public Health Service, *Preliminary Report on Survey of Regional Organization*, p. 21.

7. Roemer and Morris, p. 918.

8. Herbert G. Vaughn, Jr. (for the Committee of Interns and Residents of the New York City Municipal Hospitals), *Hospital Organization and Patient Care: A Survey of the New York Municipal Hospital System with Proposals for Increased Efficiency of Service* (New York, 1959; mimeographed), p. 10.

9. Letter from Kenneth B. Babcock of the Joint Commission on Accreditation of Hospitals to Herbert E. Klarman, February 24, 1959.

10. Leonard S. Rosenfeld and Henry B. Makover, *The Rochester Regional Hospital Council* (Cambridge, Mass., 1956), p. 107.

11. Academy of Medicine of Cincinnati and the Greater Cincinnati Hospital Council, *Joint Policy on Emergency Admission to Hospitals* (Cincinnati, Ohio, June 25, 1959; mimeographed).

12. Hospital Council of Greater New York, "Need for a Teaching and Research Hospital at State University College of Medicine, Brooklyn," its *Bulletin*, XIII, No. 2 (March–April 1958).

12. TRENDS IN INCOME, 1934–57

1. Arthur W. Jones and Francisca K. Thomas, *Report of the Hospital Survey for New York*, III (New York, 1938), pp. 321–36, 446–71.

2. *Ibid.*, p. 315.

3. Eli Ginzberg, *A Pattern for Hospital Care* (New York, 1949), Chapter 19.

4. United Hospital Fund of New York, *Financial and Statistical Information Relating to Member Hospitals and Hospital Statistics for Greater New York, Year 1947* (New York, 1948), pp. 3–7.

5. Ginzberg, p. 163.

6. New York City Department of Hospitals, *Statement of the Cost of Maintaining and Operating the Department of Hospitals, Year Ended December 31, 1957* (New York, 1958; mimeographed).

13. SOURCES OF INCOME OF VOLUNTARY HOSPITALS

1. United Hospital Fund of New York, Central Tabulating Service Bureau, unpublished tabulations for subscribing hospitals from New York City, 1957.

2. United Hospital Fund of New York, *Financial and Statistical Information Relating to Member Hospitals and Hospital Statistics for Greater New York, Year 1957* (New York, 1958).

3. United Hospital Fund of New York, *Sundry Financial and Statistical Information Relating to Hospitals in New York City, December 31, 1957* (New York, 1958).

4. New York City Department of Hospitals, *Statement of the Cost of Maintaining and Operating the Department of Hospitals, Year Ended December 31, 1957* (New York, 1958; mimeographed).

14. FINANCIAL POSITION OF VOLUNTARY HOSPITALS

1. United Hospital Fund of New York, *Financial and Statistical Information Relating to Member Hospitals and Hospital Statistics for Greater New York, Year 1957* (New York, 1958).

2. George J. Stigler, *The Theory of Price* (New York, 1946), pp. 306–7.

3. New York State Department of Social Welfare, *State Manual of Policies*

and *Procedures, Medical Care (Book 5)* (Albany, N.Y., amended annually as of July 1 and also as of February 1, if necessary), Chapter 541.

15. INCOME OF MUNICIPAL HOSPITALS

1. New York City Department of Hospitals, *Statement of the Cost of Maintaining and Operating the Department of Hospitals, Year Ended December 31, 1957* (New York, 1958; mimeographed).
2. Letter from Hospital Council of Greater New York to Charles F. Preusse, City Administrator, July 5, 1956.
3. New York City Department of Hospitals, *Annual Report, 1957* (New York, 1958; mimeographed), p. 36; and Department's Statement Showing Sources and Amounts of Revenue (Claimed or Collected) for Hospital Services Rendered during 1957 and 1958, prepared for Hospital Council of Greater New York, September 30, 1959 (typewritten).
4. New York City Department of Hospitals, *Statement of the Cost of Maintaining and Operating the Department of Hospitals*.
5. New York City Comptroller, *Annual Report, 1957–58* (New York, 1958), pp. 337, 340.

16. ROLE OF GOVERNMENT

1. Eli Ginzberg, *A Pattern for Hospital Care* (New York, 1949), p. 305.
2. David M. Schneider and Albert Deutsch, *The History of Public Welfare in New York State, 1867–1940*, II (Chicago, 1941), p. 20.
3. New York City Department of Hospitals, *Annual Report, 1949* (New York, 1950), pp. 88–89.
4. William F. Damrau, *The Rise of Municipal Hospital Expenditures in New York City, 1914–1954* (PH.D. Dissertation, New York University, 1957), p. 243.
5. New York City Department of Welfare, *Annual Report, 1957* (New York, 1958), p. 13.

17. ROLE OF BLUE CROSS

1. Agnes W. Brewster, "Voluntary Health Insurance and Medical Care Expenditures, 1948–58," *Social Security Bulletin*, XXII, No. 12 (December, 1959), p. 9.
2. Elmo Roper and Associates, *The Public's Attitudes toward Hospitals in New York City and Their Financing in May, 1958*, II (New York, 1959), p. 217.
3. Health Insurance Institute, *Source Book of Health Insurance Data* (New York, 1959), p. 12.
4. New York City Department of Hospitals, *Annual Report, 1940* (New York, 1941), p. 43.

5. Hospital Council of Greater New York, "Blue Cross Hospitalization Insurance in the New York City Area," its *Bulletin*, VIII, No. 1 (January, 1952); unpublished data from United Hospital Fund of New York.

6. Odin W. Anderson and Jacob J. Feldman, *Family Medical Costs and Voluntary Health Insurance: A Nationwide Survey* (New York, 1956), p. 185.

7. *Ibid.*, p. 184.

8. New York State Department of Labor, *Health Benefit Coverage of the Labor Force in New York State, Supplementary Tables* (New York, 1960), p. 3.

9. William C. Breed, Jr., *History of Associated Hospital Service of New York* (New York, 1959), p. 12.

10. Associated Hospital Service of New York, Hospital Payment Rates from Inception to Date (typewritten).

11. Harris, Kerr, Forster, and Company, Statistical and Financial Summary of Cost Accounting Studies in Twenty-Three Member Hospitals of Associated Hospital Service of New York for the Year Ended December 31, 1947 (New York, 1948), from files of Associated Hospital Service.

12. Greater New York Hospital Association and Hospital Association of New York State, *Establishment of Hospital Rates* (New York, 1951), p. 8; Herbert E. Klarman, *Suggestions for a Rate Policy for Voluntary Hospitals,* reprinted from *The Modern Hospital,* June, 1950.

13. United Hospital Fund of New York, Central Tabulating Service Bureau, unpublished tabulations for 33 subscribing general hospitals in New York City, 1958.

14. Associated Hospital Service of New York, *Twenty Second Annual Report, 1956* (New York, 1957), p. 9.

15. Laurence E. Irwin, "Efficient Use of Hospitals," *The Pennsylvania Medical Journal,* LXI, No. 6 (June, 1958), p. 743.

16. United Hospital Fund of New York, "Average Length of Patients' Stay, Voluntary Non Profit General Hospitals in New York City," its *Bulletin,* No. 247 (March 23, 1960), p. 9.

18. ROLE OF PHILANTHROPY

1. *Doctors Hospital, Inc. vs. Tax Commission of the City of New York,* Appellate Division, New York State Supreme Court, March, 1944.

2. The Hospital Survey for New York, unpublished data in possession of the Hospital Council of Greater New York.

3. Joseph Hirsch and Beka Doherty, *Saturday, Sunday and Everyday* (New York, 1954), p. 110.

4. United Hospital Fund of New York, *Statistical and Financial Information Relating to Member Hospitals and Hospital Statistics for Greater New York* (New York, 1955–59).

5. Hirsch and Doherty, p. 34.

6. *Ibid.*, p. 46.

7. United Hospital Fund of New York, *Statistical and Financial Information.*

8. Arthur W. Jones and Francisca K. Thomas, *Report of the Hospital Survey for New York,* III (New York, 1938), p. 89.

9. The Greater New York Fund, *A Memorandum Explaining How the Receipts of the Greater New York Fund Are Distributed* (New York, 1959; mimeographed).

10. Eli Ginzberg and Peter Rogatz, *Planning for Better Hospital Care* (New York, 1961), p. 22.

11. United Hospital Fund of New York, *Sixtieth Year Book, 1939, Supplement,* pp. 3–4.

12. New York State Hospital Study, unpublished tabulations; Archdiocese of New York, *Catholic Charities in 1958* (New York, 1959), p. 38.

13. Hospital Trustees Committee Representing the Voluntary Hospitals in New York City, *An Appeal for an Increase in the Appropriation by the City of New York to the Voluntary Hospitals for the Care of Public Charges* (New York, 1957; mimeographed).

14. Committee on Increased Rates of Payment for Public Charges in Voluntary Hospitals, *An Appeal for an Increase in the Rates Paid by the City of New York to the Voluntary Hospitals for Care of Public Charges* (New York, 1939), p. 3; Hospital Council of Greater New York, Special Committee, *Use of Tax Funds for Care of the Indigent Sick in the Voluntary Hospitals of New York City* (New York, 1940), p. 1.

19. COST OF HOSPITAL CARE

1. Associated Hospital Service of New York, "Study of Changes in Hospital Services 1937, 1947 and 1957," in its *Memoranda on Hospital Costs, Services, Reserves and Controls* (New York, 1960; mimeographed), Section 5, p. 4.

2. Hospital Survey for New York, *Report,* II (New York, 1937), p. 295.

3. John Connorton, *Statement with Regard to Application for Subscriber Rate Adjustment for Associated Hospital Service of New York,* at public hearing before Superintendent of Insurance of State of New York, New York, May 21, 1959 (mimeographed), two charts; Henry N. Pratt, *Four Key Reasons Why the High Cost of Hospital Care Is Going Higher,* reprinted from *Hospitals,* June 1, 1958.

4. American Hospital Association, *Cost Finding for Hospitals* (Chicago, 1957), pp. 29–30.

5. Ray E. Trussell and Frank van Dyke, *Prepayment for Hospital Care in New York State* (Albany, N.Y., 1960), p. 111.

6. Connorton; Pratt.

7. William F. Damrau, *The Rise of Municipal Hospital Expenditures in New York City, 1914–1954* (PH.D. dissertation, New York University, 1957), p. 145.

8. *Ibid.*, p. 202.

9. Eli Ginzberg, *A Pattern for Hospital Care* (New York, 1949), p. 60.

10. Hugh E. Luckey, *Statement*, at public hearing before Superintendent of Insurance of the State of New York, New York, June 13, 1960 (mimeographed), p. 3.

11. Damrau, p. 63.

12. Martin R. Steinberg, *Statement with Regard to Application for Subscriber Rate Adjustment for Associated Hospital Service of New York*, at public hearing before Superintendent of Insurance of the State of New York, New York, May 21, 1959 (mimeographed).

13. United Hospital Fund of New York, "Hospital Costs, Their Nature and Trends, 1947–1959," in Associated Hospital Service, *Memoranda on Hospital Costs, Services, Reserves and Controls*, Section 1, Question 9.

14. United Hospital Fund of New York, *Analysis of Financial Statements Submitted by UHF Voluntary General Hospital Members* (New York, 1948–59).

15. Ruth P. Mack, "Inflation and Quasi-Elective Changes in Costs," *The Review of Economics and Statistics*, XLI, No. 3 (August, 1959), p. 225.

16. Ray E. Brown, "The Nature of Hospital Costs," *Hospitals*, XXX, No. 7 (April 1, 1956).

17. Henry D. Lytton, "Recent Productivity Trends in the Federal Government: An Exploratory Study," *The Review of Economics and Statistics*, XLI, No. 4 (November, 1959), pp. 351–52.

18. Trussell and van Dyke, p. 159.

19. Ray E. Brown, *Forces Affecting the Community's Hospital Bill*, reprinted from *Hospitals*, September 16 and Oct. 1, 1958.

20. Eli Ginzberg in *Hearing, Joint Economic Committee, U.S. Congress, on Employment, Growth and Price Levels, Part 8*, September 28–30, October 1–2, 1959 (Washington, D.C., 1959), p. 2668.

21. Paul A. Lembcke, *Hospital Efficiency—A Lesson from Sweden*, reprinted from *Hospitals*, April 1, 1959.

22. Trussell and van Dyke, p. 158.

23. Charles D. Flagle, Ira W. Gabrielson, Abraham Soriano, and Martin M. Taylor, *Analysis of Congestion in an Outpatient Clinic* (Baltimore, Md., 1959), p. 39.

24. Robert J. Connor, Charles D. Flagle, Richard K. C. Hsieh, Ruth A. Preston, and Sidney Singer, "Effective Use of Nursing Resources: A Research Report," *Hospitals*, XXXV, No. 9 (May 1, 1961), p. 39.

25. Ray E. Brown, quoted in news item, *Hospitals*, XXXIII, No. 12 (June 16, 1959), p. 18.

26. Trussell and van Dyke, p. 126.

27. Eli Ginzberg and Peter Rogatz, *Planning for Better Hospital Care* (New York, 1961), p. 70.

28. United Hospital Fund of New York, *Financial and Statistical Informa-*

tion Relating to Member Hospitals and Hospital Statistics for Greater New York (New York, 1949–59).

29. New York City Department of Hospitals, *Distribution of Cost of In-Patient Services in General Care Hospitals, 1948 and 1958,* two charts, (photostats); New York City Department of Hospitals, *Statement of the Cost of Maintaining and Operating the Department of Hospitals for the Year Ended December 31* (New York, 1949–59; mimeographed).

30. Arthur W. Jones and Francisca K. Thomas, *Report of the Hospital Survey for New York,* III (New York, 1938), p. 109.

31. *Ibid.,* p. 301.

32. American Hospital Association, *Hospitals* (Guide Issue), annually.

33. Jones and Thomas, p. 315.

34. Ginzberg, *A Pattern for Hospital Care,* p. 163.

35. Herbert E. Klarman, *Depreciation in Hospital Accounting,* reprinted from *The Modern Hospital,* January, 1954.

36. Damrau, p. 178.

37. Letter from William C. Copeland, American Hospital Association, to Herbert E. Klarman, April 7, 1960.

38. *Ibid.;* Letter from G. Harvey Long, California Hospital Association, to Herbert E. Klarman, May 11, 1960.

39. American Hospital Association, *Hospitals,* XXVIII, No. 6 (June, 1954), Pt. 2 (Guide Issue), p. 52.

40. For a discussion of alternative treatments of this problem, see Herbert S. Levine, "A Small Problem in the Analysis of Growth," *The Review of Economics and Statistics,* XLII, No. 2 (May, 1960), pp. 225–28.

41. United Hospital Fund of New York, *Analysis of In-Patient and Out-Patient Department Income and Cost Based on Reports Submitted by UHF Voluntary General and Special Hospital Members for the Years 1958–1957* (New York 1959), Supplement IV, Financial and Statistical Analysis.

42. Howard Lee Bost, *An Analysis of Charges Incurred for In-Patient Care in General Hospitals: Implications for Protection against the Cost of Hospital Care* (PH.D. dissertation, University of Michigan, 1955), p. 53.

43. New York City Department of Hospitals, *Distribution of Cost of In-Patient Services in General Care Hospitals, 1948 and 1958.*

44. United Hospital Fund of New York, *Financial and Statistical Information Relating to Member Hospitals, Year 1958.*

45. New York City Department of Hospitals, *Statement of the Cost of Maintaining and Operating the Department of Hospitals, Year Ended December 31, 1958.*

46. *Ibid.*

47. Jones and Thomas, p. 315.

48. Ginzberg, *A Pattern for Hospital Care,* p. 163.

49. New York City Department of Hospitals, *Statement of the Cost of Maintaining and Operating the Department of Hospitals, Year Ended December 31, 1958.*

50. New York City Comptroller, *Annual Report, 1957–58* (New York, 1958), pp. 337, 340.

51. Trussell and van Dyke, p. 333.

52. United Hospital Fund of New York, *Analysis of In-Patient Service Costs Based on Reports Submitted by UHF General Hospital Members for the Year 1958* (New York, 1959), Supplement V, Section III, Financial and Statistical Analysis.

53. New York City Tax Department, List of Exempt Properties, 1958–59 (unpublished).

54. *Ibid.*

55. American Hospital Association, annual questionnaire.

56. United Hospital Fund of New York, *Financial and Statistical Information Relating to Member Hospitals, Year 1957.*

20. COMPARISONS WITH OTHER AREAS

1. Letter from Agnes W. Brewster, Social Security Administration, to Herbert E. Klarman, August 20, 1959.

2. American Hospital Association, *Hospitals* (Guide Issue), annually.

3. American Public Health Association, *Public Health and Hospitals in the St. Louis Area* (New York, 1957), pp. 117–23, 154–57; San Francisco Committee on Hospitals and Health Facilities, *Availability and Usage of Hospital Beds and Financing of Hospital and Clinic Care in San Francisco* (San Francisco, 1954), pp. 24, 28.

4. Hospital Financing Study Committee [of Philadelphia], *Report* (Philadelphia, 1955), and miscellaneous tables, 1954 and 1955 (mimeographed); Social Planning Council of St. Louis and St. Louis County, *Report of Free and Part Pay Care Given by St. Louis Hospitals* (St. Louis, Mo., 1956; mimeographed); The Hospital Council [of Baltimore], *Report to Subcommittee on Policies and Financing of Maryland's Hospital and Medical Programs* (Baltimore, 1959; mimeographed).

5. Baltimore Hospital Survey Committee, *General Hospital Facilities for the Baltimore Area, Study and Report* (Baltimore, 1958), p. 138.

6. United Community Funds and Councils of America, *Allocations and Expenditures in United Funds* (Bulletin No. 206; New York, 1959).

7. President's Commission on the Health Needs of the Nation, *Building America's Health*, IV (Washington, D.C., 1952), p. 155.

8. *Ibid.*, pp. 276–77.

9. Letter from Agnes W. Brewster to Herbert E. Klarman, August 20, 1959.

10. Fred R. Brown, *Public and Private Expenditures for Hospital Care in the United States, 1956–57* (Research and Statistics Note No. 19–1959; Washington, D.C., Division of Program Research, Social Security Administration, 1959); memorandum for Herbert E. Klarman, August, 1959.

11. Thomas Karter, "Voluntary Agency Expenditures for Health and

Welfare from Philanthropic Contributions," *Social Security Bulletin*, XXI, No. 2 (February, 1958), pp. 15–16.

12. Thomas Karter, *Public Payments to Private Hospitals and Health and Welfare Activities in 1938, 1948, and 1955* (Research and Statistics Note No. 37–1958; Washington, D.C., Division of Program Research, Social Security Administration, 1958).

13. John H. Hayes, ed., *Factors Affecting the Costs of Hospital Care* (Financing Hospital Care in the United States, I; New York, 1954), pp. 61–62.

14. Thomas Karter, "Voluntary Agency Expenditures for Health and Welfare from Philanthropic Contributions."

15. American Hospital Association, *Hospital Rates* (Chicago, annually).

21. A PATTERN FOR FINANCING HOSPITAL CARE IN NEW YORK CITY

1. Hospital Trustees Committee Representing the Voluntary Hospitals of New York City, *An Appeal for an Increase in the Appropriation by the City of New York for the Care of Public Aid Patients in Voluntary Hospitals* (New York, 1960; mimeographed), pp. 7–9.

2. Hospital Council of Greater New York, *New York City and Its Hospitals: A Study of the Roles of the Municipal and Voluntary Hospitals Serving New York City* (New York, 1960), p. 7.

3. Herbert E. Klarman, *Background, Issues and Policies in Health Services for the Aged in New York City* (New York, 1962), p. 50.

INDEX

Accreditation, 298–99

Adams, Appollonia, 542, 543

Administrator of hospital: relationship to trustees and medical staff, 273; professional background, 285–86; recruitment for municipal hospitals, 286–87

Admission policies of hospitals, 2 municipal hospitals, 44, 327, 419; definition of emergency patient, 137 voluntary hospitals: relationship to ambulance service, 60; selectivity, 119, 519

Admission rate to hospitals, N.Y.C. and U.S., 37

Admissions to hospitals, *see* Patients

Affiliated hospitals, definitions, 177, 315, 318; *see also* Teaching hospitals; Major teaching hospitals; Minor teaching hospitals

Affiliation among medical institutions, 317–24; definition, 317–18; obstacles to, 319–22; a proposal on, 322–24

Age groups, population, 16; patients in short-term hospitals, 104–9, 125–29

AHS, *see* Associated Hospital Service of New York

Alien physicians, *see* Foreign-educated physicians

Altenderfer, Marion E., 534, 537, 538

AMA, *see* American Medical Association

Ambulance service, emergency, 1, 34, 58–60

Ambulatory patients, services for, 52–55, 57–58

American Foundation, 548

American Hospital Association, 2, 35; annual questionnaire, 225, 228, 231; "Guide Issue" of *Hospitals*, 35, 263, 478; size of board, reported by, 275; as source, 542, 543, 546, 552, 554, 555, 556

American Medical Association, 2, 104–5, 112–13; "Hospital Service" issue of *Journal*, 90, 263; Bureau of Medical Economic Research, data from, 105, 113, 535, 537; Directory Department, data from, 145–47, 161, 537; Council on Medical Education and Hospitals of the AMA: *Directory of Approved Internships and Residencies*, 169, 174, 177–78, 213, changes in approval status of training programs, listed by, 198–99, suggestions for hospitals unable to qualify for internship approval, 203–4, advisory committee on internships, 205–6, as source, 537, 538, 539, 540, 541, 546; *Medical Education in the United States and Canada*, 174; other publications, 532, 533, 534, 537, 538, 539, 540, 541, 542

American Nurses' Association, 542

American Psychiatric Association, 533

American Public Health Association, 529, 534, 542, 543, 547, 548, 555

Anderson, Odin W., 536, 551

Arnstein, Margaret, 542, 544

Ashford, Mahlon, 539

Associated Hospital Service of New York (Blue Cross), 2; role in hospital economy, 5–6; effect on emergency departments, 56; and home care, 62–63; subscribers in hospitals, 93–94; tonsillectomies paid for, 114; subscribers using ward service, 103, 130–40; subscribers carrying Blue Shield, 133, 134; benefits for ward and semiprivate patients, 135; maternity cash benefits, 136; payments, as source of hospital income, 346, 421–26; payments to voluntary hospitals, 356, 363; payments to municipal hospitals, 391; role of, 415–36; service area, 415–16; payments